Water, Wastes and Health
in
Hot Climates

Edited by

Richard Feachem
Ross Institute of Tropical Hygiene
London School of Hygiene and Tropical Medicine

Michael McGarry
International Development Research Center
Ottawa

Duncan Mara
Department of Civil Engineering
University of Dundee

A Wiley–Interscience Publication

JOHN WILEY & SONS

London · New York · Sydney · Toronto

Library of Congress Cataloging in Publication Data:

Main entry under title:

Water, wastes and health in hot climates.

  'A Wiley–Interscience publication.'
  Includes bibliographical references:
    1. Sanitary engineering—Tropical conditions.
  2. Underdeveloped areas—Sanitary engineering.
  3. Tropical medicine. I. Feachem, Richard.
  II. McGarry, M. G. III. Mara, David Duncan.
  TD153.W33   628'.2   76-18946
  ISBN 0 471 99410 3

Photosetting by Thomson Press (India) Limited, New Delhi.
Printed by Unwin Brothers Limited, The Gresham Press, Old Woking, Surrey

List of Contributors

PROFESSOR D. J. BRADLEY — Ross Institute of Tropical Hygiene, London School of Hygiene and Tropical Medicine, Gower Street, London WC1E 7HT, England.

D. BROWNE — Economic Consultant, P. O. Box 21690, Nairobi, Kenya.

PROFESSOR I. BURTON — Institute for Environmental Studies, Haultain Building, University of Toronto, Toronto M5S 1A4, Canada.

I. CARRUTHERS — School of Rural Economics and Related Studies, Wye College, University of London, Ashford, Kent TN25 5AH, England.

A. J. CLAYTON — City Engineer, P. O. Box 59, Windhoek, South West Africa.

D. DONALDSON — Department of Environmental Sciences and Engineering, Pan American Health Organization, 525 23rd Street N.W., Washington, D.C. 20037, USA.

MRS LILIAN M. EVISON — Department of Civil Engineering, University of Newcastle upon Tyne, Claremont Road, Newcastle upon Tyne NE1 7RU, England.

DR R. G. FEACHEM — Ross Institute of Tropical Hygiene, London School of Hygiene and Tropical Medicine, Gower Street, London WC1E 7HT, England.

DR A. JAMES — Department of Civil Engineering, University of Newcastle upon Tyne, Claremont Road, Newcastle upon Tyne NE1 7RU, England.

DR. B. R. LAURENCE — Department of Entomology, London School of Hygiene and Tropical Medicine, Gower Street, London WC1E 7HT, England.

DR M. G. McGARRY — International Development Research Centre, P. O. Box 8500, Ottawa KIG 3H9, Canada.

M. G. MANSURI — *Department of Civil Engineering, Sardar Vallabhbhai Regional College of Engineering and Technology, Surat 395001, Gujarat, India.*

DR D. D. MARA — *Department of Civil Engineering, University of Dundee, Dundee DD1 4HN, Scotland.*

PROFESSOR G. V. R. MARAIS — *Department of Civil Engineering, University of Cape Town, Rondebosch, Cape Town, South Africa.*

PROFESSOR M. B. PESCOD — *Department of Civil Engineering, University of Newcastle upon Tyne, Claremont Road, Newcastle upon Tyne NE1 7RU, England.*

J. PICKFORD — *Department of Civil Engineering, University of Technology, Loughborough, Leicestershire LE11 3TU, England.*

PROFESSOR R. N. SHELAT — *Department of Civil Engineering, Sardar Vallabhbhai Regional College of Engineering and Technology, Surat 395001, Gujarat, India.*

M. R. SHEPHARD — *13 Walton Street, St. Albans, Hertfordshire, England.*

PROFESSOR H. I. SHUVAL — *Environmental Health Laboratory, The Hebrew University—Hadassah Medical School, P. O. Box 1172, Jerusalem, Israel.*

DR G. J. STANDER — *Chairman, Water Research Commission, P. O. Box 824, Pretoria 0001, South Africa.*

MRS ANNE U. WHITE — *Institute of Behavioural Science, University of Colorado, Boulder, Colorado 80302, USA*

DR ANNE WHYTE (*formerly* KIRKBY) — *Institute for Environmental Studies, Haultain Building, University of Toronto, Toronto M5S 1A4, Canada.*

Preface

Most people who read this book will be familiar with the magnitude of the public health engineering crisis in developing countries. They will appreciate that 86 per cent of the rural population lack an adequate water supply and that 92 per cent lack adequate facilities for excreta disposal. They will know that only 28 per cent of the urban population have water-borne sewerage facilities and that 29 per cent have no sanitation facilities of any kind. Added to this already catastrophic situation there is the ever-present problem of the population explosion. Seventy million new human beings were added to the world population during the year 1976 (equal to the population of Bangladesh) and most of these were added to the populations of countries who could least afford them. The developed countries now have fertility rates which are close to replacement levels and so it is the poor countries who have to provide food, housing, water and sanitation for most of these 70 million new people.

The ability to combat this situation must lie in the developing countries themselves because it surely cannot lie elsewhere. However, external forces can play a supporting role in assisting the developing countries to improve the conditions for their masses. These external aids are of two types; organizations with money (donors) and organizations with ideas (universities, and voluntary organizations). This book is written by people who feel they have ideas to offer. The ideas are offered humbly in the knowledge that some may not prove to be of use. However, the editors of this volume strongly believe that original thinking and research into the problems of water and wastes in hot climates are urgently needed and this book is intended to present current work of this type and to stimulate future work.

There appears to be a sterility of thought amongst those, such as commercial consultants and international agencies, who could generate new methods and techniques; and this has led to a remarkable lack of progress in such fields as urban excreta disposal technology. The editors have therefore sought contributors capable of assessing their subjects critically and writing without fear of being innovative. This policy has resulted in a volume which contains much that is new and much that will not be found in conventional texts on public health engineering. The editors have included some material which is as yet unproven by practical application and which may prove controversial. Indeed there is controversy within the book itself—for example, Carruthers and Browne (Chapter 8) warn of the hazards of self-help programmes while McGarry (Chapter 10) extols their virtues. The magnitude of the problem requires that there should be active debate and disputation and it is our hope that those sections of this book which do not have immediate application will at least prove to be provocative.

The Editors
March, 1976

There can be no solutions
without political solutions

Contents

I HEALTH AND WATER QUALITY

II WATER SUPPLIES FOR LOW-INCOME COMMUNITIES

III INSTITUTIONAL DEVELOPMENT

V EFFLUENT RE-USE AND RECLAMATION

I

Health and Water Quality

1

Health Aspects of Water Supplies in Tropical Countries

DAVID J. BRADLEY

1.1 THE NEED FOR UNDERSTANDING HEALTH ASPECTS

Domestic water supply in temperate countries is in a fortunate position. The chief ground for its provision is stated to be improvement of the public health, but people are prepared to pay an economic price for good water readily available, which rarely costs much of their income in any case. So the health aspects do not need to be looked at critically from an economic viewpoint and water is provided of a quality such that risk of disease is minimal.

In the tropical developing countries the position may be quite different in the following ways:

(1) People are often too poor to pay for a supply providing completely safe water through a multiple tap system in the home.
(2) Governments or agencies providing funds will require clearer evidence of the health benefits to be expected, since their hope of financial returns will be smaller.
(3) The funds made available may be inadequate for an ideal water supply so that difficult choices between differing incomplete sorts of improvement have to be made. If these decisions are not made consciously, the situation usually arises where a very few people get excellent water supplies and the vast majority do very badly indeed.
(4) The diseases related to water supplies are more numerous, more important and more diverse in the tropics than in temperate lands and effects of improved supplies are more complex.

For all these reasons the engineer, and also the administrator, need to have a much clearer understanding of the diseases related to water and the health consequences of improved supplies if they are to make the best use of the funds made available to them. This chapter aims to provide such information, mainly in terms relevant to the sorts of water improvement possible, but with comments on specific diseases appended for those who wish to know more about them. We first set the water-related diseases into the general picture of tropical health.

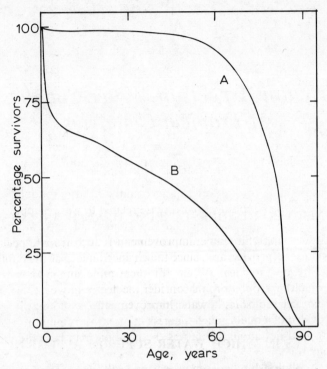

Figure 1.1 Human survival curves in (A) industrialized and
(B) developing societies

Human health in most tropical developing countries is poor. We can measure it by when people die and the sorts of disease from which they suffer. If we compare the likely fate of one thousand babies born alive in a poor developing country and a rich industrial one, their survival is as shown in Figure 1.1. In the rich country a few babies, perhaps 24 out of the thousand, die shortly after birth, and then the vast majority survive through childhood and early adult life with only occasional tragedies from cancers such as leukaemia and from road accidents. Most people survive into their fifties when mortality from diseases of the arteries becomes appreciable and there is a rapidly increasing death rate among people in their seventies and eighties. These relatively affluent people all enjoy excellent water supplies and sewerage systems and water-related disease is in consequence rare, except for a possible effect of water softness on heart disease.

By contrast, the picture in the developing country is much more gloomy. Of the thousand babies, a quarter may fail to reach their fifth birthday. One hundred and fifty of these die in the first year of life and perhaps another seventy in the second. The second year's death rate may be a hundred times that seen in the industrial country. Two causes of these deaths predominate: infectious diseases and malnutrition. Throughout childhood and adult life the chances of death from infections remain much higher than in richer nations, and relatively few people survive into old age at all. How many of the deaths are due to water-related diseases? A large number, probably 5%–10% overall in many places, and particularly among very young children when malnutrition and infection work together tragically: intestinal infections related to water increase malnutrition, and it in turn predisposes to severe infections.

The position among the sick in hospital is similar. Infections are far commoner among in-patients, both surgical and medical, than in a rich country, and many are related to water, about 10% usually. The same picture is seen among the out-patients who crowd round the few medical care facilities available. They show less intestinal but more skin infections than the in-patients, but still over 10% of water-related conditions.

So we see in the tropical developing country a large amount of misery, sickness and death due to infectious disease related to water supplies, which is prevented by the multiple household tap systems of safe water in richer countries. The way in which water improvements reduce disease depends on the particular diseases involved and, since the engineer and local authority may be unable to provide the ideal system for the people unless they completely neglect most of the population, we consider the degree to which infections may be reduced by different sorts of water improvements.

1.2 THE WAYS IN WHICH WATER SUPPLIES AFFECT HEALTH

Some sort of relationship between water and health has been recognized from the time of Hippocrates, if not earlier, in the association of marshy places with fevers, and many unsophisticated communities in the tropics have similar views and are very discriminating in their choice and use of water.

Snow (1855) was the first to show a precise relation of a disease to water in his well-known studies of cholera, and he was closely followed by Budd who demonstrated the spread of typhoid *through* water supplies. Later in the nineteenth century a different type of relation to water was shown by Manson in 1877 for filariasis and Ross for malaria. Both infections were shown to be transmitted by mosquitoes, whose larvae live in and are dependent on surface water. Before that, guinea worm, and subsequently schistosomiasis or bilharziasis, were shown to depend on freshwater invertebrates for their spread. The relation of personal hygiene to health had been recognized for many years and 'cleanliness is next to godliness' is very much a nineteenth century maxim, though only relatively recently have a series of epidemiological studies shown that the details of *access* to water determine the incidence of several infective diseases. Furthermore, the supplies of water available greatly influence facilities for disposing of human excreta and these in turn affect the spread of many important diseases.

So water affects disease in many ways. These may not all be apparent to someone who reads a standard text on water supply, and a far more limited view is usually taken. How did this come about? And can we continue to keep to this limited range in thinking about and planning water improvements?

Those infections which are spread by an insect, snail, or other cold-blooded organism, or which undergo development in the soil, need a fairly warm temperature if they are to complete the stages of their life spent outside man. They are rare in most temperate lands so that they are not a major problem for the planner or water engineer in those relatively cold countries. Also in these countries, income has been sufficiently high for people to pay for the convenience of water piped into their homes and the problem of access to water has been solved on grounds of amenity rather than health. The preoccupation of the water engineer has thus been to prevent the carefully constructed piped water supply also acting as a source of infection because of pollution. His great worry has been over water *quality* and this is naturally reflected in the books on water supplies, most of which are written for, and by, people from temperate countries.

In the tropics, we cannot safely take such a limited view. Such vector-borne diseases as malaria, schistosomiasis, guinea worm and yellow fever are either terrible scourges of, or threats to, many tropical populations. The hazards from bad water are thus much greater. Poverty is much more serious for many tropical areas; in the rural areas—where most people live—and around the edges of the cities, which are the fastest-growing communities, most people cannot afford a conventionally good water supply at present, and the choice in the short run may be between doing nothing and providing a somewhat improved supply. If an ideal water system is not possible, there are options as to what needs should be met by the partial improvements. To make the right decisions we need again the broad picture of water-related disease. So, because of these two tropical characteristics—warmth and poverty—a wider view than in temperate lands is necessary.

So far, only *infections* related to water have been mentioned. The chemical quality of waters also affects health. Some groundwater has very high fluoride levels which may affect bone growth adversely, while various types of chemical pollution of surface waters may occur. However, such chemical risks are on a small scale compared with the hazards from microbial pollution of water in the tropics. Most waters with harmful concentrations of salts are so unpalatable as not to cause a health risk. This chapter therefore concentrates on infective disease.

1.3 CLASSIFICATION OF WATER-RELATED INFECTIONS

Between 20 and 30 different infective diseases may be affected by changes in water supply. They are usually classified, by the microbe causing them, into viral, bacterial, protozoal and helminthic diseases. But this is not very helpful in considering effects of improved water supplies. What affects them is the mode of spread, and it is more useful to have four main categories:

(a) Infections spread through water supplies—water-borne diseases.
(b) Diseases due to the lack of water for personal hygiene—water-washed diseases.

(c) Infections transmitted through an aquatic invertebrate animal—water-based diseases.

(d) Infections spread by insects that depend on water—water-related insect vectors.

The structure of this reclassification is shown in Table 1.1. and is discussed in greater detail elsewhere (Bradley, 1974; White, Bradley and White, 1972). The categories are explained below.

In temperate lands there is a preoccupation with the health effects of polluted water. Here, and throughout this chapter, pollution refers to the access of mammalian, and especially human, faeces to the water. Faecal pollution means that, if those who pollute the water are suffering from intestinal infections, those who drink the water will ingest the organisms and may also get the infections. The big worries for municipal water supplies in temperate and tropical countries are that faecal pollution may allow the organisms which cause such diseases as typhoid, where the infecting dose of bacteria to someone who drinks the water is extremely low, to be spread through the water supply and cause a large outbreak of typhoid among the many people who drink the water. Such infections can clearly be accurately described as *water-borne* diseases, where the pathogenic organisms are carried passively in the water supplies, and they are prevented by attention to water *quality*.

If people have very little water, either because there is extremely little water available or because it is so far away in a well that the effort to bring much of it to the home is very great, then it may be impossible to maintain reasonable personal hygiene. There may be too little water for washing oneself, or food utensils or even clothes. Remaining unwashed not only allows skin infections to develop unchecked but also makes it easier for intestinal infections to spread from one person to another on dirty fingers. In practice, these are an important

Table 1.1 Classification of infective diseases in relation to water supplies

Category	Examples	Relevant water improvements
I Water-borne infections		
(a) Classical	Typhoid, cholera	Microbiological sterility
(b) Non-classical	Infective hepatitis	Microbiological improvement
II Water-washed infections		
(a) Skin and eyes	Scabies, trachoma	Greater volume available
(b) Diarrhoeal diseases	Bacillary dysentery	Greater volume available
III Water-based infections		
(a) Penetrating skin	Schistosomiasis	Protection of user
(b) Ingested	Guinea worm	Protection of source
IV Infections with water-related insect vectors		
(a) Biting near water	Sleeping sickness	Water piped from source
(b) Breeding in water	Yellow fever	Water piped to site of use
V Infections primarily of defective sanitation	Hookworm	Sanitary faecal disposal

group of diseases in the tropics and may be called the *water-washed* infections as they result from lack of water for washing or personal hygiene. Clearly their prevention depends on availability, access to, and *quantity* of domestic water rather than its quality.

In the tropics there are some worm infections which are not spread passively from person to person in the water. The parasite eggs or larvae which reach water are not directly infective to man, but *are* infective to specific invertebrate water animals, chiefly snails and crustaceans. They undergo development within these intermediate hosts from which, after a period of days or weeks, further larvae mature and may be shed into the water. These larvae are infective to man who is infected by drinking or contact with the water. Such worms, whose transmission is based upon an aquatic organism, may be called *water-based* infections and rather specific action to remove the intermediate hosts from the water, or other special action, is needed to make the water safe.

Lastly, there are many tropical infections spread by biting insects. Most of these, most notably the mosquitoes, breed in water bodies, sometimes as small as household domestic water containers. Yet other insects capable of transmitting disease, the tsetse flies, in some cases only bite near water, to which those lacking piped supplies must of necessity come. These *water-related insect vectors* may sometimes be affected by improvements in domestic water supplies.

It is not possible to separate water-related diseases completely from those affected by sanitation, nor is it desirable to attempt that. All the water-borne and some of the water-based diseases depend on faecal access to domestic water sources. The chain of transmission may be broken by safe disposal of faeces as well as by protection of the water supplies. Even some of the water-washed intestinal infections may be reduced if better sanitary conditions reduce soiling of the hands. There are a few infections, of which the human hookworm is most important, where sanitation is much more important than water because transmission is from faeces to soil and by direct penetration back through the human skin. The same applies to several East Asian worms whose eggs escape in the faeces but infective stages reach man encysted in fish and in other articles of food.

Sanitation affects some vectors too, in that some mosquitoes specifically favour flooded pit-latrines as breeding sites (see Chapter 15). Bringing better water supplies into such an area without sanitary disposal of waste water will make the situation worse, not better. There are therefore additional problems of *sanitation* and of *waste-water disposal*.

We now consider these categories in greater detail, going to the specific infections. By comparing these with the prevalent diseases in an area where water improvements are planned, a guide to priorities when funds are limited may be built up, and this is developed further towards design criteria in Chapter 5 for water supplies, while practical guidelines for handling wastes to reduce infectivity are set out in Chapters 13 and 14. The borders between domestic and other water in the developing tropics are sometimes blurred, and these other

Table 1.2 Main infective diseases in relation to water supplies

Category	Disease	Frequency	Severity	Chronicity	Percentage suggested reduction by water improvements
Ia	Cholera	+	+ + +		90
Ia	Typhoid	+ +	+ + +		80
Ia	Leptospirosis	+	+ +		80
Ia	Tularaemia	+	+ +		40?
Ib	Paratyphoid	+	+ +		40
Ib	Infective hepatitis	+ +	+ + +	+	10?
Ib	Some enteroviruses	+ +	+		10?
Ia, IIb	Bacillary dysentery	+ +	+ + +		50
Ia, IIb	Amoebic dysentery	+	+ +	+ +	50
Ib, IIb	Gastroenteritis	+ + +	+ + +		50
IIa	Skin sepsis and ulcers	+ + +	+	+	50
IIa	Trachoma	+ + +	+ +	+ +	60
IIa	Conjunctivitis	+ +	+	+	70
IIa	Scabies	+ +	+	+	80
IIa	Yaws	+	+ +	+	70
IIa	Leprosy	+ +	+ +	+ +	50
IIa	Tinea	+	+		50
IIa	Louse-borne fevers		+ + +		40
IIb	Diarrhoeal diseases	+ + +	+ + +		50
IIb	Ascariasis	+ + +	+	+	40
IIIa	Schistosomiasis	+ +	+ +	+ +	60
IIIb	Guinea worm	+ +	+ +	+	100
IVa	Gambian sleeping sickness	+	+ + +	+	80
IVb	Onchocerciasis	+ +	+ +	+ +	20?
IVb	Yellow fever	+	+ + +		10?

waters are further considered in Chapter 2. The more important relevant infections are set out in Table 1.2.

1.4 WATER-BORNE DISEASES

The classical water-borne diseases are due to highly infective organisms where only rather few are needed to infect someone, relative to the levels of pollution that readily occur. The two chief ones have a high mortality if untreated and are diseases which a community is very anxious to escape: typhoid and cholera. Both are relatively fragile organisms whose sole reservoir is man.

These two diseases occur most dramatically as the 'common source out-break' where a community water supply gets contaminated by faeces from a person suffering from, or carrying, one of the infections. Many people drink the water and a number of these fall ill from the infection at about the same time.

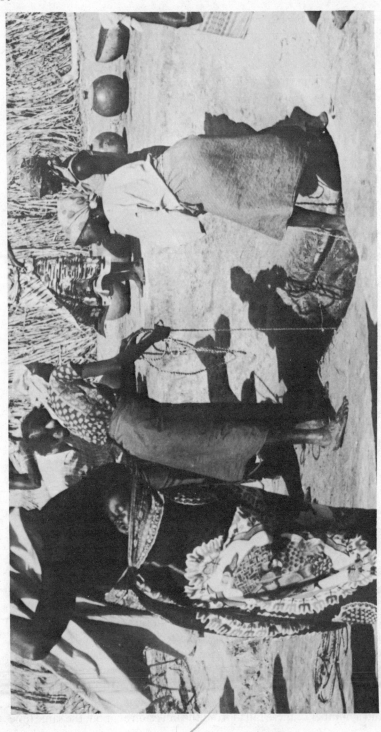

Villagers in northern Nigeria collect water from a polluted well. The ground around the well mouth has subsided so that the well now lies in a hollow. All surface drainage flows into the well and will carry with it pathogens contained in human and animal faeces. Cholera and schistosomiasis are endemic in this area and diarrhoeal disease is a major cause of infant mortality. Guinea worm is also endemic and a well such as this provides a perfect route for the transmission of the relevant parasite: *Dracunculus medinensis* (photograph: R. G. Feachem)

It is this sudden appearance of a cluster of cases combined with their severity that makes these illnesses so feared. This description also shows how the route of spread of these diseases is determined epidemiologically, by working back from the simultaneous cases to the water or other item which they had shared. Now, by and large, big groups of people tend not to share really very heavily polluted water to the point where it is obviously foul. But small rural family groups may be forced to use such water. There will be too few of these people using a source to be able to see a clear common source outbreak of further diseases that depend on very heavy contamination. Therefore it is difficult to incriminate the water supplies because of the limitations of the epidemiological method. The limits of what are occasionally water-borne diseases are much less certain therefore, but are steadily extended as our knowledge grows. Infective viral hepatitis has only in recent years been shown unequivocally to be sometimes water-borne, for example. It is also important to realize that epidemiological conclusions are not universally applicable in this matter: in temperate countries typhoid is almost exclusively water-borne; in the tropics this is less often so and evidence of water spread in the rural tropics is often absent. Therefore the simple summaries in so many temperate water textbooks often need modification in the tropics.

Typhoid is the most cosmopolitan of the classical water-borne infections. In man it produces a severe high fever with generalized systemic, more than intestinal, symptoms. The bacteria are ingested and very few are sufficient to infect. During the first week of illness they may be detected in the blood and are absent from the excreta, but subsequently they occur in large numbers in the faeces, originating from ulcers in the small bowel. These ulcers may perforate through into the abdominal cavity, with fatal consequences unless surgical aid is available. There is a considerable typhoid mortality in developing countries, though early diagnosis and adequate therapy with expensive antibacterial drugs can greatly reduce this. Prevention by immunization is possible. Reactions are rather common, the actual vaccine is not expensive and protection lasts for several years following a course of immunizations, though it is incomplete. The typhoid patient is usually too ill to go out polluting the water and is not infective prior to falling sick. However, a small proportion of those who recover clinically continue to pass typhoid bacteria in their faeces for months or years; these carriers are the source of water-borne infections. Gallstones predispose to the carrier state as the bacteria persist in the inflamed gall bladder. In the tropics, lesions of *Schistosoma haematobium* in the bladder also act as nidi of infection, producing urinary typhoid carriers, whilst rectal schistosomiasis combined with typhoid leads to a persistent severe fever lasting many months. Typhoid bacteria survive well in water but do not multiply there. They are removed by standard slow sand filtration and killed by chlorination (see Chapter 9).

Cholera is in some ways similar to typhoid, but its causative bacteria are more fragile and the clinical course is extremely dramatic. In classical cholera the onset of diarrhoea is sudden and its volume immense so that the untreated victim has a high probability of dying from dehydration within 24 hours or little more. The infective dose is quite large, but pollution levels in endemic areas are very high with immense faecal volumes full of bacteria, and in dense human populations. Within a few days the classical cholera victim of South-East Asia is dead or non-infective. With the now almost cosmopolitan El Tor strain, which has a lower mortality, convalescent carriers occur and numerous other people are infected without becoming ill so that the chance of spread is increased. Treatment of cholera is by replacing the fluid lost using intravenous infusions or oral saline mixtures. Immunization is protective but only for a few months so that improved water and sanitation is the most useful control measure.

Several other infections are water-borne but are less important than typhoid and cholera. Leptospirosis, due to a spirochaete, has its reservoir in wild rodents which pollute the water. Leptospires can penetrate the skin as well as being ingested. They produce jaundice and fever, called 'Weil's disease', which is severe but not common.

A protozol infection, giardiasis, which may produce diarrhoea, is common in the tropics and has been shown in some temperate country outbreaks to be water-borne. The route of transmission in the tropics is unclear. Amoebiasis has a similar epidemiological picture and is more important. Several amoebae infect man. *Entamoeba histolytica* gives rise to prolonged dysenteric symptoms (diarrhoea with blood) and in some cases may produce large abscesses of the liver and other viscera. Spread is from one person to another by the resistant cystic stage of the amoeba and this has sometimes been demonstrably water-borne though often it may pass from faeces to mouth via food or dirty hands.

A large group of enterobacteria related to typhoid may cause diarrhoea or dysentery. The most important, of the genus *Shigella*, can be spread through water supplies, but often are not. In the last two years, the role of a new group of viruses, the rotaviruses, as causes of childhood diarrhoea is beginning to emerge. The mode of transmission is not yet known, but most high intensities of diarrhoeal diseases have been associated with defective water supplies.

1.5 WATER-WASHED DISEASES

All the infections that can be spread from one person to another by way of water supplies may also be more directly transmitted from faeces to mouth or by way of dirty food. When this is the case, the infections may be reduced by the provision of more abundant or more accessible water of unimproved quality. This applies particularly to the diarrhoeal diseases due both to bacteria and to viruses as well as protozoa. The most thorough studies, of *Shigella* infections in the southern United States, have shown that simply making water more available tends to roughly halve the frequency of infection (Hollister *et al.*, 1955; Stewart *et al.*, 1955).

The diarrhoeas are the most important water-washed diseases in tropical areas. They are responsible for vast amounts of morbidity in people of all ages

(Van Zijl, 1966) in South America and South-East Asia particularly, (Scrimshaw, Taylor and Gordon, 1968) and along with malnutrition, measles and malaria are very important in the very high child mortalities of those areas where between one-eighth and one-third of all children born may not reach their fifth birthdays. The diarrhoeal diseases are responsible for the majority of the economic losses ascribed to water-related diseases in many countries. They result from a range of infectious agents but fall to a low incidence under good hygienic conditions.

The second main group of water-washed diseases are infections of the body surface, the skin and the eyes. Though rarely shortening life, they make many people miserable. 70% of pre-school children in Ankole, Uganda, for example (Cook, 1967) had either skin ulcers infected by bacteria, or scabies due to a small mite that burrows in the skin, or fungus infections of the skin. More water, together with improved personal hygiene are needed to reduce the frequency of these infections. They may give some guide to the public health worker as to the hygienic state of a community. In the extreme circumstances of the New Guinea highlands, Feachem (1973) found that over 90 per cent of the people suffered from skin infections at some time each year and the prevalence at any one moment, as in Ankole, was high enough to be measured on a village-sized sample.

The question immediately arises as to what is an adequate volume of water for hygienic purposes. Unfortunately no accurate answer is available. It seems clear from epidemiological data (White, Bradley and White, 1972) that a few litres is not enough and that several hundred litres is more than adequate, but this is a great range. In practice it appears that, unless water is piped into the home, water use is not at the optimal level for health. A shower or bath needs to be of sufficient volume to remove dirt and then soap without becoming too concentrated a solution of either, and similar considerations apply to the washing of clothes and pots. When supplies are very short, the successive re-use of water for washing people and utensils may be worse than substituting sand for cleaning dishes.

The eye infections are related to water availability also, and are a particular problem in arid countries where the drying effect of the air on the conjunctiva is combined with dust and sand and the scarcity of domestic water. A specific infection of the eye, due to a virus-like microbe, is trachoma, which may lead to inflammation, turning in of the eye lashes and subsequent opacity of the cornea producing partial or complete blindness. Many other bacteria may follow the trachoma agent and their relative roles in producing the frequent chronic eye lesions of the tropics is variable. Trachoma itself produces much less damage where water supplies are adequate (Pratt-Johnson and Wessels, 1958).

1.6 WATER-BASED DISEASES

Water-based diseases are all worm infections. Several are due to flukes or trematodes whose larvae depend on aquatic snails. The eggs pass from excreta to water and the larvae emerging from the snails may be ingested with domestic water directly or on food plants or animals which acquire encysted larvae from the water. By far the most important, however, the schistosome worms, can bore their way directly through the human skin and they are therefore a hazard to all in contact with infective water, whether for domestic use or not. It is thus not only necessary to provide domestic supplies but also to persuade people to keep out of the water at transmission foci. In spite of some scepticism regarding the efficacy of water supply improvements as a control measure, Jordan and his colleagues in St. Lucia (unpublished reports) have found this approach highly successful. The broader aspects of schistosomiasis are considered in Chapter 2.

Guinea-worm infection or dracunculiasis is transmitted through cyclops, a minute crustacean, and has a wide but patchy distribution in Africa and Asia. The adult worm lies beneath the skin, often of the leg. It matures near to the rainy or planting season usually, and the posterior end of the female comes to lie beneath a blister usually on the lower leg. When water is spilled upon the leg the blister bursts and many guinea-worm larvae are freed, and if they are washed into a well or pond containing cyclops the life cycle can continue. To complete it, people have to drink water containing infective cyclops. It follows that prevention may be by standard water treatment processes, or much more simply by preventing water flowing back into wells after it has been spilled. This is achieved by an outward-sloping concrete collar around the top of dug wells and these have been highly successful in parts of Nigeria in eradicating the infection.

The importance of guinea worm is great: it produces arthritis of joints adjacent to the active worm and effectively disables those infected for a couple of weeks, which, because of the timing of the infection, fall at the short planting season. Since in affected villages the prevalence may exceed 70%, the economic consequences are grave.

1.7 WATER-RELATED INSECT VECTORS OF DISEASE

The many mosquitoes and other vectors of infection that breed in water are considered in the next chapter, but in a few cases there is a particular connection with domestic supplies.

In rural areas the journey to fetch water may bring women into the preferred habitat of *Glossina* or *Simulium*. The former genus, of tsetse flies in Africa, has several members confined to riverine bush so that people get bitten when going to the few residual waterholes in the dry season when man–fly contact is most concentrated. They can transmit human sleeping sickness, a chronic lethal infection if untreated, and may be controlled by selective bush clearing near the water point.

Of much greater importance is the urban problem of water storage jars acting as breeding sites for the 'yellow fever mosquito' *Aëdes aegypti*. This occurs throughout the tropics not only where water has to be fetched to the house and stored, but also where an intermittent piped supply makes for larger storage jars, not limited by the carrying capacity of the family. Such containers are the preferred habitat of *Aëdes aegypti*. It carries several virus diseases from person to person. In the Caribbean and West Africa yellow fever, a very severe and often lethal jaundice, is the best known. Of perhaps greater current importance is dengue, an acute influenza-like illness of short duration which is endemic in many Asian cities. Under conditions of intense dengue transmission, cases of the more severe dengue haemorrhagic fever with an appreciable mortality begin to occur, possibly due to the superimposition of one strain of dengue on an individual with antibodies to another strain leading to bone marrow damage so that the blood does not properly clot. The mosquitoes can be killed by putting a suitable insecticide, of very low human toxicity, into the water containers (see Chapter 15).

1.8 DISEASES OF DEFECTIVE SANITATION

It is already clear that many diseases in the water-borne, water-washed and water-based categories depend on access of human wastes to water or people's mouths, so that they all may be reduced by measures aimed at improving waste disposal as well as water supply. Some theoretical reasons have been advanced (Macdonald, 1965) for water being more likely to be effective than sanitation against some water-based diseases; but the chief practical reason is that the use of new water supplies presents far fewer difficulties than does persuading people to use new sanitary facilities.

A number of infections, however, are only affected by the latter—human hookworms penetrate the skin from damp contaminated soil, and certain flukes encyst in food items unaffected by changes in water supply. The hookworms are a major problem in the damper tropics. They live in the small intestine and cause major blood losses into it, acting as a cause of anaemia, especially in populations where dietary iron is low or poorly absorbed. The less tropical of the two species may be spread by penetration of the mucous membrane of the mouth when water containing the larvae is drunk; but the more tropical one, *Necator*, can be prevented by sanitary disposal of faeces, or by the wearing of shoes alone.

The common roundworm or *Ascaris* lays very numerous eggs which escape in the faeces and mature in the ground before becoming infective to man if ingested. They usually get in on fingers or food and both water supply and sanitation reduce transmission. The adult worms are often over 10 cm long and they divert food from the human host, give rise to various abdominal symptoms and occasionally produce intestinal obstruction. *Ascaris* has a relatively cosmopolitan distribution as does *Trichuris*, a smaller worm that is of less significance to public health.

The various flukes whose eggs escape in the faeces and which gain access to man in or on inadequately cooked food include *Paragonimus*, the lung

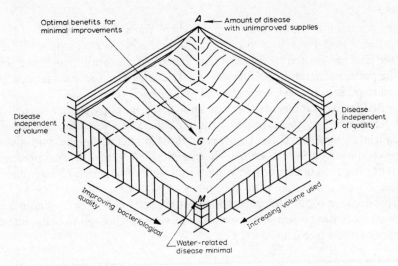

Figure 1.2 The generalized relation between volume and quality of water supplies and the burden of water-related disease. *A* is the amount of disease with unimproved supplies. At *M*, water-related disease is minimal. At *G*, optimal benefits are obtained for minimal improvements

fluke of South-East Asia and parts of West Africa, two liver flukes, and *Clonorchis* another South-East Asian parasite causing extensive liver damage. All can be controlled by thorough cooking of food or by sanitation—either standard sewage treatment approaches (Chapter 14), or leaving faeces in pit latrines, or adequate storage at appropriate temperatures prior to their use as an agricultural fertilizer (Chapters 18 and 19).

1.9 CONCLUSION

The relative importance of water-borne and water-washed diseases will affect supply priorities. The interrelation of these is represented in Figure 1.2. We have indicated that increases in water use are generally beneficial up to the level at which water is piped, with a single tap and shower, into the compound or house, and that this last step is probably a crucial one. Water quality effects are more dependent on the number of people using a common source. Any faecal pollution in a large urban distribution system carries the threat of a large epidemic; but in small village systems the probability of pollution with a pathogen is reduced by the smaller potentially contaminating population, and the size of any resulting epidemic is also much smaller, so that in situations of limited funds a lower relative priority can be given to completely unpolluted supplies. Again this will depend on the environment: bacteriological quality is more pressing in a Bangladesh village in a classical cholera area than in an isolated village in Tanzania, and is crucial in the urban situation.

It is hoped that this analysis of the health effects of water improvement, while providing no comforting but misleading rules-of-thumb for the administrator or engineer, may give some insight into the diseases he hopes to prevent and thus provide a rational basis for planning water improvements. Chapter 5 takes up the argument and shows how an understanding of water-related disease can be employed in the design, planning and evaluation of water supplies.

1.10 REFERENCES

Bradley, D. J. (1974). Water supplies: the consequences of change. In: *Human Rights in Health* (Ed. K. Elliott and J. Knight). Amsterdam: ASP North-Holland; 81–98.

Cook, R. (1967). *The Ankole pre-school protection programme, Kampala, Uganda* (mimeographed).

Feachem, R. G. (1973). *Environment and Health in a New Guinea Highlands Community.* Ph.D. thesis. Sydney: University of New South Wales.

Hollister, A. C., Beck, M. D., Gittelsohn, A. M. and Hemphill, E. C. (1955). Influence of water availability on *Shigella* prevalence in children of farm labor families. *American Journal of Public Health*, **45**, 354–362.

Macdonald G., (1965). The dynamics of helminth infections with special reference to schistosomes. *Transactions of the Royal society of Tropical medicine and Hygiene*, **59**, 489–506.

Pratt-Johnson, J. A. and Wessels, J. H. W. (1958). Investigation into the control of trachoma in Sekhukuniland. *South African Medical Journal*, **32**, 212–215.

Snow, J. (1855). *On the Mode of Communication of Cholera.* 2nd ed. London: J. Churchill.

Scrimshaw, N. S., Taylor, C. E. and Gordon, J. E. (1968). *Interactions of Nutrition and Infection.* World Health Organization, Geneva.

Stewart, W. H., McCabe L. J., Hemphill, E. C. and Decapito, T. (1955). Diarrhoeal disease control studies. IV. The relationship of certain environmental factors to the prevalence of *Shigella* infection, *American Journal of Tropical Medicine and Hygiene*, **4**, 718–724.

Van Zijl, W. J. (1966). Studies on diarrhoeal diseases in seven countries by the WHO diarrhoeal diseases advisory team. *Bulletin of the World Health Organization*, **35**, 249–261.

White, G. F., Bradley D. J. and White A. U. (1972). *Drawers of Water: Domestic Water Use in East Africa.* Chicago and London: University of Chicago Press.

2

The Health Implications of
Irrigation Schemes and Man-made Lakes
in Tropical Environments

DAVID J. BRADLEY

2.1 INTRODUCTION

If the aim of domestic water supplies is to improve human health, it should at least be the intention of those who build dams and irrigation schemes not to make matters worse than they were before. Sadly, this has frequently not been the case and where hydroelectric reservoirs have been concerned, the inhabitants of the lake area have often suffered while the benefits have been felt elsewhere. Increasingly, people realize that this ought not to be so. If such tragedies are to be avoided it is necessary for engineers, administrators and industrialists to appreciate potential health hazards well in advance and to take steps to prevent them, from the planning and design stage through to the operation of the completed system. Too often, health problems are dealt with by a series of 'fire-brigade' operations which are expensive, too late and relatively ineffective, with more value for public relations than health promotion. This is particularly true of the problems of the people living near lakes and irrigation schemes; the health of those who construct the dams has been much better looked after in recent years. Here we consider the determinants of health in water development projects and the action needed to maintain health, particularly in terms of the engineering and administrative aspects.

The components of water development projects may be thought of as water, people and time, with all the infections which are spread through, or because of, the water to the people during the time available. The water for the development comes from somewhere. Usually there is need to store it. A dam is built and the water builds up as a lake or reservoir behind it. A spillway for excess water is provided. If water is to be used for irrigation there will be a network of canals of gradually decreasing size as far as the fields themselves, which may be periodically inundated, especially for rice culture. Except where the water is of exceptionally low mineral content, as on the Gezira in the Sudan, there will also need to be a progressively increasing series of drains, returning the excess water to the river further downstream. Each of these water bodies has its health hazards.

The second component, people, are too easily neglected by the planners of water developments. Some people live in the area of proposed inundation; usually others will come in to do the construction work; a third group may undertake irrigated farming while fishermen will arrive to exploit the fish harvests of the new lake.

The third element, of time, is mentioned because those who make policy and engineers are mainly involved in the initial stages of water impoundment and irrigation; they play a relatively small role after it has been running for a decade. They are therefore faced with a rapidly changing scene with several as yet unpredictable components, so that there will be a sequence of health situations each requiring plans and action, not just one.

The medical authorities may be less than helpful. Too often their advice may tend to resemble that given to the man about to be married ('don't') and this may be economically and, even more, politically unacceptable. To prevent schistosomiasis, measures of channel lining may be suggested which are financially impracticable. Some intermediate position has to be adopted, but this does not mean following the calculations of one notable engineering company who allocated x funds for dam construction and $0.01x$ for social matters including relocation of a large population. If the expected profits allow no more than 1% for social overheads including health, the project is not economically sound! Human welfare is the object of water development and can best begin at the construction site. We now consider the sequence of health hazards and preventive action, and then go into greater detail on the control of some diseases notoriously prevalent in water development situations. The sequence is considered in relation to a very basic water development plan: design, construction works, production of a dam producing a lake, displacement of people, and introduction of irrigation.

2.2 HEALTH PROTECTION FOR PROJECT STAFF AND LABOURERS

A plan is made—the health components that should be considered in it will become clear as we progress—and construction begins. But to prepare the plan a feasibility study and a survey are needed. This should have a medical component as well as geological, engineering, economic and social expertise. At present, such surveys are often carried out by professional staff normally resident in temperate lands, and health activities begin by providing them with sound advice (e.g. Ross Institute, 1974), relevant protective immunization and prophylactic medicines. Immunization against smallpox is still legally required to enter many countries, though the risk of infection is currently confined to Ethiopia. Against poliomyelitis and tetanus immunization is essential; against typhoid and cholera it is highly desirable, and an injection of gamma globulin to reduce the risk of hepatitis is even more so in the view of most authorities. Yellow fever, though absent from India, is a hazard in Africa and Central America and the vaccine is safe and long-lasting as well as being legally required for entry to several countries. Prophylaxis against malaria is imperative for most tropical countries and expert advice should be taken before omitting it. There is more malaria about than a few years ago and official statements from a country may be over-optimistic about the risk. The choice of chemoprophylactic medicine is easy for most places; but where chloroquine-resistant malaria is prevalent in parts of South-East Asia and South and Central America, the choice is much more difficult. Two things must be remembered in leaving the tropical site: to maintain malaria prophylaxis for four weeks afterwards and, if you become ill, to tell your doctor where and when you were abroad. Much of the preceding advice has relevance not only to the visitor from a temperate climate but also to the urban tropical professional whose life may have been almost equally protected from the endemic infections of the rural tropics.

Returning to construction of a dam and related hydraulic works, the labourers are very often from an area some way from the site. If from the hills, they may lack immunity to malaria, or from the local strain of it at least, and suffer severely from it. This has been a notable feature of many water development projects but ought not to occur with modern chemotherapeutic protection and the basic anti-mosquito measures to be practised around the construction workers' settlement. Recent constructions on the Zambezi at Kariba (Webster, 1960) have been notable for their safety from malaria compared with the terrible happenings in the first attempt at Panama and in the Indian Sarda canal project. Less tropical hazards of the construction force have been more intractable: trauma, alcoholism and venereal disease. A specific risk of dam construction on rapidly flowing rivers is onchocerciasis (or 'river blindness') and staff are intolerant of the risk and also the painful nuisance biting of the vector *Simulium* or buffalo-gnat. Fortunately, local insecticidal control is usually feasible at reasonable cost as discussed below. General hygienic measures at the construction camp are as important as special action. A safe water supply and adequate sewage disposal are essential, and it is desirable to site the camp some way from the water to minimize risks. Usually, after construction ends the site tends to develop into a sizeable town for the area, which is an added reason for providing sound water and sanitation. Benefits to the contract staff (who may be quite demanding) will carry over to help the displaced local people who tend to settle there. This is the time to lay a basis for a healthy future.

2.3 HEALTH RISKS TO DISPLACED PEOPLE AND IMMIGRANTS

A less happy group are the displaced residents of the area of inundation. Until recently, the traumatic process of relocation was rarely considered with sympathetic imagination and, to the misery of being moved, perhaps unavoidably, was added the wholly preventable physical hunger from inadequate planning for the relocated people's food supplies. Malnutrition will increase the severity of infectious diseases, whose transmission will be increased by the aggregation of displaced people together. Again, the physical planning of their new villages, preferably off the shoreline of the new lake, requires attention and their domestic water supplies need construction and maintenance.

The second group are immigrants. When a man-made lake is created, the displaced inhabitants often are not the ones to exploit the often highly-productive waters, and fishermen from elsewhere migrate in, bringing parasites such as the schistosomes from their home areas. Where irrigation follows, the farmers or their labourers (as in the Gezira) may be immigrants also. Two types of health hazard result. The immigrants may bring parasites whose transmission is facilitated by irrigation and thus increase the problems for residents and themselves. Conversely, and more often, the immigrant farmers may be from an over-populated hill area and lack immunity to such diseases as malaria so that, during the early stages of development when food is short, and the success of the project least assured, a malaria epidemic may reduce productivity and cause grave disease in a malnourished and highly susceptible group.

We have laid emphasis on the general disease problems of starting water developments because they are relatively easy to control by basic public health action—water, sanitation, vector control around settlements, simple medical services and forethought about nutrition and social dislocation—before moving on to the specific hazards related to water development.

2.4 VECTOR-BORNE DISEASES

The special problems relate to infections transmitted by invertebrates which live or breed in water. Snails transmit schistosomiasis and some other worm infections; the small biting flies called buffalo-gnats, blackflies or *Simulium* transmit onchocerciasis; and mosquitoes may transmit a whole variety of pathogens of which the malarial parasites, arbovirus fevers and filariasis are the most important.

Mosquitoes

There are very many mosquito species. The larvae of all of them develop in water but the choice of water bodies tends to be very specific. Some breed in temporary puddles, others in cans of water, others around the edges of large water-bodies where they are shaded by emergent vegetation, and so on. It follows that any water development project is likely to reduce the habitats for some mosquitoes whilst greatly increasing those for others. The effects on disease transmission require some expertise to predict. Further, since the areas of surface water in man-made lakes and irrigation schemes may be too large for blanket coverage with insecticides, the best control methods will need to be specifically adapted to the species incriminated—an approach known as species sanitation. Its relevance may be illustrated from the man-made lakes of America and Africa.

The most notable early example of engineering working hand-in-hand with disease control was in the Tennessee Valley. There new dams had led to malaria epidemics until special measures to control the locally relevant mosquito, *Anopheles quadrimaculatus*, were designed. It was found that frequent variation of the water level could 'strand' the larvae and by building-in this type of variation, using siphons and other means, the mosquito populations were kept very low. By contrast, the same approach applied to the man-made lakes of Africa such as Lake Volta in Ghana, even had it been mechanically feasible (which it is not, owing to the vast size of the lake), would have greatly increased the number of malaria vectors, since *A. gambiae*, the great vector in Africa, preferentially breeds in the unshaded transient puddles that would have resulted from an oscillating shoreline.

The mosquitoes divide into two main groups and only the anophelines (the other group are the culicines) can transmit malaria. Even these vary greatly in their ability to spread it efficiently. To transmit any one of the four species of human malaria parasite, a mosquito must bite someone with the stages of parasite infective to the insect (and these are much less common than the stages that make people ill and that are more usually diagnosed under the microscope); it must survive the twelve or so days necessary for the malaria parasites to develop in the mosquito and to reach its salivary glands; and the mosquito must then bite a susceptible person. These are quite stringent requirements and from them there follow the three features of a mosquito which make it a serious malaria vector: a long life, frequent biting of man rather than other animals, and a high density. It can be shown mathematically that the last feature, high numbers of mosquitoes, is less important than the other two in affecting malaria transmission, so that although numerous mosquitoes are an unpleasant nuisance, they are not a good guide to malarial risk.

A further epidemiological aspect needs comment. In very malarious places with highly efficient vectors, all the indigenous inhabitants become infected with malaria very early in life and gradually develop an immunity, not complete or absolute, but enough to reduce the amount of overt clinical disease in older children and adults, even though the price of such immunity may be the death of 10%–20% of all babies from malaria. Under these circumstances, the amount of clinical malaria seen is determined by human immunity rather than mosquito transmission, and a rise in mosquito population may cause no further deterioration in human health. This applies above all to sub-Saharan Africa where the highly stable malaria transmitted by *A. gambiae* will not be too much affected by water developments. However, the apparent safety of the indigenous adults must not be allowed to conceal the intense danger to non-immune immigrants.

Irrigation projects may have a great effect on malaria vectors. In particular, rice cultivation with its increase of standing water may support in Africa considerable breeding of *A. gambiae* among the young rice (Surtees, 1970b) with a later influx of the other major vector *A. funestus* as the rice grows taller and shading of the water increases.

Irrigation affects culicine mosquitoes as well as anophelines, and Surtees (1970a) has distinguished six ecological effects of irrigation development which will tend to affect mosquito populations. They are:

(a) simplification of the habitat,
(b) increased surface water,
(c) a rise in the water table,
(d) changes in the flow of water,
(e) microclimatic changes towards wetter and cooler conditions,
(f) human settlement.

The direction of population change is hard to predict in irrigation systems. Usually, but not always, there will be an overall increase in numbers and the species composition will change. These effects are not confined to the tropics and, on the Camargue in Southern France, irrigation has been associated with lowered water salinity, increase of the mosquito *Culex modestus* and the consequent 'overflow' of West Nile virus from birds (the most usual host) to horses and man (Hannoun *et al.*, 1964).

The rise of the water table generally has a major consequence for human settlements around the irrigated areas. Latrines are often of the vertically bored hole or pit type. If these penetrate the water table, the resulting slurry of sewage and highly polluted water provides an ideal breeding ground for *Culex fatigans*, a cosmopolitan nuisance mosquito which in many tropical countries transmits human filariasis.

Enough has been stated to show the complexity of water development effects on mosquito-borne disease, and the need for expert advice from an early stage. What are the main features of the three major relevant disease groups, and how do they relate to the vectors?

Malaria

Malaria, transmitted by anophelines, produces an acute illness in those not previously exposed to it. The high periodic fever may be fatal, if untreated, and this clinical pattern is seen not only in Europeans but also in immigrants from non-malarious highland tropical areas and populations exposed to relatively short-lived inefficient malaria vectors. The longer-lived vectors have already been discussed.

Arboviral infections

The viruses spread by mosquitoes are, with the exception of O'nyong nyong, carried by culicines. There are many of them, usually with 'reservoirs' of infection in birds or mammals other than man, but under changing ecological circumstances infection may 'spill over' into man. A few are largely spread from man to man, the most important being yellow fever, though this depends chiefly on a domestic mosquito. Most arboviruses produce an acute fever of short duration which totally incapacitates the sufferer who is immune after recovery. Death is

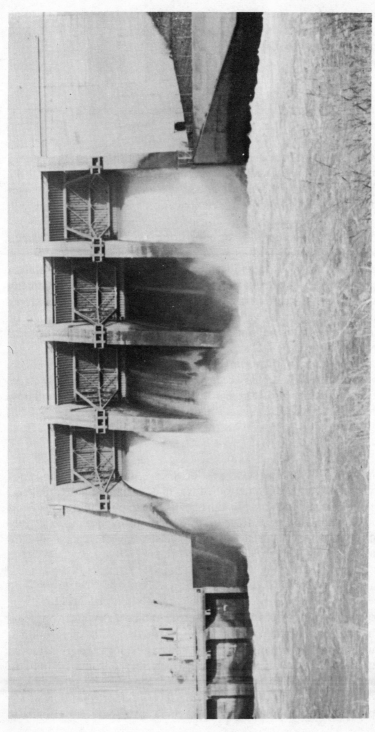

The Kainji Dam on the River Niger in Nigeria, completed in 1968, has created a 1250 km² lake. Onchocerciasis, a very prevalent disease in the area prior to dam construction, has been substantially reduced by the drowning of the breeding grounds of the vector, *Simulium damnosum*. Schistosomiasis is prevalent in some communities bordering the lake but snail populations may have been limited by seasonal variations in water level and the turbidity of the lake water. However, snail populations and the incidence of schistosomiasis, are increasing and present a special hazard in the areas irrigated by the lake water (photograph : R. G. Feachem)

relatively rare except in yellow fever, but a group of these viruses produce encephalitis with mental changes, with residual effects in a proportion of those infected. These arbovirus encephalitides are well documented in Asian irrigated areas (Simpson *et al.*, 1970).

Filariasis

Human filariasis, mainly spread by anophelines in Africa and culicines in Asia, is a chronic infection by one of two worm species which develop in the lymphatic system and release vast numbers of small larvae into the blood. These microfilariae vary in behaviour over the world, some only circulating at night when the relevant vector bites. Obstruction to the lymphatics causes fluid to accumulate in the limbs or the external genital organs, resulting in great swelling of the legs (elephantiasis), or of the scrotum (hydrocele) as well as many less dramatic changes. Since this pathology takes years to become apparent, action is required to control transmission long before clinical problems arise.

Onchocerciasis

In tropical Africa and parts of South and Central America onchocerciasis or river blindness is found, transmitted by *Simulium* flies. The disease results from a filarial worm which forms subcutaneous nodules and produces vast numbers of microfilariae which invade the skin rather than the bloodstream and persist for years so that cutaneous microfilarial populations steadily build up. A reaction to these destroys skin elasticity sometimes leading to pendulous folds of skin at the groins and also produces intolerable itching. Secondary infection of the resultant scratch marks may make matters worse. The microfilariae also invade the eyes leading, in intense infections in the savannah regions of Africa particularly, to blindness. Up to a quarter of adults may be blind in some affected villages.

The *Simulium* vector, whose bites are painful in themselves, breeds in rapidly flowing water. The main species group involved has larvae that attach to rocks in torrents and rapids so that immense numbers breed in the great rivers of Africa. Water developments have a large effect, usually beneficial. When a river such as the Volta or Nile is dammed, the upstream lake drowns the rapids and waterfalls with consequent loss of *Simulium*. Hazards arise from the spillways which reproduce suitable torrential conditions, though where control of discharge is not predetermined by hydrological needs, a regime to control breeding may be possible.

A side-effect of major dams is that they facilitate downstream control, as is illustrated by the Owen Falls dam at the head of the White Nile. The direct discharge through the dam is controllable and at the sluice gate violent turbulence occurs. A pipe is built into the dam so that insecticide can be added to the discharge. The turbulence ensures mixing and the insecticide is carried downstream. *Simulium* larvae are efficient filter feeders and remove particles under 1 micrometre in diameter selectively. When insecticide suspension size is correctly chosen the consequences are highly selective and a concentration of one part of DDT in 40 million of water sufficed to remove *Simulium* from some 70 miles of downstream Nile rapids.

The development of *Simulium* is rapid, as low as 5 days sometimes, so that intermittent discharges can rapidly constitute a hazard; and the flight range of the fly in tree cover can be many miles.

Schistosomiasis

If onchocerciasis is a disease of torrents, schistosomiasis is the disease of more slowly flowing waters. Whereas *Simulium* is not an irrigation hazard, schistosomes are *the* hazard of irrigation. This is partly because freshwater snails and irrigation engineers have similar ideas of what is ideal. There are three main schistosome species: *Schistosoma haematobium*, *Schistosoma mansoni* and *Schistosoma japonicum*, occurring respectively in Africa and the Middle East, in Africa and South and Central America including the Caribbean, and in East Asia and the Philippines. *S. haematobium* inhabits the blood vessels around the bladder while the other two species invade the intestinal venous drainage. Disease results not from the small adult worms but from their eggs and the hosts' reaction to them. The 'successful' eggs escape into the urine or faeces causing transient tissue damage and blood loss which may be noticed by the patient; but those eggs which do not escape produce inflammatory micronodules in the viscera. Many get swept from the intestine to the liver where similar granulomas result. Each adult worm lives for many years and the female lays hundreds or even thousands (in the case of *S. japonicum*) of eggs daily. So damage tends to be insidious and cumulative, as in filariasis. The short-term effects are merely unpleasant: blood in the urine, which needs to be passed frequently, episodes of diarrhoea with blood, and some abdominal pain; though there are repeated clinical accounts of general lassitude and debility in many patients of European origin. Severity is related to worm load, in turn depending on the intensity of transmission. Human acquired immunity occurs but it is incomplete and not well understood at the community level as yet. A proportion of those infected get grave late effects, in the case of *S. haematobium* damage to the urinary tract, destruction of one or both kidneys and, rarely, bladder cancer. *S. mansoni* may produce liver fibrosis resulting in bleeding from the oesophagus, and coma. The proportion of people getting these complications to an irreversible degree remains uncertain. What is clear is that those with schistosomiasis are at risk, and the higher the worm load the greater the risk. Moreover, water development in the tropics generally increases the degree of transmission greatly and measures are needed to combat this.

Can the hazards of schistosomiasis be predicted at the design stage? In general, they can: almost without exception, where an irrigation scheme or man-made lake has been constructed in an area where schistosomiasis occurs, it has led to an outbreak and increased endemicity. The transition from intermittent (river flood annually) to perennial irrigation in Egypt results in a tenfold rise in urinary schistosome prevalence together with the start of an *S. mansoni* problem. Detailed prediction is unreliable. Schistosomiasis was forecast for Volta Lake in Ghana and occurred, but the intermediate snail host was quite unexpected. The preventive measures to be taken are therefore of a more general nature, though subsequent control after a problem has arisen may be more specific. Action must be based on the transmission cycle.

Eggs in the excreta perish unless they promptly reach water so that sanitary facilities can prevent this. Theoretical models and some inconclusive rather detailed fieldwork suggests this is unlikely to be an efficient control method; but clearly sanitation has many merits in control of other diseases and deserves attention. Eggs reaching water hatch to release ciliated larvae which die unless they reach and penetrate an appropriate freshwater snail within a few hours. Development in the snail takes around a month, after which numerous free-swimming larvae are shed daily throughout the remainder of the snail's fairly short life. The larvae penetrate the unbroken skin of anyone who enters the water for up to two days (usually less) after they have been shed. Within a minute they have shed their locomotory tails and entered the skin or the mucous membrane of the mouth. Maturation, accompanied by migration within the human body, takes two or three months and worm life can exceed 25 years though 3–8 years may be more usual values.

The three further approaches to limiting transmission are therefore: reduction of snail populations, limiting human water contact, and killing worms by treatment of those infected. The last has been difficult due to drug toxicity and expense, though an inexpensive treatment for *S. haematobium* (metrifonate) is now becoming available and the more expensive single injection of hycanthone for *S. mansoni* has been widely used though its delayed toxicity is still disputed. The engineer must consider the other two approaches.

At the design stage, settlements need to be sited away from the infective watercourses and provided with their own domestic water supplies drawn off from the main intake where possible, or adequately treated. Essentially, it must be easier to get at safe than unsafe water, both for consumption and for washing clothes. This siting applies to both irrigation and man-made lakes, though if fishing is a major occupation it may be unrealistic to suggest other than lakeside villages.

In irrigation design, overhead sprinklers without runoff are safest, but health considerations can rarely dominate a decision between those and canals. The latter may be fenced near settlements or piped where this is feasible. Drainage ditches usually support larger snail populations than canals. In canal construction, lining and flow rate are crucial. A smooth surface is less attractive to snails and rapid flow dislodges them, and in Japan concrete linings have been used to reduce snail numbers and water seepage at the same time. Canal maintenance can also reduce snail populations. Vegetation harbours snails and lowers water velocity though, in the absence of rigid safety discipline, the canal cleaners may be at heavy risk of schistosomiasis. The amphibious habits of the snail hosts of *S. japonicum* pose special problems.

The water management possible in an irrigation scheme may make chemical control of snails feasible. Two molluscicides are usefully available. Niclosamide will kill snails and their eggs when 1 part per million is maintained for 8 hours in the water, while *n*-trityl-morpholine is effective against the snails at a lower concentration still, though it is not ovicidal. The aim is to achieve thorough penetration of the irrigation system by application at a limited number of canals. Design features such as night storage dams may impede this; and where coordination between the irrigation authority and health personnel is lacking, it may be impossible. Peasant irrigation schemes where central authority is limited also make difficulties. Aerial application of molluscicide has been used in large irrigated areas.

Molluscicides properly applied are effective in greatly reducing snail numbers. The proportionate effect on transmission of schistosomiasis is much less, but satisfactory control has been obtained in several parts of the world and this has been shown to be profitable in narrowly economic terms in sugar estates in Tanzania (Fenwick, 1972).

Man-made lakes are more difficult in that the volume is too vast for mollusciciding and this is also true of the periphery. Good solutions are lacking but some improvement is obtained by siting settlements near exposed rather than vegetated beaches, weed clearance near settlements, jetties and landing places, and provision of water supplies, sanitary facilities and piers. If water contact sites are extremely regular and focal, as on Lake Volta, focal mollusciciding may be attempted.

Biological control of snails has been much discussed. The only methods feasible to attempt now are the use of fish populations known to eat snails and the introduction of competitor snails, especially of the genus *Marisa*, which in Puerto Rico compete for food and in other ways with *Biomphalaria* which transmits schistosomiasis. However, the introduction of exotic species to new countries or continents can only be undertaken as part of a most carefully controlled long-term research programme.

Reduction of water contact is clearly not feasible for fishermen and irrigation workers. More can be done for their families by provision of water supplies suitably designed, with local involvement in planning and construction.

In summary therefore, water developments raise numerous health hazards. Total prevention of these may be unfeasible or far too expensive; but by highly skilled study of each situation it is usually possible to reduce the disease problems considerably at reasonable cost.

2.5 REFERENCES

Fenwick, A. (1972). The cost and a cost–benefit analysis of a *Schistosoma mansoni* control programme on an irrigated sugar estate in northern Tanzania. *Bulletin of the World Health Organization*, **47**, 573–578.

Hannoun, C., Panthier, R., Mouchet, J. and Eouzan, J. P. (1964). Isolement en France du virus West-Nile a partir de malades et du vecteur *Culex modestus* Ficalbi. *Comptes rendus hebdomadaires des seances de l'Academie des Sciences, Paris*, **259**, 4170–4172.

Ross Institute. (1974). *The Preservation of Personal Health in Warm Climates*. London: Ross Institute of Tropical Hygiene.

Simpson, D. I. H., Bowen, E. T. W., Platt, G. S., Way, H., Smith C. E. G., Peto, S., Sumitra Kamath, Lim Boo Liat and Lim Teong Wah. (1970). Japanese encephalitis in Sarawak: virus isolation and serology in a land Dayak village. *Transactions of the Royal Society of Tropical Medicine and Hygiene*, **64**, 503–510.

Surtees, G. (1970a). Effects of irrigation on mosquito populations and mosquito-borne diseases in man, with particular reference to ricefield extension. *International Journal of Environmental Studies*, **1**, 35–42.

Surtees, G. (1970b). Control of mosquitoes breeding in ricefields. *Journal of Tropical Medicine and Hygiene*, **74**, 255–259.

Webster, M. H. (1960). The medical aspects of the Kariba hydro-electric scheme. *Central African Journal of Medicine*, **6**, supplement to no. 10, 1–36.

An extremely full account of topics raised in this chapter is given in:

Stanley, N. F. and Alpers, M. P. (1975). *Man-made Lakes and Human Health*. London: Academic Press.

3

Microbiological Criteria for Tropical Water Quality

LILIAN M. EVISON *and* A. JAMES

3.1 INTRODUCTION

Micro-organisms are very widely distributed in nature and so commonly find their way into most natural waters. The microbial flora of natural waters therefore reflects their history of accessibility to colonization so that underground waters tend to contain mainly soil micro-organisms whilst surface waters have a much more diverse flora. The nutrient status of the water is also important in determining growth or die-off and this balance is affected by other environmental influences such as temperature and light intensity.

The abundance and diversity of micro-organisms may, therefore, be used to give an integrated picture of conditions in a natural body of water which may serve as a guide to the suitability of the water for fish and other animals or as a means of classifying waters for general recreational or amenity purposes. Micro-organisms are most widely used as a guide to water quality in connection with drinking waters. Here the concentration of certain intestinal indicator organisms is used to determine the degree of health risk from consuming the water and to monitor the effectiveness of the treatment process in reducing microbial numbers so that the risk is reduced to acceptable levels.

The use of micro-organisms for determining water quality does not differ fundamentally in tropical situations from the techniques employed in temperate zones. The differences are mainly in emphasis and, to some extent, in interpretation. Water-related infections are much commoner in tropical countries and the diversity of infections is considerably greater. The hygienic aspects of water quality therefore merit greater attention, particularly since the levels of faecal contamination in drinking sources are often high.

The resultant stress on the value of micro-organisms in the examination of water supplies in tropical countries has tended to overshadow their importance in other aspects of water quality. This review tends to reflect this imbalance because the majority of published work deals with micro-organisms in the context of water supplies for drinking. However, an attempt is made to redress the balance by taking a comprehensive view. The use of micro-organisms in setting water quality objectives for both abstracted and natural waters is covered and viral, bacterial, algal and animal parameters are considered.

3.2 MICROBIOLOGY OF NATURAL WATERS IN HOT CLIMATES

The microbiology of tropical waters is still largely unexplored. Economic pressures have dictated that control of water pollution for amenity or recreation has not had the same priority as water supply and therefore the scientific study has not been stimulated as in temperate countries. Such studies that have been carried out have concentrated on the medical aspects of disease spread by associating with natural waters or with the exploitation of fisheries, since these are of commercial interest. Also, spectacular developments of aquatic macrophytes have diverted interest from the more subtle mysteries of the microbiological changes. As pointed out by Blum (1956), there are many parts of the world where one lacks basic information on the species present.

Our understanding of the physical and chemical background of tropical waters also contains unexplained areas. The stability of thermal stratification in tropical lakes and reservoirs merits further study. The extent to which stratification occurs in large tropical rivers has yet to be established and its effect on the river life has not been investigated.

Because of the lack of information on microbiological processes in tropical waters there has been a tendency to use criteria derived from temperate investigations in an uncritical manner. A five-day BOD test on river water in the Nile at Khartoum, for example, may be useful for comparison of organic concentration with rivers in other parts of the world but gives a false indication of the potential uptake in that river due to differences in temperature and retention time.

Lakes and reservoirs

The assessment of water quality in lakes and reservoirs is most often concerned with measurements of the plankton in terms of either standing crop or energy flux. This is particularly true in tropical lakes and reservoirs where high light intensities and high temperatures favour primary production. Under these conditions plankton production may affect water quality in several respects:

(a) for abstraction for supply where algae may cause clogging of the filters or tastes and odours in the water;
(b) for amenity, since large concentrations of algae cause the water to become very turbid and in extreme cases, such as Ethiopian crater lakes, can produce large floating masses of decaying algae;
(c) for fishing in two ways: firstly the amount of primary production largely determines the size of fishery that a water body can support and secondly large algal growths affect the dissolved oxygen concentration of the water owing to their respiration and photosynthesis; also the dead algae constitute the principal food for benthic bacteria and so affect water quality in the lower layers of the lake.

There has been surprisingly little work on the species composition of the phytoplankton in tropical lakes and reservoirs. Gessner (1955) showed that although there are a large number of common species of worldwide distribution, there are also a large number of algae which are purely tropical. In general terms it has been shown that blue-green algae are more thermophilic (e.g. Hutchinson, 1964) and might be expected to dominate but the balance between diatoms, green algae and blue-greens depends upon many factors. A study of plankton in some Indian lakes by Seenayya (1971) showed that different groups were most affected by different factors (Table 3.1); these results indicate that many tropical and subtropical lakes show clear seasonal variations in the dominant types of algae. Often, as Dor (1974) showed in Lake Kinneret, seasonal changes are connected with the drier summer period which favours blue-greens (high temperatures and relatively high salinities) and the cooler, wetter winter which favours diatoms (lower temperatures and lower salinities).

Other hydrological factors may be involved. A characteristic of the Great Lakes of Africa is their large volume in relation to inflow—for example, Lake Victoria, which has a retention time of over 1000 years (Beachamp, 1969). This makes the water quality in the lake very stable. But smaller tropical lakes and most reservoirs have a smaller volume in relation to inflow and thus respond more sensitively to droughts and floods in the feeder streams; for example, Rzoska and Talling (1966) showed that the Sennar reservoir on the Blue Nile had a phytoplankton picture strongly influenced by the annual flood which caused algal washout. More complex hydrological cycles occur in some tropical lakes such as Lake Chilwa. Morgan and Kalk (1970) found a six

Table 3.1 Environmental factors favouring the dominance of different algal groups

Group	Favourable environmental factors
Volvocales	Dilution by short spells of rain
Chlorococcales	High concentrations of organic matter and phosphorus
Desmids	Prolonged periods of sunshine, high concentrations of dissolved solids and iron
Euglineneae:	
Euglena haematodes	Low degree of organic pollution and carbon dioxide
E. clavata *E. inflata* *E. oxyuris* *Lepocinclis ovum* *L. caudata* *Phacus acuminatus* *P. orbicularis* *P. onyx*	High degree of organic pollution, carbon dioxide and ammonia
Trachelomonas plantonica *T. hispida* *T. hirsuta*	High concentration of iron
T. armata	High concentration of iron and alkaline conditions

year cycle in this lake during which it reduced in volume and increased in salinity from 250 mg/l up to 1700 mg/l. This caused a change in dominant algae from the greens to the blue-greens. Also, in reservoirs like Volta Lake the hydrology is strongly affected by releases of water for hydroelectric power generation which in turn disturbs the phytoplankton balance.

From the above examples it is clear that the composition of the phytoplankton in tropical lakes and reservoirs is often the result of several interacting factors and that for many lakes the composition and the factors have yet to be established. With this background it is not possible to use algal composition as a guide to the pollution status of these water bodies. There are difficulties in assessing the degree of eutrophication in other ways. Marshall and Falconer (1973) found primary hourly production rates of up to 1500 mg O_2/m^3 in a Rhodesian lake affected by sewage discharge compared with 500 mg O_2/m^3 in similar lakes with no discharges. However, where control situations are lacking and it is not possible to make this type of comparison, the concentrations of chlorophyll-a and the rates of primary production can only be used as a guide because they tend to be higher than in temperate waters owing to the higher temperatures and light intensities. These types of measurement are most useful in connection with fish production. Marshall and Falconer suggested that supersaturation with oxygen in the epilimnion might be used as a criterion of eutrophication. In the Rhodesian lakes that they studied this was a permanent (diurnal and annual) feature of eutrophic lakes; but in other tropical or subtropical bodies of water it may be a seasonal feature and therefore less useful. It is, however, a more accurate indication of eutrophication than anaerobic conditions in the hypolimnion. The stratification of tropical lakes and reservoirs has been studied extensively and Talling (1969) has shown that this thermal and, to a lesser extent, chemical stratification is a permanent or semi-permanent feature. The reasons for the stratification are not clear but may be connected with increase in density difference per degree of temperature that occurs higher up the temperature scale. Ganapati (1973) showed that the change from 29 °C to 30 °C caused a change in density two-and-a-half times greater than that from 14 °C to 15 °C. Conditions in the hypolimnion of a tropical lake are markedly different from those in a temperate hypolimnion. The temperatures are usually in the range 22 °C–30 °C which gives a rate of decomposition of 4–9 times that at 4 °C. This, together with the often permanent nature of the stratification, gives rise to anaerobic conditions in nearly all tropical hypolimnions. This criterion of eutrophic conditions in temperate lakes is therefore of little value in the tropics.

There are other aspects of the pollution of tropical lakes and reservoirs for which other types of micro-organisms are more appropriate. Some smaller bodies suffer from organic pollution problems and these can occur as localized difficulties in the larger lakes and reservoirs. As noted above, the dissolved oxygen concentration can give a false impression. Bacteria have not been reported as being used in tropical waters but it seems reasonable that the C_{14} uptake technique of Hobbie (Hobbie, 1969) could be used for assessment.

Alternatively some Indian studies (Arora *et al.*, 1965) suggested the use of the protozoan fauna for classification, as follows:

(a) heavily polluted—characterized by *Codosiga, Metopus, Frontonia and Gonostomum*;
(b) mildly polluted—characterized by *Arcella, Diflugia, Acineta* and *Paranema*;
(c) clean—characterized by *Vampyrella, Chilomonas, Tetrahymena, Podophyra.*

Rivers

The problems of quality assessment in tropical rivers has received even less attention than that in lakes and reservoirs. Generally rivers do not present the same potential for the development of fisheries or major water supply and the main interest has been for amenity, for irrigation and for smaller supply schemes. Despite this lack of investigation there has been sufficient work on tropical rivers to show that they present a variety of interesting assemblages of micro-organisms which differ considerably from temperate communities because of edaphic factors. Much further work will be needed in this field before microbiological criteria can be applied but the following survey shows some of the advances that have been made in understanding relations between environments and communities and ways of using the results to classify conditions.

One of the striking factors of large tropical rivers is not just the immense size and length but that owing to topography the majority of the course is at a very low gradient. As a result, in rivers like the Nile, Amazon, Indus, etc., flow velocities are generally very low. This, together with the considerable depth and high turbidities, causes phytoplankton dominance over benthic algae. In such rivers benthic algae are either completely absent or present for only part of the year and pollution assessment needs to be based on the composition of phytoplankton communities.

Another result of the deep slow stretches is the development of thermal stratification. Hickling (1961) found stratification in a wide variety of tropical rivers from Brazil, Guyana, Sumatra and Zambia. He attributed this to the great depth and slow flow but Imbevore and Visser (1969) found a similar phenomenon in the River Niger at a point where it was only 6 m deep and moving at an average velocity of 0·8 cm/second. The results were as follows:

	pH	Temperature (°C)	DO	Na	Fe	PO_4	Chlorophyll-*a*
Surface	6·34	31·0	0·90	0·22	0·004	0·05	0·30
4 m below	6·47	32·0	1·20	0·16	0·005	0·07	0·41

(all concentrations in milliequivalents/litre)

They show a surprising degree of chemical stratification which is obviously having some biological repercussions which would need to be considered in sampling.

Temperatures in tropical rivers are consistently high (often up to 35 °C) compared with temperate rivers where they vary annually from 0 °C–5 °C to 20 °C–25 °C. The lack of any pronounced annual cycle of temperature largely eliminates the seasonal algal cycles found in temperate rivers. As pointed out by Gittleson and Ferguson (1971) the uniformly high temperatures cause an absence of cold-loving organisms like *Bodo caudatus* and restricts the microfauna to warm-loving species like *Paramoecium caudatum* or thermally tolerant organisms like *Aspidisca lynceus*. For the microflora the situation is more complicated because, as Patrick (1954) showed, there are some algae for which temperature is critical but for many others the light intensity is more important.

The hydrology of tropical rivers and their planktonic flora is often strongly influenced by the annual or twice-yearly flood. These floods arise from snow-melt (e.g. the Nile) or from the seasonal nature of tropical rainfall, i.e. monsoon (e.g. the Irrawaddy). The resulting period of scour and high turbidity not only damages the benthos but also affects the plankton very markedly. Holden and Green (1960) found that the plankton of the River Sokoto was dominated by water level. During the flood period the volume of water entering the river is so great that both chemical and algal concentrations are reduced. They considered that the plankton reduction was due to dilution, together with reduction in the concentration of nutrients (particularly SO_4) to growth-limiting levels. Talling and Rzoska (1967) found that in the Blue Nile concentrations of plankton were very low during the July–October phase of high floods, owing to the adverse conditions of rapid flow and high turbidity. The period from November to January is one of increasing algal population leading to maximum crops in February and March. During April the numbers are once more reduced owing to the emptying of the Sennar Reservoir upstream and the consequent reduction in retention time. They were unable to find a cause for a secondary maximum which occurred during May and June before the flood.

Floods also affect the composition of the plankton as well as the overall concentration. Imbevore (1970) showed that in the River Niger the water during the major flood was so turbid that photosynthesis was limited to the top metre. The plankton during this period was dominated by diatoms whereas during the secondary flood period and the dry season the main planktonic algae were blue-greens.

For algae the ionic composition of the water is of prime importance in determining growth rates and this is especially significant in tropical rivers. Because of the intense nature of the rainfall many tropical soils have been thoroughly leached and consequently the runoff contains rather low concentrations of inorganic ions. A comparison of the ionic content of world rivers was made by Livingstone (1963). He showed that the average content of tropical rivers like the Amazon (50 mg/l as total dissolved solids) was much lower than the world average (120 mg/l TDS). The nature and extent of the deficiency obviously depends upon the soil type in the catchment; for example Holden and Green (1960) found that SO_4 was limiting to algal growth, whereas in the Blue Nile Talling and Rzoska (1967) concluded that nitrogen was limiting the growth of *Melosira*. However, in all cases the deficiency was more pronounced during the wet season, thus increasing the amplitude of seasonal variation in algal numbers.

The complexities in the use of population control in the algal communities of tropical rivers are obviously considerable. This creates difficulties in the use of algae to classify the pollution status of rivers. Work of this sort has been carried out in temperate rivers notably by Fjerdingstad (1964). Unfortunately our present level of knowledge and limited understanding of tropical rivers make it impossible to apply such a sophisticated classification as that developed for temperate rivers by Fjerdingstad. Some studies have been carried out on Indian rivers by Venkateswarlu (1970). He concluded that the algal composition was controlled by the following factors:

(1) Temperature

(a) Species favoured by low temperature and high DO: *Ancanthes minatissima*.
(b) Species favoured by high organic concentration and high temperature: *Nitzschia obtusa*.
(c) Species favoured by high organic concentration and low DO: *Synedra ulna*.
(d) Species favoured by high DO and low organic content: *Gomphonema sphaerophorum*.
(e) Species favoured by high temperature: *Caloneis silicula*.
(f) Species favoured by low temperature: *Acanthes exigna*.
(g) Species adversely affected by high temperature: *Spirogyra* spp.

(2) Current

Species adversely affected by fast currents: *Caloneis silicula*.

(3) Nitrates

(a) Species favoured by high nitrates: *Cymbella microcephala*.
(b) Species favoured by low nitrates: *Cyclotella meneghiniana*.

(4) Total iron

Species favoured by low iron: *Navicula pygmaea*.

Generally, however, studies on tropical rivers have been much less detailed, as is typified by a study of a South African river polluted with discharges from gold-mining. Hancock (1973) showed that as a result of the increase in pH and ionic content there was an increase in algal biomass and also a change in dominance from diatoms to greens to blue-greens. Similarly Venkateswarlu and Jayanti (1968) in a review of river pollution studies on Indian rivers, concluded that micro-organisms were useful indicators. But they were only able to suggest a simple classification into the following two groups:

(a) clean water—presence of *Pandorina*, *Eudorina*, *Volvox* and absence of ciliates;

(b) polluted water—absence of *Pandorina*, *Eudorina* and *Volvox* and presence of *Beggiatoa*, *Oscillatoria* and ciliates.

The above remarks have been entirely directed to the use of algae for classifying tropical rivers. Other micro-organisms do not appear to have received attention except for the health aspects. These are only briefly considered below, as micro-organisms seem to be of limited utility; but reference should also be made to Section 3.3 of this chapter and Chapters 1 and 2 for a more detailed treatment of health hazards.

The health hazards from natural waters arise in two ways. Firstly they are due to the transmission of infections by entering the water or using recreational facilities on river banks. Bilharzia (schistosomiasis) is the greatest hazard. Microscopic examination of the water for the presence of cercariae is not used for assessing this type of risk. Where the water is accidentally ingested microbiological examination may be of value and some tropical equivalent of the bathing water standards used in USA (coliforms: 1000–10 000 per 100 ml) may prove useful. Because of the higher endemic levels of salmonella infections the risk of disease spreading through polluted bathing waters is obviously greater. There is also a chance of other disease like guinea worm, amoebic dysentery, hookworm infections, etc. being transmitted via recreational waters. However, the epidemiological significance of this mode of transmission has yet to be established and it is doubtful if microscopic examination of water or routine culturing would serve any useful purpose.

The second type of health hazard arises from the consumption of shellfish grown in polluted waters. There do not appear to have been any comprehensive studies of this subject in tropical countries. In the absence of any contrary indications it is suggested that standards recommended in Holden (1970) be adopted (<5 *E. coli*/ml shellfish flesh). Shellfish may also concentrate toxic algae from the overlying water, and where 'red tide' blooms of particular dinoflagellates occur the shellfish can cause severe neurotoxic poisoning in humans. The factors which give rise to red tides have not yet been fully elucidated, but they seem to be stimulated by high temperatures and excessive nutrients (Wood, 1974). The present standards are based on determination of toxins directly in the shellfish flesh rather than identification of algae in the seawater itself. Shellfish samples from the major fishing grounds can be screened by a mouse bioassay method (McFarren, 1959); safe upper limits of 'mouse units' have been specified (Ayres and Callum, 1975).

3.3 MICROBIOLOGY OF ABSTRACTED WATERS IN HOT CLIMATES

Surface and underground sources are used for a variety of different purposes wherever human habitations occur. In temperate climates water is usually in plentiful supply and can be abstracted from unpolluted underground sources

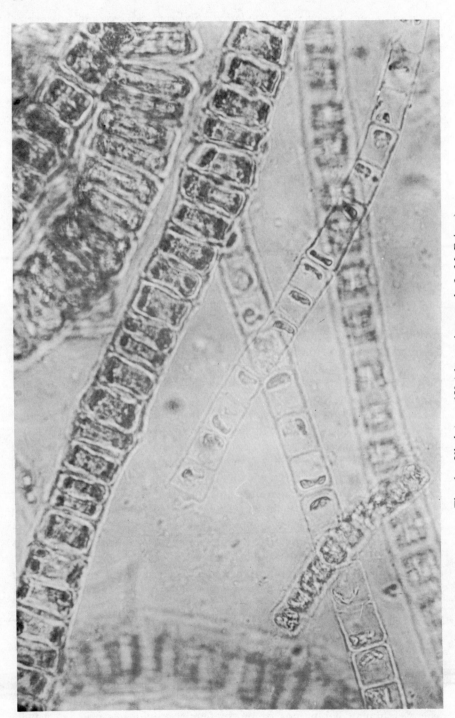

The alga *Ulothrix*, × 650 (photomicrograph: L. M. Evison)

or fairly clean surface waters. In hot climates the sources of water are very much more restricted, often extremely variable in quantity and of low microbiological quality. Water is required by the community for many purposes, principally for drinking and general domestic use, and for irrigation of crops where rainfall is very low and intermittent. A recent survey (WHO, 1973a) showed that only one half of the urban population in developing countries have a drinking water supply in their houses, and only 12% of rural dwellers have reasonable access to safe drinking water. This factor, together with the inadequate waste treatment facilities and the generally low level of personal hygiene leads to very high levels of enteric disease. In developing countries the incidence of typhoid fever, bacillary dysentery, amoebiasis, infectious hepatitis and other enteric infections that may be transmitted by water is often 10 to more than 100 times that in the more advanced of the developed countries (WHO, 1968). Epidemics of cholera are also relatively common in these countries. Other diseases such as schistosomiasis, ankylostomiasis and ascariasis are usually endemic and, although these are not water-borne disease in the accepted sense of the word, they fall into the related categories proposed by White *et al.* (1972) and Bradley (see Chapter 1).

The presence of faecal material in water presents the most immediate hazard to health, since faecal material from either human or animal sources may contain pathogenic micro-organisms. Diseases transmitted by faecal material may be caused by viruses, bacteria, protozoa or metazoa. In temperate climates water-borne diseases are usually bacterial, and the microbiological tests for water quality reflect this tendency, but in hot climates viral, protozoal and metazoal diseases may frequently be water-borne so more consideration must be given to these other micro-organisms.

Indicator bacteria

It is calculated that bacteria constitute over 30% of the total wet volume of faeces and counts of 10^{10} anaerobes and 10^8 aerobes per gram wet weight of faeces are regularly reported. Counts of intestinal bacteria can therefore be used to give a very sensitive test of the extent of faecal pollution of water. Several hundred different species of bacteria have been reported from the faecal microflora, for example Moore and Holdeman (1974) observed 113 distinct types of bacteria in the faeces of 20 clinically healthy Japanese–Hawaiian males. The majority of bacteria excreted in faeces are part of the normal intestinal flora and are adapted to intestinal conditions (high optimum growth temperature, high nutritional requirements and low requirement for oxygen). The bacterial flora of the human intestine is influenced to some extent by the diet and ethnic factors of the population studied. A study of the faeces of subjects in Europe, America, India, Japan and Uganda (Drasar, 1974; Hill *et al.*, 1971) gives some insight into the effect of diet and socio-economic changes on the intestinal flora. The Europeans and Americans lived in modern cities on typical western diets, while the Indians, Japanese and Ugandans

Table 3.2 Faecal microflora of different human populations*

Diet	Country	Mean log$_{10}$ no. of bacteria/g of faeces						
		Enterobacteria	Enterococci	Lactobacilli	Clostridia	Bacteroides	Bifidobacteria	Eubacteria[†]
Largely carbohydrate	India	7·9	7·3	7·6	5·7	9·2	9·6	9·5
	Japan	9·4	8·1	7·4	5·6	9·4	9·7	9·6
	Uganda	8·0	7·0	7·2	5·1	8·2	9·4	9·3
Mixed Western	England	7·9	5·8	6·5	5·7	9·8	9·9	9·3
	Scotland	7·6	5·3	7·7	5·6	9·8	9·9	9·3
	USA	7·4	5·9	6·5	5·4	9·7	9·9	9·3

*Reproduced from Drasar (1974) by permission of the Society for Applied Bacteriology.
[†]Numbers estimated on the basis of isolates identified.

lived in simple rural communities with largely carbohydrate diets. The results (Table 3.2) illustrate that for most groups of organisms the distribution pattern is remarkably similar in the six groups. In all groups anaerobic organisms (*Bacteroides*, *Bifidobacterium*, *Eubacterium* and *Clostridium*) greatly outnumber the facultative bacteria and the greatest geographical variation in numbers is found in the enterococcus group.

Bacteriological tests for the detection of faecal pollution of water have developed using non-pathogenic groups of bacteria selected on the basis of the following criteria:

(a) numerous in faeces but not other materials;
(b) counted by means of simple, reliable tests;
(c) more resistant than pathogens to physical and chemical inactivating agents;
(d) unable to grow in conditions outside the intestine.

The organisms which have been found to fulfil most of these criteria, at least in temperate climates, are the coliform, faecal coliform (or *Escherichia coli*), faecal group D streptococcus and *Clostridium perfringens* groups. In hot climates problems arise because of physiological changes in the organisms which alter the selectivity of the tests and enable at least some organisms to grow outside the intestine. As Table 3.2 shows the geographical variation in groups is probably not as significant as some authors have suggested.

The coliform group includes organisms now classified in the genera *Escherichia*, *Citrobacter*, *Klebsiella* and *Enterobacter*. Because several of these species are regularly found in unpolluted soils and water the standard test for these organisms cannot be said to indicate specific faecal pollution. It is also reported frequently that coliform numbers in water can increase quite significantly, especially in warm polluted waters (Deaner and Kerri, 1969; Evison and James, 1974; Dutka, 1973). Coliform regrowth conditions can be expected to occur regularly in polluted tropical waters where temperatures exceed 20 °C but it is not yet established whether pathogenic organisms such as *Salmonella typhi* will regrow under the same conditions.

In recent years the faecal coliform test has replaced the coliform test as a more specific indication of pollution. *Escherichia coli* is exclusively faecal and constitutes over 90% of the coliform flora of the human intestine. It is most easily distinguished from other coliforms on the basis of its growth at 44 °C on media normally used for coliform determination. Unfortunately, in tropical waters there are many more coliforms of the klebsiella and citrobacter groups which can grow at 44 °C (Katugampola and Assim, 1958; Moussa, 1965; Evison and James, 1973) and the sanitary significance of these organisms has not yet been established. There have also been isolated reports of regrowth of *E. coli* associated with rotting vegetation at elevated temperatures (Robertson *et al.*, 1966; Taylor, 1972). The faecal coliform test must still be taken as the most sensitive and specific indicator of faecal pollution at present available.

Faecal (group D) streptococci are occasionally used as indicator organisms, especially where confirmation of dubious *E. coli* results is required. They have also been recommended for the examination of tropical waters (Mather and Ramanthan, 1966; Sastry *et al.*, 1969). Although the organisms show little tendency to regrow, their rapid death rate in temperatures greater than 20 °C seems to diminish their value as indicators in tropical waters (Evison and James, 1974). The spore-forming anaerobe *Clostridium perfringens* which is sometimes used for the detection of intermittent pollution is adequate for this purpose in both temperate and tropical waters. Another anaerobe, *Bifidobacterium*, has also been tentatively proposed as an indicator of faecal pollution, based on its high numbers in faeces (see Table 3.2) and its limited ability for regrowth in tropical waters (Evison and James, 1974).

Tests for the indicator organisms mentioned above are all fairly simple to perform and can be carried out on a routine basis by technicians with only basic microbiological training and facilities. The technical details of the tests and media recommended are fully described and illustrated in Mara (1974).

Pathogenic organisms

Patients with overt symptoms of disease can excrete enormous numbers of pathogenic organisms. Animals can also harbour pathogens and excrete them, and sometimes apparently healthy humans act as carriers of typhoid and cholera organisms and excrete these intermittently. The nature of pathogens makes them dangerous in the hands of unskilled operators. Routine examination of waters for pathogenic organisms is unnecessary, but when epidemics occur, or attempts are made to eliminate endemic disease, it is important to be able to quantify and identify the causative organism, so at least one central laboratory in every country should be suitably equipped and staffed to isolate pathogenic organisms from water.

Human viruses excreted in faeces may be transmitted through water by faecal contamination. This group includes the infectious hepatitis virus, enteroviruses (poliovirus, coxsackie virus, and ECHO viruses) adenoviruses and reoviruses. These are extremely infectious agents, and the ingestion of only one or two virus particles can give rise to clinical infection. Several viral diseases are common in hot climates. Of these infectious hepatitis and poliomyelitis are the most important, but viruses may also be responsible for epidemics of gastroenteritis and respiratory infections. The largest viral epidemic attributed to a polluted water supply occurred in Delhi, India, during 1955–56 when over 20 000 clinical cases of infectious hepatitis were reported. During this outbreak there was no parallel increase in enteric bacterial diseases, suggesting that the municipal water treatment had been sufficient to remove bacterial pathogens but not the more resistant infectious hepatitis virus (Geldreich, 1972).

Large numbers of viruses can be readily isolated from sewage especially in hot climates. Results quoted in Berg (1973) showed that more than 11.000 plaque-forming units per litre could be isolated from sewage from communities in the lower socio-economic levels in Israel. Even after great dilution in river water, viruses are still detectable downstream of sewage outfalls and at water intakes. Because of their simple structure, viruses are able to survive longer than bacteria in natural waters. Factors such as strong sunlight, heavy bacterial predation and elevated temperatures reduce the survival time to some degree, but survival times of 9 weeks have been reported for enteroviruses in farm pond waters at 20 °C (Geldreich, 1972). The ability of viruses to survive for long periods in water increases the ratio of viruses to indicator bacteria and makes it difficult to relate indicator counts to potential health hazards.

Many bacterial pathogens are common in waters in hot climates. The most important of these are salmonellae and shigellae which give rise to widespread typhoid, paratyphoid and bacillary dysentery, and vibrios which give rise to severe epidemics of cholera. Typhoid and paratyphoid fevers are common in many countries of the Far East, Middle East, Eastern Europe, Central and South America and Africa. The causative organisms are more easily isolated from water, food and faeces than other pathogens and can be related to numbers of indicator bacteria. Data quoted in Dutka (1973) shows that there is no constant relationship between salmonellae numbers and indicator bacteria. In the relatively unpolluted St. Lawrence river water, coliform:salmonellae ratios between 66000:1 and 650:1 were demonstrated; and in an outbreak of salmonellosis in Galilee some waters had ratios of 0:5 and 1:5. The survival of salmonellae can be greatly influenced by temperature and the presence of nutrients in the water. In the nutrients from sugar beet processing, especially at low temperatures, survival of salmonellae is greatly enhanced (Geldreich, 1972). A recent study (McFeters *et al.*, 1974) on comparative survival rates of pure cultures of various pathogens and indicator species in membrane chambers suspended in a stable well water supply indicated the following T_{50} values:

	hours
Shigella flexneri	26·8
Sh. sonnei	24·5
Sh. dysenteriae	22·4
Enterococci	22·0
Coliform bacteria	17·0
Salmonella enteritidis	16·0
Vibrio cholera	7·2
Sa. typhi	6·0

These experiments were conducted at 9·5–12·5 °C in a water with little or no organic material present. Under these conditions the indicator bacteria survive longer than the salmonella and vibrio cultures, but are outlived by the shigellae. There is a great need for further studies of this type to be carried out, preferably in the higher temperature ranges and with a variety of degrees of organic enrichment in order that factors affecting survival and growth of indicators and pathogens can be more fully understood in the context of tropical water pollution.

Cholera presents a particularly acute problem in tropical water examination.

The disease is endemic in India and during the early part of the twentieth century was largely confined to Asia. In 1947 a severe outbreak of cholera occurred in Egypt, and during the last fifteen years outbreaks have occurred in Iran, Iraq, Southern Europe and Africa. This increasing spread of cholera in recent years may reflect the lack of international quarantine enforcement by some countries with primitive sanitation, and the international mobility of carriers in the world population. Cholera epidemics are explosive in nature and are particularly severe in low socio-economic groups where overcrowding and low sanitary standards prevail (WHO, 1967a). A typical cholera patient during the course of his illness excretes 10–20 litres of stool containing 10^8–10^9 vibrois per millilitre and is thus able to contaminate a wide area, including water sources, if he is not hospitalized. Although the vibrios may persist for only a short time in the grossly polluted aquatic environment, faecal contamination from victims and carriers can reinforce their population in water. Vibrios can be isolated from rivers and canals in India with ease, both in epidemic and non-epidemic periods, so surveillance for cholera in water and faecal specimens should be instigated, particularly in developing countries which are more susceptible to epidemics.

Amoebiasis is a disease caused by parasitic protozoa and is known to affect at least 10% of the world's population. The disease is particularly prevalent in tropical countries—for example, it has been reported to affect 83% of the general population in Egypt although 30% infection rate is much more usual in developing countries with poor sanitation (WHO, 1969). *Entamoeba histolytica* is the only one of the six colon-inhabiting amoebae known to be pathogenic to man. In the intestine the organisms are in the form of trophic amoebae (trophozoites) which grow and divide by binary fission. When the trophozoites encyst they become immobilized and are carried out with the faeces, and can then be transmitted either by direct contact or more often by contaminated water to another host. The cysts of *E. histolytica* are able to survive for long periods especially in a humid environment, although they are rapidly killed by temperatures above 55 °C. It has been reported that cysts of *E. histolytica* may persist in good quality water for at least 153 days at 12–22 °C (Geldreich, 1972). In all reported outbreaks of amoebiasis sewage-contaminated water supplies have been the major identified source of infection, either because of inadequate treatment, contamination of the supply in the distribution system or contamination of the water after it has been drawn (WHO, 1969).

Parasitic worms such as *Taenia saginata* (the beef tapeworm) and *Ascaris lumbricoides* (the roundworm) are infectious agents which affect more than 50% of the population in high incidence areas. Infections may occasionally occur from drinking water but are very frequently transmitted in irrigation agriculture. Ascariasis is particularly prevalent in humid areas but in dry savannahs the prevalence is generally low. Worms establish themselves in the human gut and grow to maturity—often 25 cm in length and 3 g in weight. The adult worm produces about 200 000 fertile eggs daily which are evacuated in the faeces. Eggs are able to survive for long periods, particularly in moist, shaded soil, and can also survive and develop into infective larvae in polluted waters so long as conditions do not become anaerobic (WHO, 1967b; Geldreich, 1972).

Thus it can be seen that, while the epidemic and endemic diseases prevalent in the tropics and known to be water-borne are caused by viruses, bacteria, protozoa and parasitic worms, only bacterial tests for the examination of water are in routine use. The application and interpretation of these tests in raw and treated water for potable supply and irrigation will be considered in the following sections.

Quality of raw water for potable supply

The microbiological quality of raw waters destined for drinking water supply may be studied for any of the following reasons:

(a) the assessment of the suitability of new water sources;
(b) the routine surveillance of existing supplies;
(c) the isolation of specific pathogens in epidemic situations.

When considering any new water source for domestic supply it is essential to build up an adequate knowledge of its sanitary quality. Seasonal variations in quantitative output, chemical and microbiological quality must all be established to determine the type and degree of treatment necessary. Routine 20 °C and 37 °C total agar plate counts in addition to the coliform and faecal coliform tests are performed over a range of hydrological conditions. These tests are often supplemented with the faecal streptococcus test, especially if the faecal coliform test gives equivocal results. Animals generally excrete much higher numbers of faecal streptococci than humans, hence the ratio of faecal coliforms to faecal streptococci in a water can indicate whether the pollution is derived from human or animal sources. Ratios of faecal coliforms to faecal streptococci greater than 4·0 are strongly indicative of predominantly human contamination with the associated danger of human disease transmission. Ratios of faecal coliforms to faecal streptococci less than 1·0 are suggestive of mainly animal contamination. Where pollution is suspected to occur only intermittently, the *Cl. perfringens* test is a useful adjunct since the spores are able to survive in water for many months after the other indicator bacteria have died out. Since pathogenic organisms are so much more common in tropical waters, it is suggested that the presence or absence of viruses and amoebic cysts should also be established in the initial investigations so that adequate treatment facilities can be provided.

In temperate waters the saprophytic bacteria generally have an optimum temperature for growth of 15–20 °C which reflects the temperatures of the habitat itself. In tropical waters, especially shallow waters, the temperatures may regularly reach 30 °C or higher. Many saprophytes in tropical waters are able to grow at 37 °C so tests which use direct incubation at 44 °C are subject to less interference from these other organisms.

The microbiological quality of tropical waters ranges from excellent (mainly underground sources) to grossly polluted. Surface water sources, especially near urban areas, are usually highly polluted and dilution cannot be relied upon to improve the quality. Bradley and Emurwon (1968) show that urbanization increases the faecal coliform count from 100/100 ml to 100 000/100 ml on the Mirongo River in Uganda. In the same article they report faecal coliform counts of 1000/100 ml in unprotected springs and 128/100 ml in protected springs and dry wells. Obviously in selection of water sources the best quality supply available should be selected and suitable provision made for treatment, based on the initial examinations.

Routine microbiological analysis of water is necessary once a water treatment system has been installed in order that problems in the treatment process can be anticipated. In Section 3.2 on natural waters evidence has been presented to show that both river and reservoir sources are subject to large variations in microbiological quality. Reservoirs in the tropics are particularly prone to algal blooms. These may affect the water supply by causing problems in filtration or by the taste and odour they impart to the water. Filtration problems are especially associated with diatoms such as *Asterionella*, *Melosira* and *Cyclotella*, along with green algae like *Chlorella* and *Closterium*, and become severe when algal counts exceed about 100 cells per millilitre. Tastes and odours are produced by species of *Synura*, *Uroglena*, *Anabaena*, *Anacystis* and *Aphanizomenon*. Algal blooms also give rise to secondary effects since when they die they can form food for fungi and coliforms, so that the bacteriological quality of the water from tropical reservoirs is less stable than in temperate reservoirs. River water quality is also extremely variable, and the bacteriological quality can deteriorate rapidly owing to surface water runoff following rain carrying large quantities of animal and human faeces into the rivers (Feachem, 1974).

The bacteriological tests used for the routine assessment of water sources should reflect the presence of faecal material so the coliform and faecal coliform tests are most often used for this purpose. Their tendency to regrow in tropical waters may lead to an overestimation of pollution but this is preferable to underestimation and complacency. Cox (1964) recommends the type of treatment necessary for raw waters based on their coliform count and these suggestions should be followed for any supply to a large population. WHO (1971) suggest that in small (untreated) community supplies it should be possible to achieve less than 10 coliforms/100 ml and no faecal coliforms. This standard may be unnecessarily strict in the tropics in view of the capacity of coliforms for regrowth and the ability of *Klebsiella* and *Citrobacter* species to grow at 44 °C. There is a need for sound epidemiological surveys to establish whether this standard is justified.

Quality of treated water for potable supply

The coliform and faecal coliform tests have been successfully used as the primary standard for drinking water quality for many years. In raw sewage these organisms are present in concentrations of 10^6-10^7 per millilitre. If, therefore, they do not exceed 1 per 100 ml in drinking water the level of faecal contamination must be less than 1 part in 10^8 or 10^9, giving very little risk of disease transference. Desirable water quality standards for treated water entering the distribution system and for samples of water in the distribution system are given in WHO (1971) and should be aimed at for all piped drinking-water supplies. Wherever raw water supplies can be expected to contain mainly bacterial pathogens the coliform and faecal coliform standards give an adequate margin of safety.

However, the shortage of water in hot climates sometimes means that authorities are forced to abstract water from heavily polluted sources for supply to urban communities. For example, in times of drought the water supply for Agra, India, consists almost entirely of partially treated sewage from New Delhi, 190 km away (WHO, 1973b). In such situations the distinction between water treatment and wastewater reclamation becomes very slight. The problem of removal of pathogens from heavily polluted water is particularly important; pathogenic viruses, bacteria, protozoa and metazoa are almost certain to be present although the counts of indicator bacteria cannot be relied on to give an accurate estimate of pathogen counts. The water treatment processes adopted must be designed to remove all pathogens from water, not just bacterial pathogens which are perhaps most easily dealt with. Disinfection with chlorine can certainly not be relied upon as the sole treatment. Sen and Jacobs (1969) showed that chlorinated, unfiltered water from the Hoogly River distributed to hydrants in Calcutta contained pathogenic vibrios and salmonellae in at least 5% of samples, and protozoa and viruses are known to be more resistant to disinfection than bacteria.

The water treatment selected must be appropriate to the particular raw water source; and the physical, chemical and microbiological quality of the water must be taken into account in determining the necessary combination of unit processes. In relation to pathogenic organisms the following points should be borne in mind. Storage of water as a preliminary step is a simple and cheap means of reducing the pathogen concentration where land values permit this. Larger organisms such as *Ascaris* and *Taenia* eggs are greatly reduced in number by settlement and some settlement of amoebic cysts occurs. The infective cercariae of schistosomiasis are also unable to survive for longer than 2 days without a host. Viruses and pathogenic bacteria are reduced in numbers, particularly in strong sunlight which damages the nucleic acids of the organisms.

Slow sand filtration, rapid gravity filters, and flocculation all remove microorganisms to a variable extent (Holden, 1970), but at least some pathogenic viruses, protozoa and bacteria may survive to the disinfection stage. Disinfection of water is generally achieved by chlorination, which has been applied very much on a rule-of-thumb basis. A vast literature on the chemistry of chlorination and the kinetics of disinfection of a range of micro-organisms has now accumulated and it is possible to adopt a much more rational approach to the problem of pathogen removal. Carrell Morris (1970) presented evidence that spores and amoebic cysts are most resistant to disinfection, viruses have intermediate resistance and enteric bacteria are least resistant. He made the point that specific free chlorination rather than combined chlorination should be employed for virus and other pathogen inactivation. Data from Chang (1971) gives the following residuals (mg/l) of disinfectants for 99·999% destruction of pathogens in 10 minutes at 25 °C :

	Amoebic cysts	Enteric bacteria	Enteric viruses
HOCl	3·5	0.02	0·40
NHCl$_2$	6·0	1·2	5·0
NH$_2$Cl	18·6	4·0	20·0

Thus it seems advisable that breakpoint chlorination to a minimum of 3·5 mg/l HOCl should be maintained for 10 minutes when treating a heavily polluted water source. Clearly enteric bacteria will be too sensitive to chlorination to give an accurate indication of the extent of viral and protozoal removal. It is therefore suggested that spore-forming bacteria such as *Bacillus* or *Clostridium* should be used to determine the adequacy of treatment where heavily polluted waters are used for potable supply.

Quality of water for irrigation

Irrigation of crops in hot climates is an increasingly common practice to meet the food requirements of the world's population. Water is often abstracted directly from rivers and used for spray and furrow irrigation. In countries where water is in particularly short supply sewage effluents are disinfected and then used for irrigation. Where polluted waters or treated effluents are used for crops which are consumed by humans without further processing there is a danger of disease transmission, although this is often ignored, and the physical and chemical qualities of irrigation water are often the only criteria of suitability. The relationship between contamination and disease is not so straightforward with irrigation water as it is for drinking water. Much depends upon the time elapsing between contamination and consumption and the rate at which the pathogens die off. Sunlight is damaging to all pathogens, so if a sufficient time is allowed to elapse between stopping irrigation and harvesting the crop the hazard to health may be much reduced. Studies on the survival of *E. coli* on the surface of leaves and the unbroken skin of fruit and vegetables indicate times ranging from less than 6 to more than 35 days (McKee and Wolf, 1971). There is no equivalent survival data for pathogens, so it is difficult to determine the minimum interval to be recommended between irrigation with polluted water and harvesting.

Existing standards for irrigation waters are most usually based on coliform counts, and standards vary with the country and the type of crop irrigated. As a guide it can be assumed that only a limited health risk would result from the unrestricted irrigation of agricultural crops with sewage effluents having a bacterial quality of less than 100 coliform organisms per 100 ml (WHO, 1973b). (See also Chapter 19.)

3.4 CONCLUDING REMARKS

We have attempted in this review to emphasize the particular features of tropical waters which are important for microbial (especially algal) growth, and have shown that it is not possible to assess raw water quality by the same criteria that are used in temperate waters. Differences in species composition and complex hydrological conditions require that criteria applicable to tropical waters are established, though basic research in this field is very limited at present.

In abstracted waters the problem of water quality criteria is complicated by the high incidence of disease in tropical developing countries, by the resistance to disinfection of viruses, amoebic cysts etc., and by the unsuitability of several of the standard bacteriological tests. Standards for water quality have largely been based on experience from waters in temperate, more developed countries. There is still a real need for research into the suitability of the various tests and for sound epidemiological studies to establish realistic standards which can be applied in developing countries.

3.5 REFERENCES

Arora, H. C., Krishnamoorthi, K. P. and Shrivastava, H. N. (1965). Biological characteristics of water quality. In: *Proceedings of a Symposium on Problems in Water Treatment*, Nagpur: CPHERI, pp. 186–205.

Ayres, P. A. and Callum, M. (1975). A monitoring programme for paralytic shellfish poisoning on the northeast coast of England. *ICES Publication No. CM 1975/K:29.* London: Ministry of Agriculture, Fisheries and Food (Fisheries Improvement Committee).

Beauchamp, R. S. A. (1969). Hydrological factors affecting biological productivity: A comparison between the Great Lakes in Africa and the new man-made lakes. In: *Man-Made Lakes* (Ed. L. Obeng). Accra: Ghana Academy of Sciences, pp. 91–93.

Berg, G. (1973). Reassessment of the virus problem in sewage and in surface and renovated waters. *Progress in Water Technology*, **3**, 87–94.

Blum, J. L. (1956). The ecology of river algae. *Botanical Review*, **22**, 291–341.

Bradley, D. J. and Emurwon, P. (1968). Predicting the epidemiological effects of changing water sources I. *East African Medical Journal*, **45**, 284–291.

Carrell Morris, J. (1970). Disinfection of water supplies. In: *Water Treatment in the Seventies, Proceedings of a Symposium, Reading, Jan. 1970*, London: Society for Water Treatment and Examination, pp. 160–176.

Chang, S. L. (1971). Modern concepts of disinfection. *Journal of Sanitary Engineering Division, ASCE*, **97** (SA5), 689–707.

Cox, C. R. (1964). *Operation and Control of Water Treatment Processes*. Geneva: World Health Organization.

50

Deaner, D. G. and Kerri, K. D. (1969). Regrowth of faecal coliforms. *Journal of American Water Works Association*, **61**, 465–468.

Dor, I. (1974). Considerations about the composition of benthic algal flora in Lake Kinneret. *Hydrobiologia*, **44**, 255–264.

Drasar, B. S. (1974). Some factors associated with geographical variations in the intestinal microflora. In: *The Normal Microbial Flora of Man* (Ed. F. A. Skinner and J. G. Carr). London: Academic Press, pp. 187–196.

Dutka, B. J. (1973). Coliforms are an inadequate index of water quality. *Journal of Environmental Health*, **36**, 39–46.

Evison, L. M. and James, A. (1973). A comparison of the distribution of intestinal bacteria in British and East African water sources. *Journal of Applied Bacteriology*, **36**, 109–118.

Evison, L. M. and James, A., (1974). Bifidobacterium as an indicator of faecal pollution in water. *Paper Presented at 7th International Conference on Water Pollution Research, Paris, September*.

Feachem, R. (1974). Faecal coliforms and faecal streptococci in streams in the New Guinea Highlands. *Water Research*, **8**, 367–374.

Fjerdingstad, E. (1964). Pollution of streams estimated by benthal phytomicro-organisms. *Internationale Revue der gesamten Hydrobiologie*, **49**, 63–87.

Ganapati, S. V. (1973). Ecological problems of man-made lakes of South India. *Archive für Hydrobiologie*, **71**, 363–380.

Geldreich, E. E. (1972). Water-borne pathogens. In: *Water Pollution Microbiology* (Ed. R. Mitchell). New York: Wiley-Interscience, pp. 207–241.

Gessner, F. (1955). *Hydrobotanik I*. Energiehaushalt. Veb. Deutsch. Ver. Vissensch., Berlin, pp. 5, 6, 53–54, 61, 70, 75, 81, 87–88, 90–92, 99.

Gittleson, S. M. and Ferguson, T. (1971). Temperature-related occurrence of protozoa. *Hydrobiologia*, **37**, 49–55.

Hancock, F. D. (1973). Algal ecology of a stream polluted through gold mining on the Witwatersrand. *Hydrobiologia*, **43**, 189–229.

Hickling, C. F. (1961). *Tropical Inland Fisheries*. Longmans: London.

Hill, M. J., Drasar, B. S., Aries, U., Crowther, J. S., Hawksworth, G. and Williams, R. E. O. (1971). Bacteria and aetiology of cancer of large bowel. *The Lancet*, 16th January, 95–100.

Hobbie, J. E. (1969). A method for studying heterotrophic bacteria. In: *A Manual on Methods for Measuring Primary Production in Aquatic Environments*, Oxford: Blackwell, pp. 146–151.

Holden, M. J. and Green, J. (1960). The hydrology and plankton of the River Sokoto. *Journal of Animal Ecology*, **29**, 65–84.

Holden, W. S. (1970). *Water Treatment and Examination*. London: J. & A. Churchill.

Hutchinson, G. E. (1964). *A Treatise on Limnology*, Vol. 2. New York: Wiley.

Imbevore, A. M. A. (1970). Chemistry of River Niger in Kainji Reservoir area. *Archiv für Hydrobiologie*, **67**, 412–431.

Imbevore, A. M. A. and Visser, S. A. (1969). A study of microbiological and chemical stratification of the Niger River within the future Kainji Lake area. In: *Man-Made Lake* (Ed. L. Obeng). Accra: Ghana Academy of Sciences, pp. 94–102.

Katugampola, D. S. and Assim, T. H. (1958). Coliform organisms in domestic water supplies in Ceylon. *Ceylon Journal of Medical Science*, **9**, 95–101.

Livingstone, D. A. (1963). Chemical composition of rivers and lakes. *Professional Papers 440-G*, US Geological Survey, pp. 1–64.

McFarren, E. F., (1959). Report on collaborative studies of the bioassay of paralytic shellfish poison. *Journal of Association of Agricultural Chemists*, **42**, 263–271.

McFeters, G. A., Bissonnette, G. K., Jezeski, J. J., Thomson, C. A. and Stuart, D. G. (1974). Comparative survival of indicator bacteria and enteric pathogens in well water. *Applied Microbiology*, **27**, 823–829.

McKee, J. E. and Wolf, H. W. (1971). *Water Quality Criteria*. Publ. No. 3-A. The Resources Agency of California, State Water Resources Control Board.

Mara, D. D. (1974). *Bacteriology for Sanitary Engineers.* Edinburgh: Churchill-Livingstone.

Marshall, B. E. and Falconer, A. C. (1973). Eutrophication of a tropical African impoundment. *Hydrobiologia*, **45**, 109–123.

Mather, R. P. and Ramanthan, K. N. (1966). Significance of enterococci as pollution indicators. *Environmental Health*, **8**, 1–5.

Moore, W. E. C. and Holdeman, L. V. (1974). Human faecal flora: The normal flora of 20 Japanese–Hawaiians. *Applied Microbiology*, **27**, 961–979.

Morgan, A. and Kalk, M. (1970). Seasonal changes in the waters of Lake Chilwa (Malawi) in a drying phase (1966–68). *Hydrobiologia*, **36**, 81–103.

Moussa, R. S. (1965). Type distribution of coliforms isolated from faecal and non-faecal habitats. *Indian Journal of Medical Research*, **53**, 629–637.

Patrick, R. (1954). A new method for determining the pattern of the diatom flora. *Notulae Naturae*, **259**, 1–12.

Robertson, J. S., Croll, J. M., James, A. and Gay, J. (1966). Pollution of underground water from pea silage. *Monthly Bulletin of the Ministry of Health*, **25**, 172–179.

Rzoska, J. and Talling, J. F. (1966). Plankton development in relation to hydrobiology and reservoir regime in the Blue Nile. *Verhandlungen der Internationalen Vereinigung Limnologie*, **16**, 716–720.

Sastry, C. A., Aboo, K. M. and Rae, M. N. (1969). Incidence of coliforms and enteroccocci in natural Waters. *Environmental Health*, **11**, 32–40.

Seenayya, G. (1971). Ecological studies in the plankton of certain freshwater ponds of Hyderabad, India. *Hydrobiologia*, **37**, 55–85.

Sen, R. and Jacobs, B. (1969). Pathogenic intestinal organisms in the unfiltered water supply of Calcutta and the effect of chlorination. *Indian Journal of Medical Research*, **57**, 1220–1227.

Talling, F. (1969). The incidence of veritcal mixing and some biological and chemical consequences, in tropical African lakes. *Verhandlung der Internationaken Vereinigung Limnologie*, **17**, 998–1012.

Talling, G. F. and Rzoska, J. (1967). The development of plankton in relation to the hydrological regime in the Blue Nile. *Journal of Ecology*, **55**, 637–662.

Taylor, E. W. (1972). Report on the results of the bacteriological, chemical and biological examination of London waters 1969–1970. *Report of the Metropolitan Water Board*, **44**, 22–23.

Venkateswarlu, T. and Jayanti, T. V. (1968). Hydrobiological studies of the River Sabarmati to evaluate water quality. *Hydrobiologia*, **31**, 442–448.

Venkateswarlu, V. (1970). An ecological study of the algae of the River Moosi, Hyderabad (India) with special reference to water pollution IV. Periodicity of some common species of algae. *Hydrobiologia*, **35**, 45–65.

White, G. F., Bradley, D. J. and White, A. U. (1972). *Drawers of Water.* Chicago: Chicago University Press.

WHO (1967a). WHO expert committee on cholera. *Technical Report Series No. 352.*

WHO (1967b). Control of ascariasis. *Technical Report Series No. 379.*

WHO (1968). Water pollution control in developing countries. *Technical Report Series No. 404.*

WHO (1969). Amoebiasis. *Technical Report Series No. 421.*

WHO (1971). *International Standards for Drinking Water*, 3rd ed.

WHO (1973a). Community water supply and sewage disposal in developing countries (end of 1970). *World Health Statistics Report*, **26**, 720–783.

WHO (1973b). Reuse of effluents. *Technical Report Series No. 517.*

Wood, P. C. (1974). The discharge of sewage from sea outfalls into the North Sea. In: *Discharge of Sewage from Sea Outfalls* (Ed. A. L. Gameson). Oxford: Pergamon Press, pp. 1–7.

4

Surface Water Quality Criteria for Tropical Developing Countries

M. B. Pescod

4.1 INTRODUCTION

In these days of widespread interest in the environment and in the preservation of its quality, it is timely to consider the implications of water quality criteria as they relate to tropical developing countries. The need for rational surface water quality goals, consistent with the environmental and economic conditions in developing countries, is apparent when one considers their importance relative to investment in water pollution control. The stringency of water quality standards will largely determine the costs of achieving the standards and, thus, society's investment in pollution control measures. In developing countries, environmental pollution control projects must compete for the national budget with high-priority development projects and in the past they have not performed well in this respect. Municipal and industrial wastewaters are largely being discharged without treatment into surface receiving waters throughout the developing world and examples of gross pollution are ubiquitous. These conditions must and will change and it is the engineer's responsibility to ensure that public funds appropriated for controlling the quality of the environment are applied in the most efficient way to manage and allocate the resource.

Neglect of this could neutralize future development gains if a society has to pay more than is necessary for its basic water needs. Water quality criteria must be developed on the basis of sound technological considerations with an awareness of their significance in economic terms.

4.2 WATER AND WASTEWATER QUALITY CRITERIA

There are two types of quality criteria of relevance in water pollution control: the discharge, or effluent, standard and the ambient, or stream, standard. The former is interrelated with the latter in the case of a particular water system, but use of the stream standard for control purposes allows greater flexibility in managing the water resource. Whereas an effluent standard only allows flexibility within the water-use system before effluent discharge, a stream

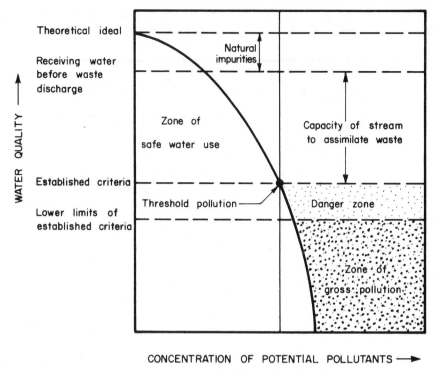

Figure 4.1 Pollution and levels of water quality (after Power, 1967)

standard encourages the same intra-system flexibility but, in addition, permits use of the stream's capacity to assimilate polluting discharges.

Figure 4.1 conveniently illustrates the possible conditions in a stream receiving polluting discharges of any nature and introduces the concept of 'safe minimum standard', the established criterion. The safe minimum standard applies to a particular water quality parameter (such as dissolved oxygen level, pesticide concentration, etc.) and is associated with a particular down-stream water use (that which is critical relative to the particular quality para-meter). However, since streamflow is stochastic, which may result in poor water quality for short periods, and because a relatively high pollutant concen-tration may be tolerated in the water use for a short duration, a danger zone occurs in which the threshold of pollution is exceeded for limited periods. To allow advantage to be taken of this zone in managing the water system, it is desirable to use statistical standards where the probability of occurrence of a given level of a particular parameter is defined. An absolute lower limit to the standard may be imposed where a poorer water quality would prevent legitimate use of the water by downstream users or result in serious economic loss, such as through fish being killed.

Implicit in this discussion is the principle that water quality criteria are necessary to protect legitimate and beneficial uses of a water resource.

Legitimate and beneficial are here used in a public sense and it is to be assumed that private interests must be subordinated to the general interests of society. However, in particular instances, management of a water resource principally to accommodate private industrial users might well be in the best interests of the public.

It is possible to plan for surface water quality to improve with development of a country by increasing the severity of the stream standard over a period of time. The initial level of the standard, however, must be selected taking into consideration the benefits and costs immediately arising out of the choice *and* with an awareness of the risk of long-term ecological damage. At the present time there are engineers and ecologists who believe that it is irresponsible to utilize even part of the assimilative capacity of the environment in disposing of polluting wastes and that all pollutants should be removed before discharges are released. This is technologically feasible but adds significantly to the costs of waste handling and disposal. Clearly, developing countries are in no position to aim at ecological perfection in pollution control, but neither should they assume that their economic state gives them licence to ignore the ecological consequences of irresponsible use of the environment. A knowledge of the importance of different water quality parameters to various water uses, and of the technology applied to achieve water and wastewater quality criteria, will allow rational decisions to be taken considering the benefits and costs of alternative schemes. Normally, this is the limit of the engineer's involvement until the implementation stage of a project, when his recommended measures are designed and constructed. Before that time, the engineer's recommendations will be evaluated and be subject to political and budgetary constraints.

Public opinion is one major factor in promoting pollution control in developed countries and the political climate for action reflects public attitudes. In developing countries, in general, public opinion has not in the past been a significant factor in environmental clean-up; it is understandable that a primarily low-income public considers subsistence more important than environmental quality. However, in recent years the pressures of urban population increases and industrialization have given rise to environmental stresses which have had considerable public impact and individual cases are given wide publicity. Political decisions are now being affected by public protest as well as by powerful public figures and national leaders in many countries, and private and public funds are being applied to pollution control projects. It is up to the engineer to prove the worth of an optimum degree of pollution control to a society by benefit–cost analysis, and thereby justify expenditure of public funds.

4.3 CHARACTERISTICS AND ASSIMILATION CAPACITY OF TROPICAL SURFACE WATERS

Tropical surface waters have certain general characteristics which make them different from most surface waters in temperate zones, with respect to their

Table 4.1 Discharges, low flow periods and silt contents of some tropical rivers

River	Discharge (m^3/s) Maximum	Minimum	Max./min. discharge ratio	Low flow* period (months)	Silt content % Max.	Min.	Average
Mekong	67·000	1250	54	—	0·31	—	0·06
Red	35·000	700	50	—	0·70	0·01	0·106
Brahmaputra	72·460	2680	27	6	0·30	—	0·12
Ganges	61·200	1170	52	7	0·3	—	0·13
Indus	31·200	490	64	—	—	—	0·33
Chao Phya	6·500	65	100	5	0·093	—	0·03
Irrawaddy	63·990	1306	49	—	—	—	—
Meghna	13·100	370	35	5	—	—	—

*Arbitrarily chosen as the continuous period during which discharge does not exceed 4 times minimum discharge.

capacity for handling waste discharges. Owing to the nature of tropical rainfall, streams usually have very high ratios of maximum to minimum discharge and low flows occur for extended periods, as can be seen in Table 4.1. Because dilution is of major importance in waste assimilation, long periods of low streamflow militate against a stream being able to accept heavy waste loads continuously without damage. Low streamflow, particularly in flat delta areas (where many major cities are located) produces little turbulence, which in turn reduces oxygen diffusion at the surface. In these low-lying plains in the tropics, wind speeds are also usually low and water surface turbulence from this source is often slight. Surface diffusion normally provides the greatest source of oxygen for biological breakdown of organic materials discharged to surface waters.

There are, in addition to these hydraulic and physical conditions, other quality characteristics which seriously affect the ability of a tropical stream to assimilate wastes, particularly those of an organic nature (such as municipal sewage) which are biologically degradable. Most important of the quality parameters which affect organic waste assimilative capacity are stream temperature, turbidity and dissolved oxygen concentration. High temperatures, commonly near 30 °C in the tropics, not only reduce the amount of oxygen which can dissolve in water, thereby minimizing the oxygen supply available to micro-organisms, but also increase the rate at which oxygen is utilized by micro-organisms. A high rate of oxygen use might result in low or zero dissolved oxygen concentration in a particular stream reach, according to the traditional dissolved oxygen sag curve, which would impair the stream's subsequent capacity to receive further polluting discharges. The high suspended load prevalent in most tropical surface waters (Table 4.1), a measure of which is turbidity, indirectly affects the oxygen supply available to micro-organisms by preventing the transmission of sunlight through a significant depth of water. Photosynthetic plants, mainly planktonic algae, which can supply significant quantities of oxygen under optimum conditions are thus deprived of their activating energy and do not act as a significant oxygen source (Pescod, 1969).

4.4 MAJOR WATER USES AND QUALITY CONSTRAINTS

It is a generally accepted concept that water resources should be developed on a multi-purpose basis; but rarely has water quality been considered in the planning of water schemes in developing countries. The major water uses for which large schemes have been designed are power, flood protection and irrigation; water pollution control, although an important and legitimate use of a surface water, has never been seriously considered in project designs. Low flow augmentation is a recognized way of providing greater dilution for waste discharges and can often be incorporated into the planning and design of a control structure at a cost lower than the alternative of treating downstream waste discharges. With increasing urbanization, developing societies must look for rational low-cost solutions to environmental quality problems if development goals are to be achieved without destroying natural resources.

Table 4.2 lists the more important uses to which a surface water can be put and the major quality parameters which are involved in deciding its suitability for each use. The uses of a water which should be considered in arriving at quality criteria will vary with the location of the particular reach of stream being studied but some general factors will apply in developing countries at their present stage of development.

Power and flood protection

River control structures for power production, flood protection and large-

Table 4.2 Water uses and quality considerations

Water uses	Important quality parameters
Power	Dissolved oxygen, pH
Flood protection	—
Irrigation	Dissolved solids, electrical conductivity
Potable water supply	Colour, turbidity, hardness, pathogenic organisms, organics
Industrial water supply	Hardness, pH, dissolved oxygen
Navigation (transportation)	Suspended solids, pH
Fishing (commercial and subsistence)	Dissolved oxygen, pesticides, CO_2, pH, heavy metals
Recreation	Pathogenic organisms, pH
Nature conservation (wildlife and aesthetics)	—
Waste disposal	—
Saline water intrusion prevention	—

scale irrigation are usually upstream of major polluting discharge sources and can be eliminated from consideration here.

Irrigation

Irrigation of cultivated land contiguous to reaches of a river downstream of polluting sources will be a possible water use subject to quality constraints. The water quality parameter of major importance is salinity, as measured by electrical conductivity (EC) or total dissolved solids (TDS), which seriously affects crop growth when present in high concentration. A TDS level greater than 1000 mg/l might well reduce crop yields but is unlikely to occur unless either saline water intrusion into an estuary results from low freshwater discharge or if industrial effluents contain large quantities of salts. The relative proportion of sodium to other cations, as measured by the sodium-adsorption-ratio (SAR) is also important to prevent the soil from becoming more alkaline. Release of a normal municipal sewage into a watercourse will rarely affect its use as irrigation water, and may even enhance it, provided there is reasonable dilution. However, if a reach of a river is anaerobic, this may affect the oxygen supply to plants by way of the groundwater, which will be in balance with the watercourse. Direct use of municipal wastewaters in irrigation is not generally recommended and, particularly in areas where schistosomiasis is or may become a problem, careful study of the health implications of this practice is necessary.

Potable water supply

In developing countries, surface waters are still used directly for water supply without treatment. Wherever there is a significant population dependent on a stream for potable and washing water, quality criteria will need to be very strict and wastewater discharges will have to be carefully controlled, particularly from the point of view of pathogenic organisms. This implies that the quality of surface waters in developing countries should be better than that normally acceptable in more developed countries. Contrary to the conditions in western countries, giving rise to the situation where investment in water pollution control is mainly justified on the basis of recreation, fish and wildlife uses, public health may become a justifiable benefit in developing regions. If surface waters continue to be used without treatment for potable supply then this use undoubtedly will be the most demanding in terms of water quality, will result in the strictest water quality criteria, and will be the most inflexible in terms of water management. In the long term, no country can afford the luxury of maintaining potable water quality in its surface waters and, in most developing countries, any attempt to do so would be futile because of the widespread habit of free defecation in the open.

Most municipal water supplies are treated before distribution and the same raw water quality as required for safe direct use is not necessary. In fact, except for particular pollutants (such as toxic materials) which might require special treatment processes, the cost of water treatment is not highly sensitive to water quality variations resulting from municipal waste discharges (Frankel, 1965). Gross pollution with little dilution will cause special problems in water treatment but even these conditions can be overcome using conventional water treatment processes with careful control.

Industrial water supply

Industry utilizes two main qualities of water, a high quality supply, principally for steam raising, but possibly for process water, and a relatively low grade supply for cooling. In developing countries, industry has usually accepted the responsibility for treating its own high grade water supply and raw water quantity is usually more important than quality. Groundwaters are widely used for this purpose, whereas surface supplies act as the main source of the larger quantities of cooling water required. It appears, therefore, that unless a surface water is highly corrosive as a result of waste discharges, industrial use will not be a constraint in arriving at realistic water quality criteria.

Navigation

Where rivers are used by shipping and smaller craft, two water quality parameters are likely to be important. Large quantities of suspended solids discharged to streams where deposition is likely to occur might interfere with the safe passage of vessels. In tropical countries, the silt burden naturally suspended in the alluvial rivers as a result of erosion makes it highly unlikely that normal waste discharges will significantly affect the solids concentration. This will not apply in special instances, such as with discharges from tin-mining operations, when large quantities of solids are wasted. In most cases, however, suspended solids concentration could be removed as an effluent standard for discharges released to tropical streams.

The only other factor of importance in this use category is the corrosivity of the water. Normal protection applied to the hulls of steel vessels would counteract all but the severest conditions arising from waste discharges. Smaller craft in tropical countries are usually of wooden construction and raise no water quality problem.

Fishing

Game fishing can be eliminated from consideration in tropical developing countries but, in addition to commercial fishing, subsistence fishing is of great importance. The rural population of many developing countries relies to a large extent on fish as their source of protein. Tropical fresh waters support only the coarser varieties of fish, carp and catfish being prominent types, but in addition many surface breathers exist which do not rely on oxygen dissolved in the water for their survival. Even in a temperate climate, coarse fish can tolerate lower dissolved oxygen concentrations than game fish and so the stream standard for this quality parameter should be less restrictive than in colder countries. Also, since a significant proportion (often more than one third) of the freshwater catch in tropical countries are surface breathers, even when extreme pollution creates anaerobic conditions in a reach of stream all fish will not be killed. However, adverse conditions might well affect the general ecology of a stream, causing a break in the food chain and resulting loss of fish at the upper trophic level. Alternatively, the migratory and spawning habits of fish might be affected by poor water quality and production might suffer.

Little published work is available on tropical fish toxicity or the effects of pollutants on tropical stream ecology, but many examples of reduction of fish catches over the years of pollution build-up have been cited by fishermen. Until more research is carried out on the tolerance of tropical freshwater species to polluting materials care should be exercised in the choice of stream standard so that this important food supply is protected.

Recreation

Recreational uses of a surface water resource, such as swimming, boating, water-skiing, etc., are less justifiable reasons for controlling water pollution in developing countries than in developed countries. People generally have much less time for recreation and little money to spend on it, their concern being rather for improving living standards at a more mundane level. In tropical countries, the recreational habits of the people also differ from those in temperate countries, and poor surface water quality will affect these habits less. It is still a common sight to see young bathers enjoying the delights of a heavily-polluted canal or stream without worrying about the water quality, and perhaps they have the more appropriate attitude when one considers that epidemiological evidence of the danger of swimming in polluted water is very slight. This is not the case, however, where water-related parasitic diseases are prevalent. In addition, the high solids burden in most tropical streams camouflages quality shortcomings which might otherwise prove objectionable. If a surface water is of suitable quality to support fish and if schistosomiasis is not a problem it is more than likely that recreational uses will not be affected in tropical developing countries.

Nature conservation

Waterways in tropical countries are much more a part of the life of the people than in temperate regions, but their aesthetic value takes second place to more pragmatic uses. This is in part due to the fact that most tropical rivers look alike, being red-brown in colour due to suspended silt, but is also a result of the low aesthetic sensitivity of people whose primary objective is to improve their standard of living above the present low level. Economic development of a country will certainly change this situation but aesthetic enjoyment of a surface water will not be a justifiable benefit to offset the costs of water pollution control in developing countries for some time. Preservation of wildlife is a cause supported more in developed countries than in developing regions, but even so, with respect to the water habitat, the reasons for supporting fishing and the quality criteria thereby adopted will normally be adequate for this purpose as well.

Waste disposal

If the wastes from an urban area exceed the capacity of a watercourse to receive them without serious damage (such as complete dissolved oxygen depletion) then this use must compete with other justifiable uses for priority. The benefits of preserving a particular quality level must more than balance the costs of achieving it, say by waste treatment, for a net gain to accrue to society. Complete freedom to discharge city wastes to a surface water without control will normally eliminate it from being applied to most other uses and, although this may be justifiable under certain circumstances, it must be a decision taken in the full knowledge of its implications in economic and social terms. Too often in developing countries has a town exploded into a large city in very few years, with gradual but predictable deterioration of surface waters, and without any thought having been given to controlling the situation.

Saline water intrusion prevention

Low flow augmentation, which increases the minimum freshwater flow in a river, has been a planned purpose of some river control structures in developing countries. Where valuable agricultural land is irrigated or where a large city's water supply is taken from the tidal reach of a river, it is important to ensure low salinity at points of abstraction. Some river control structures have been designed with these purposes as a secondary consideration, and waste dilution has been improved fortuitously.

4.5 RATIONAL WATER AND WASTEWATER QUALITY CRITERIA

The quality requirements of water use should be the only constraints governing the choice of stream standards for a particular surface resource, and these in turn will decide the effluent standards to be imposed. In the context of a developing country, therefore, it is advisable to be as lenient as possible by choosing that quality level which is just suitable for the predominant use of the surface water. A rational stream standard developed in this way will produce the most flexible effluent standards and allow the cost of water pollution control to be minimized and, often, justified. In no case should an arbitrary water quality objective be suggested as the basis of a management scheme, because any technical and/or economic optimization techniques subsequently applied and related to that objective will not then achieve a quality level governed by the controlling water use.

Basis for stream standards

From the discussion on possible water use it is clear that those uses which are likely to be the basis for stream standards in developing countries are *potable water supply*, *irrigation* and *fishing*, all other uses not being significant from a quality point of view at the present time. If a sizeable population is dependent on a surface water for its potable water supply, and if no central treatment plants provide an alternative supply, the source should be protected as much as possible for public health reasons. Under these circumstances the costs of maintaining a safe water quality must be balanced against the costs of providing alternative water supplies, or supplying other health services, to justify further investment in pollution control measures. Direct use of surface water for potable supply will occur mainly in rural areas but is unlikely to arise in metropolitan areas, or along the estuarine reaches of rivers. However, in most developing countries the largest proportion of the population live in rural areas and often rely on contaminated surface waters for their potable supply. It is unrealistic to conceive of treatment being applied to all such sources in the foreseeable future and so this enormous problem will be with the majority of developing countries for some time to come. If an alternative potable water supply is available to the population in a region, then irrigation or fishing will normally be the only other legitimate uses for which the water quality should be controlled in developing countries. Irrigation is the largest water use in tropical developing countries and may sometimes be the only basis for stream standards, where quantities are inadequate for crop production or where there are saline or poorly-drained soils. Municipal sewage does not contribute much towards salinity on discharge to a river, but industrial wastes and irrigation return waters can increase salinity to a significant level. The benefits of limiting salinity will be relatively easy to calculate with present information but the costs of control will normally be high and often prohibitive. In rural areas it will be difficult to evaluate the economic benefits of improving water quality for fishing use because data on subsistence fishing are not easily acquired. However, the water quality required to support subsistence fishing will be the same as for commercial fishing. Perhaps in the future, when fish ponds are more widely operated in developing countries, the need for maintaining high water quality in many surface streams to support fish will not exist. In larger rivers and near urban centres, where commercial fishing is organized, the economic losses resulting from deteriorating water quality are more easily quantifiable and, therefore, the justifiable investment in pollution control is more identifiable.

In many instances, conflicting legitimate uses of a water are compatible, such as would be the case if a reach of stream was to be used both for fishing

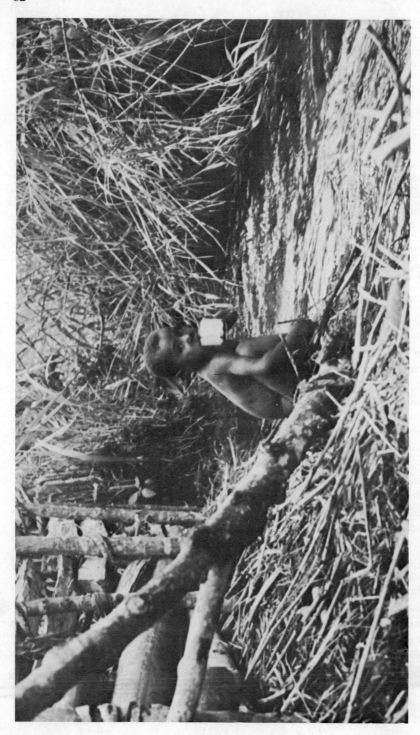

A child drinks water in the New Guinea Highlands. The stream is polluted by pig faeces and contains up to 100 *E. coli* per 100 ml (photograph : R. G. Feachem)

and municipal water supply. Occasionally, however, possible uses of the water are not compatible and society must decide which use should take precedence. This is often the case when a stream is receiving increasing pollutional loads from expanding industry and fishing begins to suffer. If the benefits of using the stream as a sewer for industrial waste discharges outweigh the damage costs, that is the economic loss of fish, then no waste treatment should be imposed through application of a rigorous stream standard. In the Ruhr in West Germany, the River Emscher has been converted into a single-purpose stream, without stream standards, used exclusively for waste dilution, degradation and carriage to serve the concentration of industry which provides employment in the region. Subsequently, the whole streamflow is subjected to primary treatment before discharge into the River Rhine, taking advantage of the economies of scale which would not have been possible in providing individual treatment plants for each waste discharge. This approach might well have wide application in developing countries, when authorities decide to plan rationally to encourage and accommodate industrial development.

Potable water supply

If potable water supply is the primary use to which a water is to be applied and if no treatment facilities are available, then a stream standard should be imposed to protect the health of the public using that supply, but only as a short-term measure. The stream standard should ensure the safety of the water for human alimentation but should not impose unreasonable quality levels. Essentially, a quality similar to the natural state of the surface water before receiving pollution is adequate. Thus, the water should not contain dangerous levels of pathogenic organisms or toxic materials but could have a relatively high solids content (turbidity) in tropical regions. Quality parameters likely to be important in developing countries and their suggested limits, equivalent to the established criterion level in Figure 4.1, are presented in Table 4.3. These reflect the quality

Table 4.3 Proposed stream standards for potable water supply

Quality parameter	Suggested level of stream standard
Faecal coliform density	Effluent quality similar to the natural state of surface water
pH	6·5–8·5
Dissolved oxygen	> 2 mg/l
Arsenic	< 0·05 mg/l
Lead	< 0·05 mg/l
Chromium (hexavalent)	< 0·05 mg/l
Cyanide	< 0·2 mg/l
Phenolic substances	< 0·002 mg/l
Chlorides	< 1000 mg/l
Total dissolved solids	< 4000 mg/l

requirements of potable water only in those aspects essential from a health viewpoint. The coliform standard suggested is based on World Health Organization (WHO, 1971) recommendations for untreated water but may be impossible to achieve in tropical streams receiving natural runoff. There is great uncertainty concerning the toxic levels to man of compounds in water and the standards imposed by WHO are necessarily conservative.

Irrigation

Irrigation use of a surface water will normally impose the least restrictive quality standards and will often allow free discharge of wastewaters. Table 4.4 lists those essential parameters which should be limited and their suggested levels. The main water quality parameter for irrigation water is the concentration of salts which causes plasmolysis of plant cells. The lethal concentration of salts varies from plant to plant, and is dependent on contact period and ambient temperature. The second problem with salts, especially those containing sodium, is the displacement of calcium ions from the soil, causing permeability to decrease. A good drainage system and proper irrigation management lower the contact period between the plant and saline water so that a well-

Table 4.4 Proposed stream standards for irrigation

Quality parameter	Suggested level of stream standard
Total dissolved solids (TDS)	Not more than 400 mg/l where there are poor drainage, saline soil and inadequate water supply. (EC less than 75 millisiemens per m at 25 °C) Not more than 1000 mg/l where there are good drainage and proper irigation management. (EC less than 175 millisiemens per m at 25 °C) Not more than 2000 mg/l where there are salt-resistant crops, good drainage, proper water management and low sodium adsorption ratio (SAR) of water. (EC less than 225 millisiemens per m at 25 °C)
Sodium adsorption ratio (SAR)	Not more than 10 where there is poor drainage. Not more than 18 where there is good drainage.
Boron	Not more than 1·25 mg where there are sensitive crops. Not more than 4 mg/l where there are tolerant crops.
Dissolved oxygen	Greater than 2 mg/l. A level of 2 mg/l should not occur for more than 8 hours out of any 24-hour period.
Faecal coliform density	Not more than 100/100 ml if the water is to be used for unrestricted irrigation. This standard may be relaxed when the crop is not intended for human consumption.

drained soil may tolerate a lower irrigation water quality. High temperature increases water consumption of plants, and this demands a better irrigation water quality than would be required in a cold climate. Besides those parameters mentioned, an excessive concentration of metal ions retards plant growth and sometimes causes death, even though the same metal ions are essential micro-nutrients in very low concentrations. The health hazards to agricultural workers and consumers of distributing irrigation waters contaminated with pathogens or parasites must also be considered in establishing quality standards.

Fishing

If irrigation use is not a consideration, the most rational controlling water use in a developing country is fishing and here the stream standards must be consistent with the local ecological conditions. The fishing industry is an important sector in developing countries as a principal source of badly needed protein in the diet. Table 4.5 lists only those quality parameters which are likely to be important to tropical freshwater fish species useful as food. The main parameters that affect fish catch are dissolved oxygen concentration, presence of toxic compounds (such as cyanide and heavy metals), temperature, the presence of non-biodegradable substances which are concentrated in the food chain (such as DDT), and substances which impart an undesirable odour and taste to the fish. The levels suggested as reasonable limits are based on information from temperate countries modified for tropical conditions and

Table 4.5 Proposed stream standards for fishing

Quality parameter	Suggested level of stream standard
CO_2	< 12 mg/l
pH	6·5–8.5
NH_3	< 1 mg/l
Heavy metals	< 1 mg/l
Copper	< 0·02 mg/l
Arsenic	< 1 mg/l
Lead	< 0·1 mg/l
Selenium	< 0·1 mg/l
Cyanides	< 0·012 mg/l
Phenols	< 0·02 mg/l
Dissolved solids	< 1000 mg/l
Detergents	< 0·2 mg/l
Dissolved oxygen	> 2 mg/l
Pesticides	
DDT	< 0·002 mg/l
Endrin	< 0.004 mg/l
BHC	< 0·21 mg/l
Methyl parathion	< 0·10 mg/l
Malathion	< 0·16 mg/l

from tropical research, but can only be considered as illustrative at this time. Research on the tolerance of local species to polluting substances and low dissolved oxygen tension needs to be carried out in each developing country before stream standards can be specified with any degree of confidence. In general, if a surface water is suitable for fish, then it is also acceptable as raw water to be treated for municipal water supply. Where a polluted stream discharges into the sea, certain quality characteristics may cause loss of marine fish and this must be taken into account in deciding on quality criteria.

Other uses

If a particular surface water in a developing country is not the only source of potable water and if irrigation and fishing cannot be justified as protected uses, there seems to be no reason to impose any but the loosest of stream standards at the present stage of development. Under these conditions, waste disposal becomes the primary use for which the resource is managed. To prevent grossly offensive conditions it seems advisable to impose a limit only on dissolved oxygen and for this to be > 0 mg/l. Otherwise, to give the maximum incentive for industrial development, no stream or effluent standards should be devised. However, the responsible authority should collect data on stream and waste flows and their quality characteristics in preparation for the time when quality management of the water resource is necessary. The authority should likewise be prepared to implement regional schemes for water pollution control whenever appropriate in the interests of development. At the present time, very few municipal areas in developing countries are sewered, so even the most basic waste disposal amenity provided to small industries in developed countries is not available. It is unreasonable to expect a small company, often in a highly competitive market, to invest in waste treatment when municipal wastes are being freely discharged without control. Nor is it logical to assume that the costs of any enforced waste treatment will not be passed on to the public in the form of increased product prices. Particularly with small industries, individual waste treatment plants are uneconomic and regional facilities provided by a controlling authority will often be the least-cost approach. This will only be the case when factories are located very close together, because the cost of wastewater transmission over long distances is high.

Effluent and stream standards

Once stream standards are decided for any reach of stream, effluent standards can easily be designed to achieve the required stream quality if sufficient data are available on the hydrometric characteristics of the stream and the waste discharges. Both stream and effluent standards should preferably be defined in terms of probability of occurrence to allow most efficient management of the water resource. The technology to achieve optimum stream quality under variable stream conditions is available and water management techniques have been developed to implement control, while at the same time allowing system flexibility.

4.6 THE TECHNOLOGY OF WATER POLLUTION CONTROL

System modelling

Once desirable water quality goals have been established in the form of stream standards, the stream system concerned must be modelled to ascertain the effects of mixing and diffusion processes on waste discharges and to allow effective utilization of the stream's assimilative capacity. A great deal of work has been carried out on stream and estuarine models, examples of which are O'Connor (1967) and Pescod and Ratasuk (1968), but a prerequisite of the usefulness of a model in practice is the availability of input data. Since hydrometric and water quality information in developing countries is often nonexistent, new data will need to be collected to test any mathematical model developed. Collection of these data is very costly, particularly if badly organized, so only essential data should be obtained. Obviously, data collection should be related to use in a model, and sampling and analysis should follow a logical design (Montgomery and Hart, 1971). Because the distribution of non-conservative substances (such as dissolved oxygen) in a stream is dependent not only on hydrodynamic effects but also on decay functions, for which the mathematical models allow, it is also necessary to study the characteristics of waste discharges and any other sources or sinks of the substances affecting the system. Probabilistic or stochastic models are available which will allow a system to be managed so as to minimize the probability of the established criterion or stream standard not being achieved. Management models, such as that described by Fan *et al.* (1971), have been developed whose aim is to enable optimum water quality in a stream to be maintained while the total cost benefit function is minimized. Development and application of models require trained scientists and engineers, which are scarce in many developing countries, and this may limit the usefulness of the more sophisticated modelling techniques in many cases.

The desirable output from a model study will be suggested effluent standards for known waste discharges or alternative water quality management possibilities. When these have been defined, the water quality control alternatives can be considered.

Water quality control methods

Treatment of wastes is not the only way of achieving stream standards and should often be the last method to be considered in developing regions because it is normally the most costly. Basically, the approach to the water quality problem must be in one or a combination of the following directions: modifying the assimilation capacity of the water resource, reducing wastes generation, or reducing wastes after generation. Not all methods are appropriate for all wastewaters and the choice will depend on the particular waste problem. Most of the methods reviewed in this section will be applicable to industrial wastes but only some to municipal wastewaters. The management choice available in handling wastes from households is very limited, because changing consumption patterns is difficult, and often treatment is the only general method for reducing these waste discharges. The more complex problem of controlling industrial wastewater discharges, which will increase as industry expands in developing countries, allows many of the following techniques to be used to advantage:

(1) Methods for modifying the assimilation capacity of a water resource:
    (a) Low-flow augmentation for increased waste dilution
      —river control structure
      —groundwater release to surface water
    (b) Reservoir design and management to prevent adverse effects of storage on quality
      —multiple outlets
      —reservoir mixing
    (c) Stream reaeration to increase oxygen supply
      —at turbines, if power generation
      —weirs
      —mobile or fixed aerators
    (d) Saltwater barriers to prevent salt water intrusion
      —injection wells
      —impermeable physical barriers
    (e) Effluent redistribution
      —regulated discharges
      —transfer to different location
      —underground disposal
(2) Methods for reducing wastes generation:
    (a) Change type of raw material inputs to process
    (b) Change production process
    (c) Change product output from process
    (d) In-plant recirculation of water
    (e) Segregation of strong waste sources
    (f) Good housekeeping
(3) Methods for reducing wastes after generation:
    (a) Materials recovery and recycling
    (b) Byproduct production
    (c) Waste treatment
    (d) Effluent re-use

Improving or making better use of the assimilative capacity of surface waters has hardly been considered in tropical developing countries. The possibilities of this approach should never be overlooked because the methods available will often be less costly to society than other alternatives. If this technique is used to achieve stream standards in a region, the associated effluent standards will be lenient.

In developing countries the potential for reducing wastes generation from industrial plants is great. Few present-day plants have been designed or are operated with any consideration of wastes, and misuse of water is widespread. With little difficulty it is usually possible for water use in a plant to be reduced, for example by changing from once-through cooling water to a recycled system, thereby reducing the quantity of waste discharged. By identifying sources of pollution, insisting on good housekeeping in a plant, and organizing maintenance to minimize leaks etc., the amounts of pollutants discharged can be minimized. Segregation of strong wastes might allow the bulk of relatively unpolluted wastewater to be discharged to a stream without treatment, reducing the investment in plant needed to treat the reduced volume of concentrated waste.

Of the methods for reducing wastes after generation, waste treatment has been used least in developing countries. Materials recovery and recycling have been practised in many industries, particularly in those processing agricultural products. Byproduct production has likewise received attention, the philosophy being not to waste any useful, or rather saleable, material. Even effluent re-use has not been neglected; in Asia in particular, wastewaters have been used for irrigation and fertilization for centuries. Waste treatment has not been popular because the costs are significant and the direct benefits to a manufacturer are zero. The industrialist generally has not considered the external damages and social costs caused by his waste discharges sufficient incentive to invest in waste treatment; but increasing pressure is being brought to bear by the authorities on industries to control their wastes.

The situation with regard to municipal wastewater treatment in many developing countries is complicated by the fact that conventional sewerage systems are not often found in cities. Without wastewater collection and transport to central plants, the cost advantages of large-scale treatment plants cannot be achieved. However, it may be necessary to think unconventionally in arriving at a solution to this problem because the capital cost of installing sewers in large cities is usually prohibitive. From the point of view of water pollution control it is as important for municipal wastewaters to receive treatment as it is for industrial wastes. Furthermore, it is only fair for the authority forcing industry to control its wastes to do the same with the municipal sewage, which will be of greater pollutional capacity than industrial wastes in most developing countries at the present time.

The combination of unit processes making up a treatment plant flow diagram will depend on the characteristics of the particular waste and the effluent standards imposed. Invariably, the costs of constructing and operating a wastewater treatment plant increase with the degree of treatment required and so the controlling authority should be careful to impose only those stream standards essential for downstream water uses. Although the technology is available to achieve any degree of clean-up, the methods adopted should suit local conditions in a particular country. In general, the choice of treatment process to achieve any effluent standard will be highly dependent on the cost of land, but it is essential in developing countries to be flexible and innovative in design. This can only be effective if authorities are susceptible to unusual solutions for controlling water pollution.

4.7 POLLUTION CONTROL POLICY ALTERNATIVES

Ideally, the water quality management system adopted must provide incentives for maintaining stream standards at the lowest cost to society, and governmental policy should be developed to provide the mechanism by which this objective can be achieved. This usually means that a public authority should be created with jurisdiction for water quality management over a wide region and that legislation be enacted giving the regional authority power to enforce regulations. Private water users and waste dischargers should have representation on the authority. In some instances river basin agencies have been empowered to plan, design, construct, operate and finance virtually all water control measures. Formation of a regional authority with power to control all discharges to and abstraction from a water resource system will at least be necessary to ensure that stream standards are maintained.

The most common method by which stream standards have been achieved in the past is by direct control of discharges through the application of effluent standards. Administratively, this is a complex procedure when there are many waste dischargers in a region because to allocate the resource in an ideal way an authority would have to have full information on the costs associated with existing and potential waste generation and disposal. In some developed countries, political support has been given to implementing water quality management schemes involving effluent standards by providing subsidies, such as rapid tax writeoffs and tax-credits, or direct grants for capital and/or operating expenses associated with waste treatment. These approaches not only act as a drain on the national treasury, an undesirable burden in developing countries, but are irrationally biased towards the construction of waste treatment plants using equipment. No incentive is given to consider the other alternatives discussed or to look for low-cost treatment systems utilizing little equipment. One of the main advantages of a regional authority is that it is able to evaluate and implement a wide range of alternatives to minimize the cost of water quality control.

Another approach to water quality management which is strongly supported by Kneese and Bower (1968) is that of providing economic incentives, in the form of *effluent charges*, to achieve stream standards. Effluent charges, based on damage costs, are levied by the authority on each unit (usually weight) of undesirable waste material discharged, taking into account hydrological variability. This technique uses indirect means to induce optimum reduction of waste discharges from municipalities and industry. Effluent standards are not imposed on dischargers but a charge is made for using the assimilative and transport capacity of the water resource, allowing each waste discharger to adjust in the most efficient way for his particular circumstances. Thus an industry or municipality could store waste temporarily, adjust inputs to a process, change or modify a production process, treat or modify wastes, change process outputs, pay the effluent charge, or adopt any combination of these approaches. To induce the least-cost solution, the initial effluent charge imposed on any reach of stream needs to be chosen carefully if it is to distribute the costs of control equitably among the polluters, but the unit charge can be changed gradually with time to reflect economic development and improved technology. One additional advantage of the charges approach is that it will normally yield a net revenue which can offset some of the costs of running the regional authority. For this approach to be effective, trained manpower is needed, and the shortage of technical personnel in many water management authorities in developing countries may limit its application to relatively few situations.

It is clear that a combination of direct and indirect controls on waste discharges and water usage may be necessary to suit conditions in a particular country. However, the establishment of a regional authority, with a competent staff including engineers, scientists, economists and other social scientists, will be able to adopt those measures which are most applicable to the local situation. Policy alternatives can be considered when relevant data are collected, and legislation drafted to allow enforcement of regulations.

4.8 CONCLUSIONS

Stream standards are likely to form the basis for water quality management in tropical developing countries in the foreseeable future. They should be carefully chosen to maintain only the minimum water quality level required for legitimate uses of the water resource. Maximum advantage should be taken of the waste assimilative capacity of receiving waters in the early stages of industrial development of a country. All possible technological alternatives in waste control should be considered in attempting to achieve desirable stream standards. A regional water authority is the most efficient administrative unit for water quality management. Effluent charges should not be overlooked as a mechanism for managing water quality in developing countries but they are likely to be suitable for application in particular situations rather than over a whole country because of trained manpower limitations. The technologist has an important part to play in supplying quantitative information on alternative water management schemes so that objective decisions can be made by public authorities, taking into consideration the local environmental and economic conditions.

4.9 REFERENCES

Fan, L. T., Nadkarni, R. S. and Erickson, L. E. (1971). Management of optimum water quality in a stream. *Water Research*, **5**, 11, 1005–1021.

Frankel, R. J. (1965). Water quality management: engineering-economic factors in municipal waste disposal. *Water Resources Research*, **1**, 2, 173–186.

Kneese, A. V. and Bower, B. T. (1968). *Managing Water Quality: Economics, Technology, Institutions*. Baltimore: The Johns Hopkins Press.

Montgomery, H. A. C. and Hart, I. C. (1971). The planning of sampling programmes with particular reference to river management. *WPR Report No. 1253*, Water Pollution Research Laboratory, Department of the Environment, Stevenage, United Kingdom.

O'Connor, D. J. (1967). The temporal and spatial distribution of dissolved oxygen in streams. *Water Resources Research*, **3**, 1, 65–79.

Pescod, M. B. and Ratasuk, S. (1968). Oxygen balance in the Chao Phya River estuary. Bangkok: *Asian Institute of Technology Research Report No. 3*.

Pescod, M. B. (1969). Photosynthetic oxygen production in a polluted tropical estuary. *Journal of the Water Pollution Control Federation*, **41**, 8, Part, 2, R309–R321.

Power (1967). Waste-water treatment. *Power Magazine Special Report*, New York.

WHO (1971). *International Standards for Drinking Water*. Geneva: World Health Organization.

II

Water Supplies
for Low-Income Communities

5

Water Supplies for Low-Income Communities: Resource Allocation, Planning and Design for a Crisis Situation

RICHARD G. FEACHEM

5.1 THE NATURE OF THE CRISIS

This chapter presents a new approach to the planning and execution of rural water supply programmes in developing countries. In order to appreciate why a new approach is necessary one must examine recent statistics prepared by the World Health Organization (WHO, 1973) which depict the community water supply situation in 91 developing countries at the end of 1970. The rural population (defined in accordance with each country's own rural–urban distinctions) of the countries surveyed amounted to 72% of the total population of those countries. Of this rural population, 1·11 thousand million people or 86%, were without 'reasonable access to safe water' (reasonable access is defined as being that 'a disproportionate part of the day' is not spent in water fetching; safe water supply 'includes treated waters or untreated but uncontaminated waters such as from protected boreholes, springs and sanitary wells'; WHO, 1973). Considered by region, the numbers and percentages of people without reasonable access to safe water were as follows:

Africa	136·0 million	89%
Americas	92·1 million	76%
Eastern Mediterranean	139·5 million	82%
Europe*	23·3 million	56%
South-East Asia	661·7 million	91%
Western Pacific	59·0 million	79%
All regions	1111·6 million	86%

This chapter is based in part upon a paper entitled 'Water supplies for low-income communities in developing countries', published in the *Journal of the Environmental Engineering Division*, American Society of Civil Engineers, **101**, 687–702, October 1975.

*This region includes only three developing countries surveyed: Algeria, Morocco and Turkey.

In 1972 the World Health Assembly set a new target of 25% of the rural populations of developing countries to have reasonable access to safe water by 1980. This target was amended for the American Region where higher targets were set because of the existing superior water supply situation in that region. To reach these targets, 241 million people (well over the total population of the USA) must be provided with a water supply by 1980. Even if this is achieved, which seems unlikely at present, the water supply development will still not keep pace with population growth in rural areas of developing countries. If by 1980 the number of people without an adequate water supply is to be equal to the number in that position in 1971 (1·11 thousand million), then 297 million people have to be supplied by 1980. In other words, merely to keep the number unserved constant, it is necessary to provide water for a population equal to over five times that of the United Kingdom by 1980. It would not, I feel, be overstating the case to describe this ever-worsening situation as a crisis.

5.2 THE NEED FOR DEFINED GOALS

Part of the solution, if indeed there is a solution to this problem, must lie in efficient and rational resource allocation and planning for water supply developments. The resources concerned include not only water itself, but also the financial and human resources needed to design, implement and maintain a water supply programme. However, rational planning presupposes the existence of closely defined and agreed objectives and it is necessary to examine whether we have such objectives for low-income water supplies.

In the design of any civil engineering structure, a purpose or goal is always implicit in the designer's deliberations and is very often explicitly stated. For instance, the purpose or goal of a bridge is not merely to maintain a structure above an obstacle but might be to provide the means for specified people and goods to cross a specified obstruction at a specified rate within certain topographical and environmental constraints. Similarly, the purpose of a building might be stated as the provision of a specified indoor environment in which specified people may undertake specified activities. Clearly civil engineers, sometimes in collaboration with architects, have always designed bridges and buildings with these, or similar, goals in mind. However, in the provision of water supply for low-income communities there has not usually been any closely defined goal or purpose in mind, other than to have water flowing out of the end of a pipe.

In the design of water supply systems for high-income communities in the developed countries, the question of goals and purposes has been avoided simply because a certain high-level provision of water services has come to be regarded as essential. However, for the great majority of the world's population who live in rural communities or low-income urban slums, with grossly inadequate access to safe water, there is no possibility that available financial and human resources will provide them with this high level of water provision to which the people of North America and Europe have become accustomed.

Because there is no immediate prospect of providing a significant proportion of low-income communities with high-grade water facilities, it is necessary to examine closely the goals of water supply in order that scarce resources may be allocated in the most efficacious and rational manner.

As with any engineering endeavour, a water supply has various levels of goals from the immediate and short-term to the diffuse, complex and long-term goals. Table 5.1 sets out a scheme of possible goals for a water supply development in a low-income community in a developing country. Under 'immediate aims' are listed the improvements to water which, in some combination, will from the basis of the design. For a high-grade water service in a prosperous community the immediate aims have become established as high quality, abundant quantity, complete availability and total reliability. However, it has been pointed out that these aims are unattainable for the majority of the population of developing countries and so some combination of improvements in quality, quantity, availability and reliability must be decided upon for the purpose of design. In order to decide on which combination of improvements is appropriate to a particular case it is necessary to examine the potential benefits from a water supply and so asses the degree to which different improvements will realize different levels of benefit. In this way the improvements with the most impact, at a given cost, can be determined and the anticipated cost-effectiveness of alternative schemes can be compared.

Table 5.1 lists three stages of potential benefits or goals. These are organized partly chronologically in that Stage I benefits are likely to be realized before Stage II which will usually precede Stage III. They are also arranged according to the extent to which external, or complementary, development inputs and initiatives are necessary to achieve the stated benefits. Table 5.2 lists the basic complementary inputs necessary to achieve the immediate aims, and the three stages of benefits, and it will be seen that Stage I complementary inputs are both more limited and more likely to be forthcoming that those for Stage II. Stage III complementary inputs are very wide-ranging and involve many governmental initiatives over which the water supply engineer will have no

Table 5.1 Aims and Potential Benefits of Water Supply Improvements

Immediate aims	Stage I benefits	Stage II benefits	Stage III benefits
Improve water: quality quantity availability reliability	Save time Save energy Improved health	Labour release Crop innovation Crop improvement Animal husbandry innovation Animal husbandry improvement	Higher cash incomes Increased and more reliable subsistence Improved health Increased leisure

Note The horizontal alignment has no significance.

control. Therefore, as one moves from left to right across Table 5.1 one not only moves chronologically but also with respect to the magnitude and feasibility of the complementary inputs which are necessary to give a reasonable chance that the stated benefit will be realized.

5.3 THE NEED FOR COMPLEMENTARY INPUTS

At this point it is useful to make a short digression to discuss the question of complementary inputs for water supply development. Over the past two decades a considerable number of evaluation studies have been conducted on water supply schemes in developing countries and nearly all of these have indicated that water supply may be a necessary, but is never a sufficient condition, for development. These studies (Carruthers, 1973; Feachem, 1973a; Saunders and Warford, 1974; White *et al.*, 1972) have stressed the fact that a water supply development must be accompanied by a carefully designed package of complementary inputs if it is to achieve its stated goals. Table 5.2 outlines possible complementary inputs associated with the realization of the benefits listed in Table 5.1 and shows how even the 'immediate aims' require specific complementary efforts which are not self-generating but require particular thought and attention. For instance the 'active community participation and support' and the 'adequate facilities for operation and maintenance'

Table 5.2 Complementary inputs necessary for the achievement of the various aims and benefits set out in Table 5.1

Aim or benefit (see Table 5.1)	Complementary inputs or prerequisite conditions
Immediate aims	Active community participation and support. Competent design. Adequate facilities for operation and maintenance. Appropriate technology utilized.
Stage I benefits	New supply used in preference to old. New supply closer to dwellings than old. Water use pattern changed to take advantage of improved quantity, availability and reliability. Hygiene changed to utilize improved supply. Other environmental health measures taken. Supply must not create new health hazards (e.g. mosquito breeding sites).
Stage II benefits	Good advice and extension services must be provided by government personnel concerned with agriculture, animal husbandry, cooperatives, marketing, education, credit etc.
Stage III benefits	Water supply development must be just a single component of an integrated rural development programme which has the active support of the local community.

are fundamental and engineers with experience in developing countries will appreciate the commonness of water supply, water treatment and sanitation schemes failing owing to lack of community support and inadequate facilities and trained personnel to ensure long-term maintenance.

5.4 THE DESIGN BENEFIT CONCEPT

How can a table of potential benefits, such as Table 5.1, be used to aid our ability to design or evaluate a water supply scheme? If the engineer can decide that specific benefits will be the goals of a proposed water scheme then three things are made possible. Firstly, the design, in other words the combination of different improvements to water quality, quantity, availability and reliability, can be selected with the specific goals in mind. Secondly, the cost-effectiveness of a design can be assessed, and compared with that of rival designs, by weighing the cost against the savings associated with the chosen design benefits. Thirdly, national and regional planning and resource allocation can proceed within the rational framework of attempting to achieve the defined goals.

It is necessary therefore for specific benefits to be selected and for these to be the 'design benefits' on the basis of which planning, design and evaluation will be conducted. These design benefits will depend on the specific scheme under consideration and need to be defined quite precisely if they are to be of any real value. Turning to Table 5.1, it is likely that the appropriate design benefits in many situations will be those listed as Stage I benefits. These Stage I benefits can be achieved in the fairly short-term future, they depend upon fewer and simpler complementary inputs than the other benefits listed and the anticipated impact of a particular design on Stage I benefits is fairly readily assessed.

Stage I benefits relate firstly to changes in the water collection journey (time and energy saving) and secondly to improvements in health. Both these benefits may lead to Stage II and Stage III benefits, but these are more distant in time and depend upon more complex complementary inputs (Table 5.2).

This recommendation, that design benefits should be time–energy savings and health improvements can be restated as a more general proposition: *that the fundamental aim of water supply improvements for low-income communities should be to reduce the cost of water to the consumer.* In other words, the generalized design benefit, with almost universal application, should be cost reduction. The cost of water to the individual is made up, as suggested by White *et al.* (1972), of the sum of:

(a) any cash payment made to the water authority, to the standpipe owner, to the watercarrier or vendor etc.;
(b) the value of the time–energy expended in collecting water where the individual lacks water supplied to the dwelling;
(c) the cost of sickness related to the use of polluted water, to the use of insufficient water or to diseases acquired in the course of water collection.

These three costs make up the total cost of water to the individual consumer. If one assumes that item (a) above is either absent (as in most rural settings) or is unlikely to be decreased by any improvements in water supply facilities, then one is left with the possibility of reducing costs by shortening the water collection journey and by improving health—in other words, by achieving the Stage I benefits outlined in Table 5.1.

The central proposition can thus be stated as follows. The fundamental aim of water supply improvements is to reduce the cost of water to the consumer and, in most cases, this will be done by adopting time–energy savings and health improvements as the design benefits. This approach, apart from its other obvious advantages, will facilitate the allocation of priorities simply by answering the question, 'which low-income communities currently bear the highest cost for water and in which communities can we affect the greatest reduction of cost to the consumer by the expenditure of x dollars per head on water supply improvements'. The answer to such a question will tell the water supply planner in which communities the hardships related to poor water are greatest and in which communities a given per capita investment by the government can produce the best return. These two sets of communities may or may not be the same.

In order to put this approach into practice it is necessary to understand fully the interactions between various water supply improvements and the nominated design benefits, namely improvements to the water collection journey and to health. These interactions will now be discussed in turn.

5.5 THE WATER COLLECTION JOURNEY

One of the most obvious and immediate impacts of a water supply scheme is to change the nature of the water collection journey. The significance of this change will depend upon the nature of the pre-existing water supply situation. In certain communities the water collection journey is short and convenient, for example in the highlands of New Guinea (Feachem, 1973b), and so any improvements in accessibility of supply will not save significant amounts of time or energy. However, there are many communities in which, during certain periods of the year or all the year, the collection of water involves a significant expenditure of time and energy and an improved supply has an obvious potential for reducing these efforts which in turn may lead to labour release and other benefits in Stages II and III of Table 5.1. Chisholm (1968) quotes West African studies which report that the Ngwa of south-east Nigeria live up to 13 km from permanent water and that, in Eastern Nigeria as a whole, half the rural population live more than 5 km from perennial streams and individuals spend up to five hours per day collecting water in the dry season. An extensive survey of water use in East Africa (White et al., 1972) has shown that water-carriers in rural areas spend a mean time of 46 minutes per day collecting water and that in some communities up to 264 minutes per day are required.

It is clear therefore that, in regions where a substantial effort is required to collect water, savings of time and energy are important design benefits for a water supply improvement. There are various possible approaches to the quantification of these design benefits and the most useful is probably to express the time and energy spent in water collection as a percentage of the total available daytime time and energy. These percentages may be calculated for the existing situation, and for the anticipated situation following the construction of an improved supply, and so a meaningful measure is obtained of the impact of the scheme on the water collection journey. Alternatively some investigators (Feachem, 1973b; White *et al.*, 1972) have placed a monetary value on the water collection journey by costing the amount of staple food required to produce the number of calories which are needed to collect water. This is attractive in that it provides a monetary value which can be fed into an overall cost–benefit equation; but it has logical weaknesses, particularly in a society based upon subsistence agriculture. Examples of the recommended approach can be cited from the New Guinea Highlands (Feachem, 1973b) where an average of only 1·6% of the total available daytime energy is spent in water collection whereas in East Africa (White *et al.*, 1972) a mean figure of 1·8% of the total available energy is reported while individual communities can expend up to 4% and individual households expend up to 14·4%.

5.6 WATER-RELATED DISEASES

The Stage I benefits listed in Table 5.1 include improved health in addition to time and energy savings and it is suggested in this paper that Stage I benefits are suitable design benefits for water supply improvements. If improved health is to be a design benefit it is desirable to have a clear understanding of the mechanisms which link different diseases to water supply and to have the ability to predict the impact, on a particular disease, which a particular water improvement scheme is likely to have. It must be stressed that these clear understandings of epidemiological mechanisms, and predictive capabilities for impact, do not exist at the present time for all water-related diseases. However, the last decade has seen considerable advance in the epidemiology and ecology of water-related diseases and we are now in a position where sufficient knowledge exists to enable improved health to be used as a design benefit. Over the next few years, research currently being planned will improve our ability to use improved health as a design benefit in a quantified and rigorous manner.

The most important single advance in understanding the relationships between water supply and disease is the reclassification by D. J. Bradley (Chapter 1) of water-related diseases into categories which relate diseases directly to water. A water-related disease is one which is in some way related to water or to impurities within water. We can distinguish between infectious water-related diseases and those related to some chemical property of the water, as, for instance, cardiovascular disease is associated with water softness (Shaper *et al.*, 1974) and high nitrate levels are associated with infantile cyanosis

(Fish, 1974). This latter type of non-infectious water-related disease is of major importance only in industrialized countries where infectious diseases have been greatly reduced. In developing countries it is the infectious water-related diseases which are important and so it is only these which will be considered here.

The classification of water-related disease proposed by Bradley rests upon four distinct mechanisms by which a disease may be water-related. These mechanisms are water-borne, water-washed, water-based and water-related

Table. 5.3 The four mechanisms of water-related disease transmission and the preventive strategies appropriate to each mechanism

Transmission mechanism	Preventive strategy
Water-borne	Improve water quality Prevent casual use of other unimproved sources
Water-washed	Improve water quantity Improve water accessibility Improve hygiene
Water-based	Decrease need for water contact Control snail populations Improve quality
Water-related insect vector	Improve surface water management Destroy breeding sites of insects Decrease need to visit breeding sites

Table 5.4 A classification of water-related diseases

Category	Example
1. Faecal–oral (water-borne or water-washed)	
(a) low infective dose	Cholera
(b) high infective dose	Bacillary dysentery
2. Water-washed	
(a) skin and eye infections	Trachoma, scabies
(b) other	Louse-borne fever
3. Water-based	
(a) penetrating skin	Schistosomiasis
(b) ingested	Guinea worm
4. Water-related insect vectors	
(a) biting near water	Sleeping sickness
(b) breeding in water	Malaria

insect vector and have been described in detail in Chapter 1 and elsewhere (Bradley, 1974; Feachem, 1975a, 1975b). Table 5.3 lists these four water-related transmission mechanisms and links them to the appropriate preventive

Table 5.5 Water-related diseases with their water associations and their pathogenic agents

Water-related disease	Category from Table 5.4	Pathogenic agent
Amoebic dysentery	1b	C
Ascariasis	1b	D
Bacillary dysentery	1b	A
Balantidiasis	1b	C
Cholera	1a	A
Diarrhoeal disease	1b	H
Enteroviruses (some)	1b	B
Gastroenteritis	1b	H
Giardiasis	1b	C
Hepatitis (infectious)	1b	B
Leptospirosis	1a	E
Paratyphoid	1b	A
Tularaemia	1b	A
Typhoid	1a	A
Conjunctivitis	2a	H
Leprosy	2a	A
Louse-borne relapsing fevers	2b	E
Scabies	2a	H
Skin sepsis and ulcers	2a	H
Tinea	2a	F
Trachoma	2a	B
Flea-, louse-, tick- and mite-borne typhus	2b	G
Yaws	2a	E
Clonorchiasis	3b	D
Diphyllobothriasis	3b	D
Fasciolopsiasis	3b	D
Guinea worm	3b	D
Paragonimiasis	3b	D
Schistosomiasis	3a	D
Arboviral infections (some)	4b	B
Dengue	4b	B
Filariasis	4b	D
Malaria	4b	C
Onchocerciasis	4b	D
Trypanosomiasis	4a	C
Yellow fever	4b	B

A = bacteria; B = virus; C = protozoa; D = helminth; E = spirochaete; F = fungus; G = rickettsiae; H = miscellaneous.

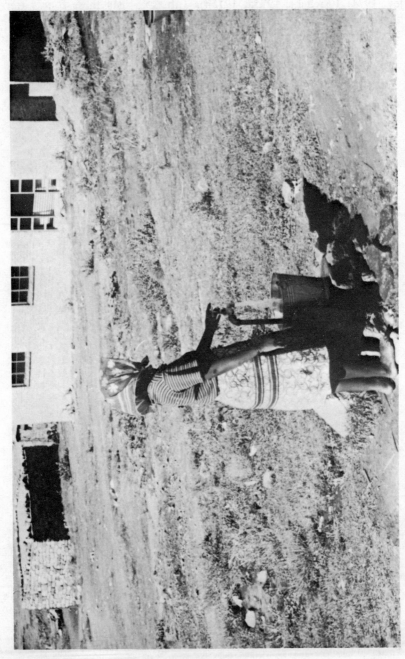

A woman in Lesotho collects water at a village tap. The water is untreated and is piped from a spring above the village. The water contains a few *E. coli* (photograph : R. G. Feachem)

strategies. In order that these concepts may be employed to assess the impact on health of a water improvement scheme it is necessary first to list the chief water-related diseases and assign them to an appropriate category. Bradley has proposed that each disease be assigned to a category which corresponds to one of the four mechanisms listed in Table 5.3. However, this leads to the problem of having all the faecal–oral diseases assigned to both the water-borne and the water-washed categories and so the categories cease to be mutually exclusive. The author therefore proposes a revised categorization, shown in Table 5.4, in which faecal–oral infections are all together in a special category which is water-borne or water-washed. Category 2 is reserved for water-washed diseases which cannot be water-borne, in other words the skin and eye infections plus diseases which are associated with infestations of fleas, lice, ticks or mites. All water-related diseases can therefore be assigned to one of the four categories in Table 5.4. Table 5.5 lists the major water-related infections and assigns them to their category in addition to linking them to their pathogenic agent.

This classification of water-related disease can facilitate the use of health improvements as design benefits and thus promote efficient resource allocation. If the principal water-related diseases in a region are identified and classified according to Table 5.4, then it is possible to identify the types of water supply improvements which will have the greatest impact on health, to consider the cost–benefit aspects of different schemes and to nominate local and regional priorities for supply development.

5.7 THE QUALITY–QUANTITY DILEMMA

It is argued in this chapter that the aim of reducing costs to the water user provides an operational strategy for the planning and design of water supply programmes. In situations where no cash payment is made for water, these costs are chiefly made up of the water collection journey and water-related disease. Improvements in the water collection journey are readily observed, quantified, predicted and analysed but this is not the case for reductions in water-related disease. Many years of epidemiological research are required before it will be possible to predict confidently the reductions to all water-related infections which will follow a specific water improvement in a given socio-environmental context. However, in general terms and using the classification of water-related disease given here, it is possible to relate water improvements to changes in community health.

The most difficult to handle, and the largest, group of water-related infections is the faecal–oral group because they are all potentially water-borne but can also be transmitted by any other faecal–oral route. Therefore, the decision concerning the correct supply design which will have most impact on a faecal–oral infection is not easily made. Suppose, in a particular community, it was known that diarrhoeal disease was almost entirely water-borne, then the appropriate strategy would clearly be to improve water quality. Suppose, on the other hand, it was known that diarrhoeal diseases were almost always transmitted by direct contact in the home, then it would be appropriate to promote water quantity and availability and to improve domestic hygiene. However, in most, if not all, real situations faecal–oral infections will be transmitted by both water-borne and non-waterborne routes and therefore improvements in both quantity and quality are indicated.

If limitless financial and human resources were available then it would be possible to design water supplies for low-income communities so that they provided abundant high quality water. However, this chapter commenced by arguing that the size of the global water supply problem is so large and the resources so scarce that it is necessary to design and plan to achieve the best possible impact with the resources available. It will not usually be possible to contemplate the perfect supply, only an improved one, and the method outlined in this chapter is designed to facilitate the choice of appropriate improvement. Improvements in water quantity and availability will affect that component of the faecal–oral disease load which is not water-borne and will also reduce the prevalence of infections in the water-washed category. Improvements in water quality will affect the truly water-borne component of the faecal–oral load and also guinea worm and schistosomiasis where these are found.

Water quantity

Current knowledge of tropical epidemiology indicates that, probably without exception, low-income communities in hot climates suffer from high morbidity due to non-waterborne faecal–oral infections and to the water-washed infections. In the faecal–oral category, diarrhoeal diseases (especially among infants) are a major cause of acute morbidity and mortality throughout developing countries and it has been indicated earlier in this chapter that much of this diarrhoeal disease may be non-waterborne. In the water-washed category, the skin and eye infections are also major causes of morbidity and, like non-waterborne diarrhoea, they are reduced by increasing the quantity, availability and reliability of the water supply almost irrespective of its quality. Therefore a general rule can be postulated that all low-income water supplies should strive to bring abundant quantities of water near to or into dwellings throughout the year.

Water quality

Improvements in water quality can affect the water-borne component of the faecal–oral load and also the transmission of guinea worm and schistosomiasis. Conventional engineering wisdom has held that all water supplies, except those using high quality groundwater sources, should be treated to improve their quality and that such treatment will pay substantial dividends in improved health. It has further been held that treatment should bring water quality standards up to those recommended by the World Health Organization (WHO, 1971) as appropriate international water quality standards. For example WHO claims that, for individual or small community supplies, water should be condemned if it is repeatedly found to contain more than 10 coliforms or 1 *Escherichia coli* per 100 ml. These standards are far too stringent for hot climates and would lead to the condemnation of the vast majority of existing water supplies in low-income communities. This conventional wisdom is highly misconceived and may well have been responsible for retarding the development of water supplies in less developed countries.

The addition of any form of treatment process to a supply design will add a major new cost factor and will increase the maintenance problems, and the risks of failure, by an order of magnitude. This is especially true of a treatment process sophisticated enough to produce water which meets WHO quality standards. There is no such thing as a simple or easily maintained treatment system and planners and designers should approach the decisions about treatment and quality with an open mind and not with the pre-judgement that treatment is necessary and WHO standards must be guaranteed. There will be those circumstances when treatment is appropriate and those when it is not; Figure 5.1 presents an algorithm of the decision-making process involved. The 'water source' in Figure 5.1 is the source selected for a proposed engineered water supply and may or may not be a source already used by the community. Figure 5.1 guides the planner or designer to one of four eventual decisions: to supply with treatment, to supply without treatment, to supply without treatment but with 48 hours storage time in the system or to abandon a supply based upon the specified water source. The factors involved in Figure 5.1 will be discussed individually.

Water quality

The quality of the best available raw water source will have an important influence on the decision to treat or not to treat. In Figure 5.1 it is suggested that a raw water source commonly containing less than *a E. coli* per 100 ml should be regarded as clean and not likely to spread water-borne infections. Therefore, with the proviso that 48 hours storage time should be incorporated into the design in regions where schistosomiasis is endemic (to allow time for all infective cercariae to die) no treatment is regarded as necessary for water of this quality. This assumes that the water source concerned is reasonably protected from subsequent faecal contamination. A water source containing between *a* and *b E. coli* per 100 ml is of good quality and should be treated if possible but supplied untreated if treatment is not feasible. A water source containing between *b* and *c E. coli* per 100 ml is of poor quality and should be treated if possible. If not, it should either be supplied untreated or abandoned according to a series of decisions set out in Figure 5.1. Water containing more than *c E. coli* per 100 ml is regarded as grossly polluted and, if treatment is not possible, it should be abandoned unless the proposed supply will not increase the number

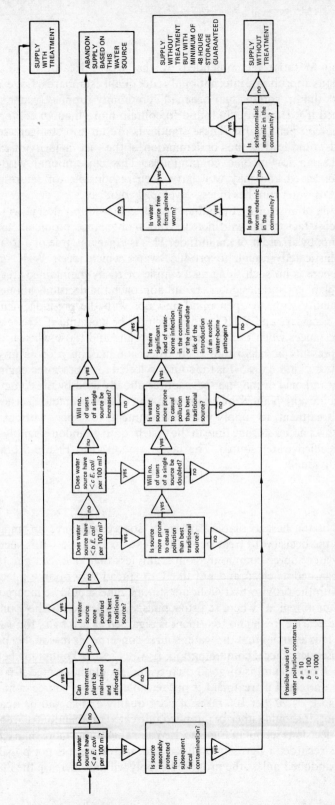

Figure 5.1 An algorithm of the decision to treat, not to treat, or to abandon a particular water source

of users of a single raw water source. In summary the quality distinctions
made in Figure 5.1 are as follows.

< a	E. coli per 100 ml	Supply untreated
a–b	E. coli per 100 ml	Treat if possible, if not supply untreated
b–c	E. coli per 100 ml	Treat if possible, if not supply untreated or abandon depending on various other factors
> c	E. coli per 100 ml	Treat if possible, if not abandon or supply untreated depending on various other factors

These quality distinctions have been expressed in the non-specific terms of a,
b and c in order that Figure 5.1 may be adapted to local conditions and may be
adjusted as our understanding of water quality and water-borne disease
increases. It is suggested that appropriate standards for many hot countries
would be $a = 10$, $b = 100$ and $c = 1000$. This would allow the untreated supply
of water containing < 10 E. coli per 100 ml and would advise the treatment of
all other water. However, where treatment is not realistic because of maintenance or financial constraints, water of inferior quality may be supplied
untreated or abandoned according to the method given in Figure 5.1. In certain
very specific circumstances, even grossly polluted water containing more than
1000 E. coli per 100 ml may be supplied untreated. These guidelines clearly
run counter to conventional practice based on WHO standards and suggest
the possibility of providing piped water supplies of known low quality in
certain circumstances. The reader should note that all standards used here are
based on the numbers of Escherichia coli (alternatively called 'faecal coliform')
and the standards used in Figure 5.1 must always be for specifically faecal
organisms. The use of a total coliform index, or any other indicator organism
which is not of wholly faecal origin, would be quite inappropriate as a measure
of the health hazard of untreated waters in hot climates.

It must be stressed that water quality has been viewed in purely biological
terms and that only water-related infectious diseases have been considered. In
areas where chemical water quality provides a serious health problem the
appropriate modifications must be made to Figure 5.1. Chemical water-related
disease problems tend to be very localized phenomena and it is not possible to
incorporate useful general statements into Figure 5.1. Obvious quality related
factors concerning guinea worm and schistosomiasis are also incorporated
into Figure 5.1.

Number of users of a single source

A major objection to the deliberate piping of poor quality water is that one
may thereby increase the risk of a water-borne epidemic. The risk must be
related to the existing risk of a water-borne epidemic by considering whether
the proposed new supply will increase the number of people who take water

from a single source. If a community of 100 people traditionally take water from a single pool and it is proposed to pipe water to the community from a stream then, assuming that the risk of faecal pollution of the pool and the stream are identical, no new risk of a water-borne epidemic is created. The risk of water-borne disease is only increased if the piped water is of poorer quality than the existing water sources, if the piped water source has greater chance of casual faecal pollution than existing sources or if the new supply will serve more people than any one existing water source. For instance, a village of 1000 people may traditionally draw water from six scattered sources and a new piped water supply would greatly increase the number taking water from a single source and would thus increase the magnitude of an epidemic resulting from the pollution of this source by a water-borne pathogen.

This concept is incorporated into Figure 5.1 in two places. Water of very poor quality ($>c$ E. coli per 100 ml) which cannot be treated is abandoned unless the proposed new supply will not increase the number of co-users of a source and the new source is at least as clean as existing sources. In this case, no extra risk is created by piping dirty water to the community and piping this water may well have an effect on the many infections related to water quantity and so be beneficial. The design is therefore based on the taking of known and specific risks in order to achieve known and specific benefits. The result of not taking these risks is to abandon the supply and so to forgo all possible benefits. A brief discussion of risk-taking designs is given in Section 5.8.

The number of co-users is also used in Figure 5.1 to decide what treatment is appropriate for waters having between b and c E. coli per 100 ml. In this case it is suggested that, unless the number of co-users is doubled, the water should be untreated rather than abandoned. If the co-users are at least doubled then the epidemic risk is such that other considerations are brought into the decision. This factor of 2 should be adapted to meet local circumstance. For instance, a region threatened by the current spread of cholera would reduce the factor of 2 to perhaps 1 or 1·5.

The comparative quality of the water source

Figure 5·1 is designed so that whenever a water source of inferior quality is under consideration, it is at least as pure as the best of the sources currently used by the community. This eliminates the possibility of piping untreated water which is actually more polluted than a traditional water source.

The comparative exposure to pollution of the water source

Figure 5·1 ensures that note is taken of the proneness to pollution of the new water source when compared to that of the existing water sources.

The water-borne disease load

Where the supply of poor quality water is contemplated, Figure 5·1 ensures that a community known to have a high load of water-borne infection is considered differently from one which has little water-borne disease.

Summary

In most, if not all, low-income communities in hot climates infections which are non-waterborne faecal–oral or water-washed will be major causes of morbidity and mortality. These disease problems will respond to improvements in water quantity, availability and reliability and therefore these improvements should always be a major focus of the design of new water supplies.

Water treatment is always preferable when the raw water source is not of excellent quality or is not protected from the risk of pollution. However, water treatment plants are often expensive and always very difficult to maintain and operate. In situations where treatment is deemed to be not feasible owing to financial or maintenance constraints, then a choice must be made between supplying water without treatment or abandoning plans for supply. Figure 5·1 provides an algorithm of the decision-making process and can be used to assist the planner or designer in his decision to treat, not to treat or to abandon. The outcome of using this algorithm will be to greatly increase the number of untreated water supplies and the number of supplies which deliver water of known poor quality. It is a risk-taking procedure which favours the acceptance of known hazards to achieve known benefits. It is in contrast to conventional practice which favours abandoning a supply programme rather than accepting a risk-taking design or causes the construction of treatment plants in circumstances where they can never be operated or maintained.

The procedure given in Figure 5·1 is an advance on current conservative and non-explicit practice but it is not presented as a total or final paradigm. It merely indicates a more rational approach which will lead to greater progress by countering the current unduly conservative design procedure. It will be modified and improved by others and, in particular, research will aid our ability to quantify the exact nature of the various risks and benefits and so will lead to the formulation of better questions to which we shall have better answers.

5·8 RISK-TAKING DESIGN

The recommended approach (Figure 5·1) is a risk-taking one and is thus in line with recent trends in all branches of civil engineering. While the general public may sleep well at night in the belief that bridges and blocks of flats are built not to fall down, that dams are built not to overflow or that treatment works will always treat to guranteed standards, the fact is that all these structures are designed with certain probabilities of failure in mind. Great advances have been made in analysing the failure risk, in quantifying the consequences of failure and feeding this information into a decision on whether the cost of incremental improvements is justified by the incremental risk reductions. Very often the consequences of failure involve loss of human life and, in such cases, a monetary value on a life has to be included in the analysis. Revell (1973) has written in connection with spillway design.

The engineer has been too reticent to place an economic value on human life or suffering. This, of course, is understandable; however, in order to make meaningful decisions such an evaluation is unavoidable. The alternative, in effect, places an infinite value on a human life, which is unrealistic. The resources of the Nation are not inexhaustible. The incremental cost between a safe dam and an extremely safe dam may be great. This difference in cost, when considered as a national resource, might save more lives or prevent more suffering if spent in some other activity such as highway or industrial safety or medical research. The committee believes that the engineering profession should delay no longer the use of monetary human values in the economics of spillway design. The courts have shown that human values are finite not infinite. Precedents in law have charted a technique to appraise this value in monetary terms. Actual awards properly adjusted to present worth provide further guidance.

Precisely similar arguments may be applied to developing country water supplies. Risks are always present and it is better that these should be explicit than concealed. Research in tropical epidemiology will increase the ability to quantify the risk of epidemics associated with particular levels of polluted water supply. As this ability develops, so it will be appropriate to use monetary values for illness and death in analyses which consider the costs and benefits of different levels of water treatment.

5·9 APPLICATIONS OF THE METHOD

This chapter will be concluded with a discussion of how the methodology outlined here may be applied to real situations. Four sets of decisions are guided by the application of the recommended approach and these will be described individually.

Planning and resource allocation

By following the method given here it is possible to plan local, regional or national water supply programmes in such a way that scarce human and financial resources are utilized most efficiently and that the potential benefits are realized. This is done by closely defining the design benefits appropriate for water supply improvements in each region or type of community. Suitable designs can then be outlined and the costs of these designs can be related to the magnitude of design benefits. Available resources for water improvement can then be allocated both in time and over space in a way which, within various political and humanitarian constraints, seeks to achieve the maximum benefit at the minimum cost. The necessary complementary development inputs can be identified and a variety of village and governmental agencies can be mobilized to ensure that the necessary supporting programmes (for example, health education) are carried out. Completed water supply programmes can be retrospectively evaluated to determine the extent to which the anticipated design benefits have been achieved. Such evaluations will then modify and guide future programmes.

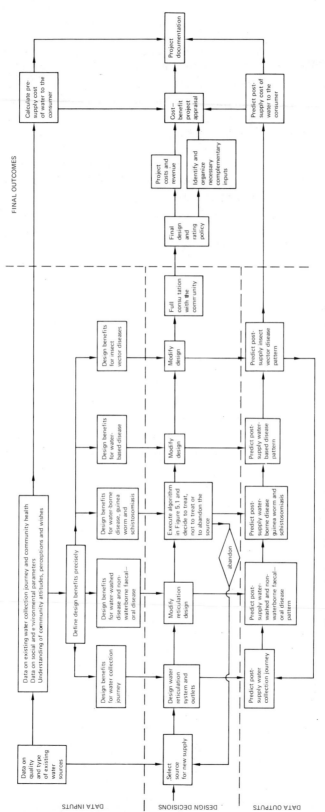

Figure 5.2 A guide to the design process for a water supply in a low-income community

Priority selection

The concept of the cost of water to the consumer provides a rational method for priority selection by identifying those communities which currently bear the greatest cost. It will often be found that it is the poorest and most underprivileged communities which bear the highest cost. It is a useful exercise for planners to categorize communities according to the nature and magnitude of their water costs and then to rank them. This ranking provides an instant check list of communities whose need for improved water supplies is the greatest. Such a listing is made more useful by quantifying the benefits which can be achieved by the spending of x dollars per head in each community type. It will then be possible to select between the high priority cases on the basis of the returns anticipated from the available investment.

Design

The approach given in this chapter has enormous implications for all aspects of the design process for low-income water supplies in developing countries. The concept of designing for precisely defined design benefits should rationalize and improve the present rule-of-thumb methods in water supply design and should lead to tailor-made designs achieving more benefits at a lower per capita cost.

The exact manner in which the recommended approach is used will be affected by the circumstances of each case. However, a general guide to design procedure is presented in Figure 5·2 showing how the various principles of the method are incorporated into an integrated design philosophy. Figure 5·2 can be modified where appropriate so that it reflects local conditions and can then be used by the water engineer to guide and rationalize his design. It can also be used by the engineer to explain and justify his design to non-technical colleagues or it can be used by the planner and administrator to encourage the engineer to relate some controversial decision to an agreed framework.

Donor support

The fourth potential use for the method recommended here is to facilitate improved communication on low-income water supply between developing country governments and bilateral or multilateral aid donors. At present, despite the current interest in giving aid to grass-roots projects which improve conditions and prospects for the rural and urban poor, there is reluctance among many donors to support domestic water supply projects. One reason for this is that water supply projects have usually not been documented with the same rigour and thoroughness as projects in other sectors (for instance, agriculture) and have not been exposed to the same degree of financial and economic analysis. Water supply sector project documents typically appear to be poorly thought out and casual in their approach to economic analysis. This results simply from the lack of an agreed framework in which a water supply project can be formulated, described and analysed and from a general lack of information on techniques for exposing water supplies to cost–benefit appraisals.

Over the last decade an almost standard format has emerged for the presentation of project documents in the agricultural and transport sectors whereas no such format has emerged for the water supply and sanitation sectors. The approach described in this chapter provides a framework in which water projects can be described, justified and rigorously analysed and this may be an important first step in encouraging greater support from aid agencies.

5·10 REFERENCES

Bradley, D. J. (1974). Water supplies: The consequences of change. In: *Human Rights in Health*. Ciba Foundation Symposium 23 (new series). Amsterdam: A. S. P.

Carruthers, I. D. (1973). *Impact and Economics of Community Water Supply*. Ashford, Kent: Wye College.

Chisholm, M. (1968). *Rural Settlement and Land Use*. London: Hutchinson.

Feachem, R. G. A. (1973a). *Environment and Health in a New Guinea Highlands Community*. Ph.D. thesis. Sydney: University of New South Wales.

Feachem, R. G. A. (1973b). The pattern of domestic water use in the New Guinea Highlands. *South Pacific Bulletin*, **23**(3), 10–14.

Feachem, R. G. A. (1975a). Water supplies for low-income communities in developing countries. *Journal of the Environmental Engineering Division, A. S. C. E.*, **101**, 687–703.

Feachem, R. G. A. (1975b). The rational allocation of water resources for the domestic needs of rural communities in developing countries. In: *Proceedings of the Second World Congress of Water Resources, New Delhi*, **2**, 539–547.

Fish, H. (1974). Nitrate and London's public water supply. *Civil Engineering*, December, 31–37.

Revell, R. W. (1973). Reevaluation of dam spillway adequacy. *Journal of the Hydraulics Division, A.S.C.E.*, **99**, 337–372.

Saunders, R. J. and Warford, J. J. (1974). Village water supply and sanitation in less developed countries. *P.U. Report No. Res. 2*, washington: International Bank for Reconstruction and Development.

Shaper, A. G., Clayton, D. G. and Morris, J. N. (1974). *The Hardness of Water Supplies and Cardiovascular Disease*. Paper presented to the International Water Supply Association Congress, Brighton, England.

White, G. F., Bradley, D. J. and White, A. U. (1972). *Drawers of Water*. Chicago and London: Chicago University Press.

WHO. (1971). *International Standards for Drinking Water*. Geneva: WHO.

WHO (1973). *World Health Statistics Report*, **26**, 720–783.

6

Patterns of Domestic Water Use in Low-Income Communities

ANNE U. WHITE

6·1 VOLUME OF DOMESTIC WATER USE

The volume of water used by the people of tropical developing countries is chiefly a function of income and material wealth, with only the highest income group having access to large amounts of safe water. The costs of that usage include the individual costs and benefits which influence behaviour and the social costs and benefits which stem from health and economic effects and influence community well-being. These two elements of cost are both associated with the volume used and with the settlement pattern of the people.

The volume of water used ranges, as is shown in Figure 6·1, from a daily mean consumption per person of a little over a litre to about 25 litres for rural consumers without tap connections or standpipes. For city or village dwellers who use public standpipes or fountains the consumption is about 10–50 litres per person daily, 15–90 litres for those with only a single tap in the household, and 30–300 litres for those with multiple taps in the house.

In most low-income communities, both rural and urban, facilities for water

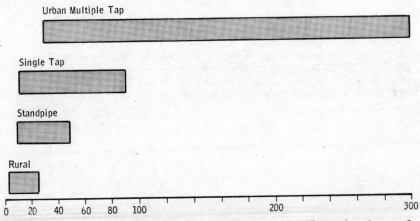

Figure 6.1 Range of daily consumption per person in litres for major classes of water use. (Borjesson and Bobeda, 1964; Feachem, 1973; Frankel and Shouvana-virakul, 1973; Teller, 1963; Roure, 1973; Warner, 1973; White *et al.*, 1972)

range from no public service at all, through public standpipes, to instances of adequate piped supply. Water that has to be fetched from a source outside the home assumes quite a different role in the day of a householder than that obtained with a twist of a wrist from a tap, and carrying water is the daily lot of most women and many children in these communities.

People on the lower end of the income scale in developing countries reside for the most part in rural areas, either in clustered communities or in scattered residences, or in city peripheries where urban services are scarce or completely lacking. In these three types of settlement water for domestic use is often costly in terms of cash or energy expenditure, and its quality varies from safe to extremely hazardous. An attempt will be made here to show how domestic water is used in these different kinds of communities, and how the characteristics of use relate to the possibilities of improving the supplies.

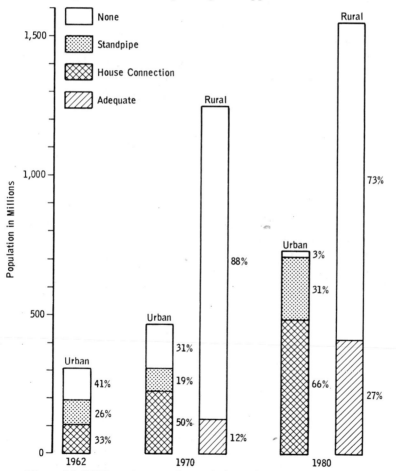

Figure 6.2 WHO estimates of population of developing countries provided with adequate water for 1962 and 1970, and target for 1980. (WHO, 1973)

6·2 THE POPULATION INVOLVED

The most complete recent estimate regarding domestic water supply in developing countries has been made by the World Health Organization (WHO, 1973), based on a questionnaire sent out in 1970 to 91 selected countries, covering about one half of the population of the world and using each country's own national definition of 'rural' and 'urban'. These estimates provide a comparison with services provided in 1962, when a smaller number of countries answered a similar questionnaire, and with the goals suggested by WHO for 1980. It will be seen from Figure 6.2 that about 31% of the urban population and 88% of the rural population of these countries did not, in 1970, have reasonable access to what WHO define as safe water, which includes treated surface water or untreated but uncontaminated water from such sources as protected boreholes, springs and sanitary wells.

6·3 SETTLEMENT PATTERNS

Patterns of water use and wastewater disposal, health risks, and the cost of obtaining water may be roughly judged from the literature and observation to vary according to the settlement pattern of people in rural areas of developing countries along the lines indicated in Table 6·1. The woman who goes to the nearby village tank in Asia may have a low cost for her water in terms of energy and time, but when the tank is used for washing clothes, people, cattle and

Table 6. 1 Characteristics of settlement and water supply

Pattern of settlement	Types of sources available	Health hazard from water	Cost (in energy or cash)
Urban peripheries	Taps	low	high
	Standpipes	medium	medium
	Vendors	high	high
	Surface—ponds, streams	high	low
	Underground—springs, wells	high	low
	Rain-barrels	high	low
Rural clustered	Taps	low	high
	Standpipes	low	medium
	Vendors	high	high
	Surface—ponds, streams	high	low
	Underground—springs and	high	low–high*
	shallow wells, deep wells	low	low–high*
	Rain-barrels	medium	low
Rural scattered	Surface—ponds, streams	high	low–high*
	Underground—springs, wells	low	low–high*
	Rain-barrels	low	low

*Depends on area—tends to be low in humid areas and high in arid areas, especially in the dry season.

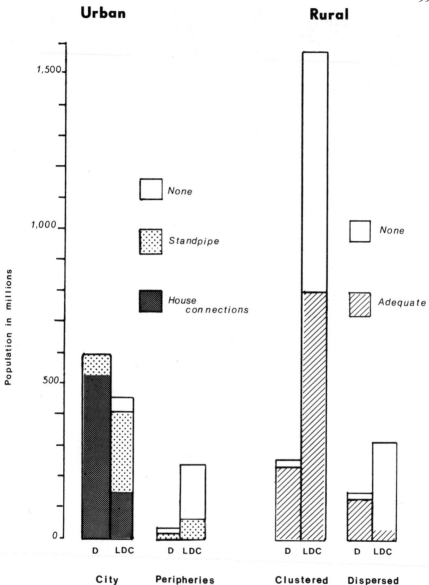

Figure 6.3 Estimated distribution of water services for the world population in 1970; developed, D, and less developed, LDC, countries (White, 1974)

cooking pots the health hazard is high. An Ethiopian woman may object to the 5 kilometres she has to walk to a borehole in the dry season, but the water she gets is not likely to be polluted with faecal bacteria. However, water carried substantial distances may well become contaminated by the time it reaches the home. Settlement patterns also affect very much the cost of possible improvements, so it is important to try to estimate how the population is distributed.

Despite statistical difficulties, a rough estimate can be made of the proportion of people in rural areas of developing countries who live in concentrated settlements, those who live in scattered or dispersed households, and those who live on the peripheries of the large cities. White (1974) has made the estimate given in Figure 6·3 which shows the distribution of water services in 1970 in the developed and less developed countries of the world according to settlement patterns. He defines classes of settlement as follows:

Cities: Organized urban areas and their satellites.
Peripheries: Disorganized shantytowns, bidonvilles, barrios, and other (one hopes) temporary living area on the immediate fringes of cities.
Rural—clustered: Settlements, primarily for agricultural purposes, of household grouped together.
Rural—dispersed: Widely scattered households lacking grouping and nuclei.

It can be seen that most of the water service developed in rural areas has gone to the clustered settlements, and that those who live in the peripheral areas of the cities have little better access to safe water than their isolated cousins in

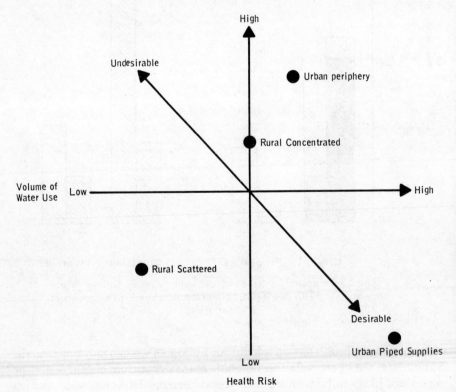

Figure 6.4 Water use and health risk

dispersed rural settlements. These figures are rough estimates which deal with the population of the whole world, including China, and therefore contain judgements about the adequacy of water services in rural areas where WHO data is not available. If China were excluded, the clustered rural population served adequately would be smaller, but still much larger than the dispersed settlement population so served.

These settlement types can be roughly grouped according to the health risks from the water used (Figure 6·4). The population of the urban peripheries may have access to a fair quantity of water from standpipes or from local streams or ponds, but their health risk from crowded conditions leading to contamination and from poor waste disposal facilities is likely to be very high. Those in rural concentrated settlements often have access to convenient supplies, depending in part upon whether they are in a humid or dry area, but because of the closeness of their neighbours and the larger numbers of people using any one source, their health risk may be fairly high, and their waste water disposal may cause problems of contamination and insect breeding. In the scattered rural homesteads, access to sufficient water may well be a problem; but when few people use each source there tends to be less health risk, and disposal of waste is much less of a problem. These are broad generalizations, for within each group sources vary, and the health risk and costs vary with them.

6·4 WATER USE IN DIFFERENT TYPES OF COMMUNITY

Rural concentrated

A 'village' is a very different entity in different parts of the world, ranging from the settlements in Peru made up of 100–200 people which contain some 16% of the rural population of that country to the villages of India, containing thousands of people, where about 80% of the rural population live. Each country has its own census definition of 'rural', and many rural villages are usually included in it. Rural regions of the developing world differ considerably in the availability of safe water (Figure 6.5), with the Americas and Western Pacific ahead of the rest of the regions, with nearly one quarter of their rural people having 'reasonable access' to safe water. This term is defined by WHO as implying 'that the housewife or members of the family do not have to spend a disproportionate part of the day in fetching the family's water needs' (WHO, 1973).

The main difference that 'reasonable access' can make to the householder is in the saving of time and energy in fetching it, for the volume she uses and her patterns of use once she gets it do not seem to change very radically unless water is available piped inside the home, with several taps, in which case the volume used does increase considerably. In Tanzania, where Warner (1973) made studies before and a year after the installation of improved water supplies which reduced the distance from the source for most households, the quantity

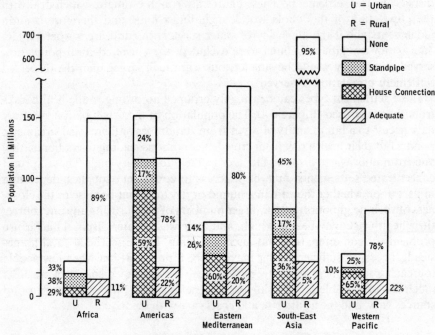

Figure 6.5 WHO estimates of population of developing countries in tropical areas with adequate water in 1970, by region (WHO, 1973)

used increased, but not by more than a few litres per capita daily. The lower the initial use, the greater the increase with the more readily available supply.

It is likely that design criteria used for rural water systems often overestimate the demand, and thus increase unnecessarily the cost of the system. In a study of 14 communities with newly installed piped supplies and without alternative supplies in north-east Thailand, ranging in size from 800–5000 inhabitants, Frankel and Shouvanavirakul (1973) found the range of consumptive figures used for design purposes to be 50–80 litres per capita daily. Actual use he found to vary from 9·6–36·8 lpcd at standpipes, and 24·4–65·2 lpcd for house connections. This led him to believe that design figures of 25 lpcd for standpipes and 50 lpcd for house connections would be more realistic.

In most of the concentrated settlements water is available within about half an hour's walk, according to what sparse information is available. This is not everywhere the case. For example, in 1969 a survey revealed that out of 576 000 villages in India, about 90 000 (16%) have no water within a radius of 2 kilometres, or have wells more than 15 metres deep (WHO, 1974). Since women with water tend to walk at about 4 kilometres an hour (White et al., 1972), their trip would take them an hour, plus considerably more energy expenditure if the water has to be lifted from a deep well.

The sources available for people in concentrated settlements are varied, and frequently there is some choice of sources. In the Americas the public fountain is usually the first step in the improvement of water supplies, and up to half the population of this type of settlement in the region may have access to them (Donaldson, 1973). Here the housewife has a trip of relatively short duration, unless she has to spend a long time in a queue waiting her turn. Other sources include various kinds of surface water such as ponds, streams and canals, or underground water from springs, hand-dug shallow wells, and deep tubewells. In some communities rainwater is collected from the roof into containers; in others this is not even considered a potential supply. Except for the tubewell, or the rain-barrel in sparsely populated areas, the sources tend to be hazardous to health unless they are protected or their water treated. They may be used for washing clothes, people and animals as well as drinking from.

As Burton (1974) points out, there is tremendous ingenuity in the ways that pre-industrial societies have devised for lifting, storing and transporting water. Devices such as the shaduf, the Archimedes screw and various animal-powered methods serve to lift the water; it can be stored in hafirs or tanks, and bamboo pipes, canals or qanats may transport it where needed. These devices exist alongside modern water supply technology and, if new systems do not seem to be workable, there is considerable evidence that people will return to the older method.

In these relatively crowded settlements wastewater, even with the limited amounts used, may become a problem. The easiest disposal is out the door, but in humid areas this may lead to pools where mosquitoes breed. Where there are open drains for wastewater, as in India, their load of human and animal waste may contaminate the groundwater (Airan, 1973).

Rural scattered

In many of the rural areas of the Americas and of Africa settlement is scattered, with the single households or small groups of households spread over a wide area. In humid areas of this type water may be readily available at short distances from the house; and even in the dryer areas there may be springs, wells, sometimes a borehole, and the variety of potential sources associated with a river— the stream itself or holes dug near the main channel. In addition there is rainwater collected from roofs or trees, or in dug ponds or tanks which last at least into the dry season. The household that is remote from neighbours may even have its own exclusive well or spring and, consequently, little contamination except from its own wastes. Such areas may also have households at the extreme limits of distance from a water source as in the Dongore area of Ethiopia where in the dry season people have to go 5 kilometres or more to the only available source (Browne, 1974).

Water fetching does much to determine the structure of the day for the woman in the household. Usually she has to go for water first thing in the morning and again during the day. A diagram of water use (Figure 6·6) at two sites in East Africa shows how it fits into a woman's use of time. At Alemi, in the Lango district of Uganda near the River Nile, the land appears

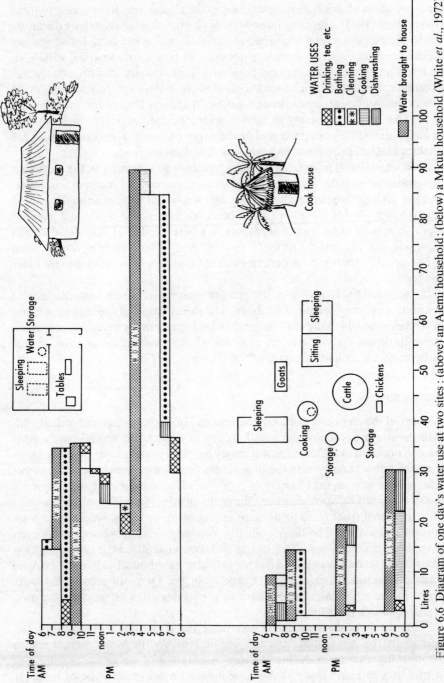

Figure 6.6 Diagram of one day's water use at two sites: (above) an Alemi household; (below) a Mkuu household (White *et al.*, 1972)

swampy; but for three months of the year the women have to dig holes in the edges of the swamp, or walk from their widely scattered households to a government borehole. The household illustrated contains six people, with only the mother and daughter carrying water. The mother made three trips this day to the borehole, one in the morning and two in the afternoon, and the daughter one. Each trip takes her only about ten minutes, although some of the family's neighbours may be half an hour's walk from any source. The trip is strenuous, for she uses a large tin container holding about 40 kilograms of water. The largest volume of water is used for bathing, although people bathe also in streams and ponds. Cooking claims the next largest volume, with enough left for dishwashing and drinking. Water is stored in a covered pot in the house.

In the second household at Mkuu, a farming community on the green slopes of Kilimanjaro in Tanzania, another family of six people uses a much smaller total volume of water. Here the mother sends her children several times a day to fetch water from the rural standpipe. The water originates in a high mountain stream. They walk about 1 kilometre to this source, as she feels the little stream running near their house is not safe to use. Outside her house she keeps a 200 litre cask in which she stores water, and into this goes water from her roof when it rains, but today it is dry. Her husband's bath, and that of a male visitor, use up the rest of the water in the cask, so she makes two trips to replenish the supply. In the afternoon she sends the children off again to the standpipe. Her drinking water she keeps in a small clay pot and feels it is safe to drink without boiling. Had there been laundry to do she would have carried more water.

In both these households, wastewater was used for livestock or dumped out on the ground.

Both these women are responsible for most of the food growing for their family, and have to fit their water carrying in with the rest of their daily tasks. In Africa today it is estimated that 80% of the women take a major part in the food production, carry 80% of the fuel supplies, and supply the labour for half of the house repairs and a third of the housebuilding (*Focus*, 1975).

Urban peripheries

For large numbers of people in the developing world the move to the city represents an opportunity for employment and a better life, aspirations not always realized. Between 1950 and 1970 the number of people in urban centres of the developing world more than doubled. Assuming that this trend continues, by the year 2000, about 43% of the population of these countries is expected to live in urban settlements (World Bank, 1971). At the same time very high unemployment in the urban areas means that these migrants have little opportunity of getting jobs, and many can only exist by urban subsistence activities such as peddling, hawking or begging. They have no place to live, and shelter is provided by ingeniously assembled cardboard, tin scraps, or other materials. City services are usually entirely lacking. There may be a few stand-

106

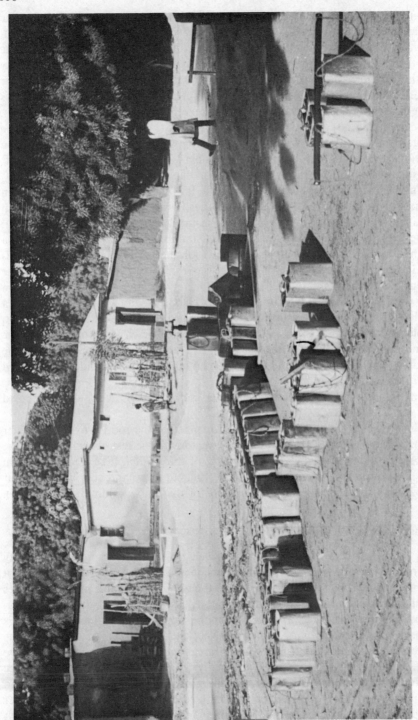

A long line of tins awaiting the re-opening of an urban standpipe in northern Nigeria (photograph : R. G. Feachem)

Table 6.2 Rate of consumption and water tariffs at the standpipe*

City	Average number of persons per standpipe	Average consumption (lpcd)	Water tariff at standpipe ($US/m³)
Upper Volta			
Ouagadougou	1850	6·5	0·3
Bobodioulasso	1550	5	0·3
Gabon			
Libreville	3300	7	0·5
Port Gentil	750	10	0·5
Lambarene	1200	2	0·5
Cameroon			
Douala	1450	8·5	0·2
Yaoundé	2250	7	0·3

*WHO/IRC (1975).

pipes, each one supposed to serve very large numbers of people, as shown in Table 6·2. In practice, it is more probable that a single standpipe serves some 500 people, as is estimated for the city of Yaoundé (Rouleau, 1975), but even this number could involve considerable waiting time at peak morning and evening hours.

Problems with standpipes include the need for guards to prevent wastage, flooding and contamination by waste water, vandalism and the failure of equipment (WHO/IRC, 1975). The person going for water has to expect a long wait in line at rush periods, and possible disappointment if the standpipe closes or breaks before she gets her turn. In this situation people have to turn to other more risky sources; rainwater, ditches, ponds, wells or streams. It is clear that they do this anyway in the wet season. In Yaoundé, Cameroon, for example, the consumption of water from the standpipes more than doubles in the dry season from January to May (Roure, 1973).

Another source is the vendor who goes from house to house selling his water from a tank with a hose or from tins on a cart. Vendors may be found in rural areas of concentrated settlement, and even occasionally serving scattered households, but they are especially common in urban areas where working people do not have the time to spend waiting at the standpipe, or where, as in parts of Asia and Africa, women do not care to be out on the streets. The costs are very high for a limited amount of water of dubious quality, and often a family buying water in this way will pay in a month as much as or more than a city dweller with a tap in his home providing a much greater quantity of safer water (Table 6·3).

Where people are crowded together, and the fight for employment often requires a clean shirt and a neat appearance, the city dweller is hard pressed to be able to pay these sums for water. Despite the cost, the urban dweller without piped supplies tends to use more water than his rural cousin in the same situation (White et al., 1972). Even where there are standpipes, the

Table 6.3 Cost of water delivered by vendor and water supply company
($US/m³)*

	Delivered by water supply company	Delivered by vendor
Upper Volta	0·3	1–1·5
Ghana	0·1†	1·25–2·5
Senegal	free	1·6 –2·4
Nicaragua	0·29	0·83–4·12

*Sources: WHO/IRC, 1975; Instituto Centroamericano, 1974.
†Estimated cost based on monthly use and levy per house.

water agency seldom provides the washing places, public baths or toilets which make life easier, as these facilities are usually not within its administrative bounds.

6·5 FACTORS AFFECTING WATER USE PATTERNS

Water use patterns have been described here in three types of settlement patterns, but it should be remembered that they are very much intermixed. The woman who carries home 40 litres of water to supply her family of four for 24 hours may be within hailing distance of a family with a tap in the house. One common characteristic of the low-income communities is that there is much more necessity for choice of source than in the higher-income areas where piped water serves almost everyone. Recently there have been some studies seeking to determine what factors affect the choice of source, the quantity of water used, and the ways in which it is used. These studies are still few in number, and do not cover the globe by any means, but there appear to be some general findings emerging.

There is considerable evidence that a woman in selecting her source picks what she considers the best quality for her family. Whether it is the Raiapu Enga of New Guinea who consciously avoid the water of one warm and turbid river in favour of two (bacteriologically) cleaner streams (Feachem, 1973), or women in the bustees of Calcutta who use tank water for washing but not for drinking (Lee, 1969), or villagers in north-east Thailand who prefer rainwater for drinking (Frankel and Shouvanavirakul, 1973), a judgement regarding quality is made. A user's criteria may be more likely to include taste, temperature, odour and appearance than considerations of bacteriological quality, but they are nonetheless real for her.

Cost, in terms of the distance walked, cash payments or time spent waiting in a queue seems an important factor in the choice of source in all areas. However, cost does not seem to determine the amount of water carried home (Browne, 1974; White et al., 1972) and there is no entirely satisfactory explanation of why one woman will struggle home with 40 kilograms of water on her head while another is content with much less. There is some evidence that the amount of water carried from a standpipe does decrease slightly with distance (WHO/IRC, 1975), but this may simply indicate that alternative sources—puddles and rain-barrels in this case—are used to a larger degree.

The volume of water used by people who carry it home seems to be associated with the number of people in the household in a variety of cultures. The larger the household, the smaller the per capita use daily (Teller, 1963; Lee, 1969; White et al., 1972). This may have something to do with the make-up of the household and who carries water; but as it also seems to hold true for the low-income families with piped water supplies in a city, it may be related to lack of access for any one individual in a crowded household to the water (Lee, 1969).

One of the major factors affecting the quantity of water used in a household is whether the washing is done at home or not. Where rural water schemes have been introduced in Latin America there are often clothes washing facilities associated with them, although in urban low income areas of Africa this is seldom the case. People often carry clothes to the source to wash them, as in the tanks available in towns in south-east Asia, or to a special spring as in Nandi country in Kenya. The closer they are to the source, the more they tend to use it for washing clothes (White et al., 1972). Warner (1973) observed that about one-fifth of the water drawn from a standpipe in a Tanzanian village was used on the spot or wasted.

Other considerations include technology—the need for a bucket, a strong arm on the borehole pump handle, or a gutter connected to the rain-barrel. A woman must also allow for the fact that when she gets to a source the pump may be broken. The normal assumption in both Bangladesh and Thailand is that 50% of the hand-pumped tubewells will be out of order at any one time (WHO, 1974) as 45% of the standpipes were in the City of Dakar in 1968 (WHO/IRC, 1975). Personal relationships may enter into the choice of source also, if on the walk to get water a woman might encounter undesirable

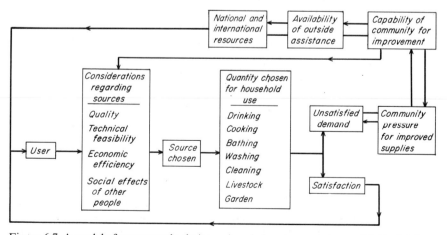

Figure 6.7 A model of water supply choice and use in low-income communities in developing countries (adapted from White et al., 1972)

contact with other people such as an irritated landowner or rival groups (White *et al.*, 1972; Feachem, 1973).

A reasonable model of domestic water choice and use might appear as shown in Figure 6·7, where the user considers water quality, technical feasibility, costs in a broad sense, including time, cash and energy, and the social relationships involved in getting the water, and selects a source. This is adaptation of a model developed by White *et al.* (1972). An earlier description of this mode of analysis was tested by Teller (1963) in Bolivia, and by Schmoyer (1967) and Olinger (1970) in rural areas of the southwestern United States, and seemed quite effective in describing the processes of choice. Water that is carried home is then used in the household in a variety of ways including drinking, cooking, washing, bathing and sometimes for livestock and garden use. These uses determine the volume needed and leave the user either satisfied with the supply of water, or not satisfied as to quantity or quality, or both. If there is dissatisfaction it may lead to the user re-examining her choices, or to community pressure for improved supplies and an examination of the capability of the community for improvement. This act of examination could result in the user getting some new information affecting her own choices of sources, or in pressure for community improvement and a search for some form of outside assistance. Possibilities here would depend on local, national and international institutional structures and resources available for this purpose. At the same time, any water supply improvement programmes or health education efforts could stimulate the perceptions of the user, who is likely to subject a new source to the same criteria she used in judging the old ones, and to either accept or reject it accordingly.

There is one break in this cycle that is not immediately apparent. In almost all parts of the world where water is carried it is the woman who does most of the carrying. It is also true that in most of the developing countries it is the man who makes most of the decisions for the family. This means that while the woman may have control over some of the considerations in choosing a source, she does not control all of them. For example, the man usually decides where a house will be placed, and rarely is it with regard to how long a walk it is to the water source. The quantity of water a woman must carry in a day is influenced very much by her husband's bath habits. In both the rural and urban situation, the woman rarely has much control over the family income, so she may be restricted as to whether she can use cash to buy water from a vendor, or to join in a community water supply improvement scheme, or whether cash investments can be made for an improved well or for gutters to catch water from the roof.

A second break in the cycle may come where unsatisfied demand for more or better water becomes translated into community pressure for improved supplies. Here the woman may be the one feeling the dissatisfaction, but seldom in the developing countries does she have a direct voice in community affairs. She may indirectly influence a town council through her husband, but she is unlikely to be able to make her priorities felt. This, of course, is true for many other areas of her life such as agriculture or food preparation where she has little access to education or to labour-saving technology.

The role of education and public information in this process is not altogether clear. As noted, dissatisfaction with either quality or quantity of water may come from the user's own perception, or it may grow out of an awareness stimulated by education and information. There is evidence that people with individual water systems tend to be satisfied with the water supply they already have, despite dubious quality, even in the highly industrialized countries (Whitsell and Hutchinson, 1973). Baker (1948) pointed out that boiling and filtering through sand were both known to the Egyptians by about 2000 BC as methods of purifying water, and that the technology for improved quality of water supplies was known in western countries long before it was in much demand. There is reason to believe that gradual stages in improving water supplies lead people to demand larger quantities and somewhat better quality. Donaldson (1973) estimates that in Latin America, for a basic water system to go from all public fountains to about 80 per cent of house connections takes about eight to ten years and a constant promotional effort. An increased desire for better service seems to lead to an increase in the willingness of the population to pay for the improvements.

The patterns of domestic water use described here cover the majority of the people in the developing countries, some 1200 million of them, who live in rural areas and on the fringes of large cities and do not have access to adequate supplies of safe water. The prospect is that their numbers will increase in the future despite current improvement programmes, which, if continued at present levels, will not keep up with population growth. This makes imperative a better understanding of the processes of choice and use that influence the acceptance of new programmes and the willingness to support ongoing systems.

Acknowledgements

I would like to acknowledge helpful comments and suggestions from David Donaldson, William B. Lord, Robert W. Kates and Gilbert F. White.

6.6 REFERENCES

Airan, D. S. (1973). Water supply and wastewater disposal in rural areas of India. *Water Resources Bulletin*, **9**, 1035–1040.
Baker, M. N. (1948). *The Quest for Pure Water: The History of Water Purification from the Earliest Records to the Twentieth Century.* New York: American Water Works Association.
Browne, D. G. (1974). *Dongore Water Supply: A Study of a N.W.R.C. Rural Well.* Addis Ababa: National Water Resources Commission, Planning and Programming Office, Ethiopia.
Burton, I. (1974). Domestic water supplies for rural peoples in the developing countries: The hope of technology. In *Human Rights in Health.* Amsterdam: Ciba Foundation, Symposium 23 (new series).

Donaldson, D. (1973). *Progress in the Rural Water Programs of Latin America (1961–1971)*. Washington, D. C.: Pan American Health Organization.

Feachem, R. (1973). *Domestic Water Use in the New Guinea Highlands: The Case of the Raiapu Enga*. New South Wales: The University of New South Wales, School of Civil Engineering, Report No. 132.

Focus, No. 5, (1975). Africa's food producers: The impact of change on rural women.

Frankel, R. J. and Shouvanavirakul, P. (1973). Water consumption in small communities of Northeast Thailand. *Water Resources Research*, 9, 1196–1207.

Instituto Centroamericano de Administracion de Empresas, Centro de Asesoramiento (1974). *Low Income Family Housing Situation, Managua, 1974* (Preliminary Report). Doc. No. NI/PL-016.

Lee, T. R. (1969). *Residential Water Demand and Economic Development*. Toronto: University of Toronto Department of Geography Research Publications.

Olinger, C. E. (1970). *Domestic Water Use in the Española Valley, New Mexico: A Study in Resource Decision-making*. Chicago: Master of Arts thesis, Department of Geography, University of Chicago.

Rouleau, S. (1975). Domestic water use in Cameroon. Unpublished paper. University of Yaoundé, Centre for Health Services.

Roure, J. (1973). Les bornes-fountaines en milieu tropical africain. Paris: BCEOM, *Informations et Documents*, 10, 2eme trimestre.

Schmoyer, R. (1967). *Decision-making in the Development of Domestic Water Systems in Powers County, Colorado*. Chicago: Master of Arts thesis, Department of Geography, University of Chicago.

Teller, C. H. (1963). *Domestic Water Use in Tarija Valley, Bolivia*. Master's thesis, Department of Geography, Clark University, Worcester, Massachusetts.

Warner, D. (1973). *Evaluation of the Development Impact of Rural Water Supply Projects in East African Villages*. Palo Alto: Program in Engineering–Economic Planning, Stanford University.

White, G. F. (1974). Domestic water supply: Right or good? In *Human Rights in Health*. Amsterdam: Ciba Foundation, Symposium 23 (new series).

White, G. F., Bradley, D. J. and White, A. U. (1972). *Drawers of Water: Domestic Water Use in East Africa*. Chicago: University of Chicago Press.

Whitsell, W. J. and Hutchinson, G. D. (1973). The forgotten water consumer. *Transactions of the American Society of Agricultural Engineers*, 16, 782–786.

World Bank (1971). *Trends in Developing Countries*.

WHO (1973). Community water supply and sewage disposal in developing countries. *World Health Statistics Report*, 26(11), 720–783.

WHO (1974). *Provision of Safe Water Supplies to Rural Communities in South East Asia*. Report of the Technical Discussions held during the WHO Regional Committee for South East Asia, Denpasar, India, 3–9 September, 1974. New Delhi: WHO Regional Office for South East Asia. SEA/Env. San./141.

WHO/IRC (1975). *Water Dispensing Devices and Methods for Public Water Supply in Developing Countries*. The Hague: World Health Organization/International Reference Centre for Community Water Supply.

7

Water Supply and Community Choice

ANNE WHYTE *and* IAN BURTON

7.1 INTRODUCTION

Water supply is a daily necessity and a key factor in human health and well-being. Yet in 1970 88% of the rural population in developing countries was estimated to be without 'reasonable access to a safe and adequate water supply' (WHO, 1972). In that year, the level of expenditure for the construction of improved supplies to reach another 10·6 million people was about $ US 138 million. Of the new systems that have been constructed within the last two decades, probably one-third are not working at all and another 30% are working only intermittently or ineffectively.

Thus the problem of rural water supply in developing countries is one that is crucial, enormous in scale, and not being solved by present strategies and solutions. This picture is supported by the World Health Organization's predictions for 1970–80. Their set target of doubling the percentage of people receiving adequate supplies in rural areas by 1980 (from 12% to 25%) requires that the 1970 rate of expenditure be more than doubled. Despite the ambitiousness of the target, it will mean that the number of people still not adequately served with water in 1980 will actually *increase* because of the increase in rural populations (Table 7.1). Furthermore, on the evidence of progress so far, the targets set for 1980 will not be met (Figure 7.1).

Of the many constraints to progress that can be seen on a global scale among

Table 7.1 Programme for rural water supply in 90 developing countries 1970–80

Type of Supply	1970		1980		Increases 1970–80	
	No.*	%	No.*	%	No.*	%
Acess to safe water	140	(12)	357	(25)	217	(155)
Without access to safe supply	1026	(88)	1081	(75)	55	(5)
Total population*	1166	(100)	1438	(100)	272	(23)

*Population in millions.

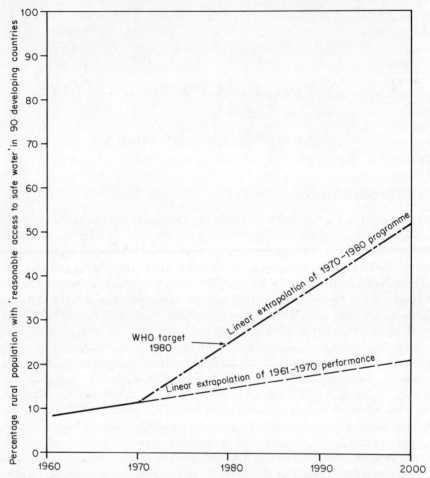

Figure 7.1 Linear extrapolations of rural populations with 'reasonable access to safe water' under 1961–70 performance and 1970–80 programme

the most frequently cited are:

(a) Insufficient national or internal funds;
(b) lack of trained manpower;
(c) weaknesses in the structure and process of national programmes;
(d) insufficient external funds;
(e) difficulties in operation and maintenance of systems;
(f) inadequate legal frameworks;

All these constraints are widespread and are generally recognized as such, so that efforts are now being made to remedy them. More national and international funds are being mobilized for rural water programmes; the training of manpower is being increased; national water authorities are beginning to restructure, and to some extent decentralize, their bureaucracies, and technical improvements are continually made to make systems more foolproof. But most of the developments outlined above are in the spirit of improving the 'delivery system' to give the consumer a better, more reliable, up-to-date product. There is another way to approach the problem and that is to consider the 'product' from the point of view of the consumer—to see what his needs and aspirations are in relation to water; how they are related to other needs and aspirations; and what type of water scheme and management system will fit in with these perceptions, or indeed can be evolved by the users themselves. The concern thus becomes focused on the user of water rather than the delivery of a water system. This philosophy has been described elsewhere as 'user-choice' (Kirkby, 1973) and it is in the same spirit that this paper examines the rural community as 'user' and suggests ways in which the user-choice approach might be implemented.

Each of the six constraints mentioned above can be mitigated or exacerbated by the attitudes and actions of people in the communities themselves. The best designed hand-pump or water pipe available, can be broken or misused by those who want to do so, or who simply do not care. The purest and most adequate supplies of water can be, and are, abandoned in favour of impure, traditional supplies. The ingenuity and resourcefulness of villagers is not only a matter of training and funding, it is also a function of commitment, price and identity with the water supply system and its objectives. It is rare to see indigenous expressions of beauty and art embellishing new water supply schemes in developing countries, yet these are indicators of where a community's heart is.

Part of the commitment and identity certainly comes about with improved awareness of the health and related benefits that biologically purer water brings. This has been the rationale behind the integration of water supply with health education programmes and the provision of medical facilities, which has been carried out with considerable success in some Latin American countries. But there are two other aspects of community commitment to using, maintaining, and even initiating, rural water schemes which are as important as perception of health benefits. These are:

(a) in selecting between alternative sources of supply, communities and individuals provide their own frame of reference and criteria for calculating sets of trade-offs;
(b) choices 'delivered' to communities are accepted with less commitment than the choices they have made for themselves.

7.2 COMMUNITY FRAMES OF REFERENCE

In bringing an improved water supply to a village, the engineer or water authorities are usually the ones who specify what the range of choice is. Even

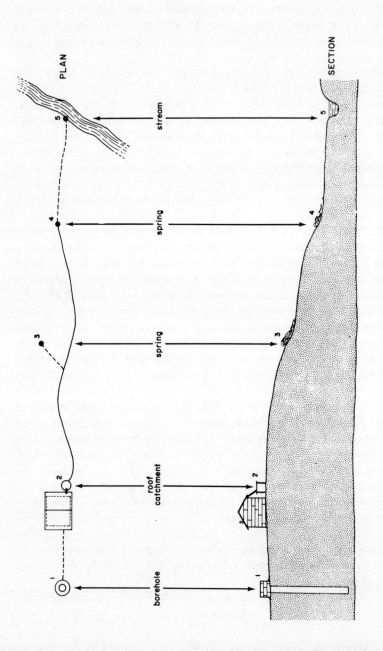
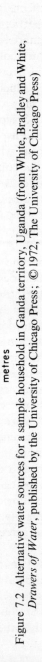

Figure 7.2 Alternative water sources for a sample household in Ganda territory, Uganda (from White, Bradley and White, *Drawers of Water*, published by the University of Chicago Press; © 1972, The University of Chicago Press)

where only one type of improvement is offered, there is generally the choice between the improved and the old, unimproved supplies. What the engineer cannot do, though he may often wish he could, is to specify the criteria by which alternative supplies are evaluated. He may inject his own criteria, such as degree of bacteriological contamination, but the overall frame of reference, and the weights given to each criterion, remain those of the individuals and communities who are to use the water.

White, Bradley and White (1972) provide a good illustration of contrasting frames of reference between the user and the government official. In their example from the Ganda territory north of Lake Victoria, a household has a choice of five nearby sources consisting of a borehole, a roof catchment system, two springs and a stream (Figure 7.2). These are evaluated by the woman of the household against four main criteria of water quality (including taste), technological feasibility and economics (mainly cost and distance or effort). Less critical but also influential is the consideration of relationships with other people in respect of using a particular source. The user's frame of reference is presented as a 5×5 perception matrix in which alternative sources are ranged against criteria in the mind of the user as she makes her decision (Table 7.2(a)). In this case, the more distant of the two springs is selected because it fulfils her quality and technology criteria and avoids the need to cross an irritable neighbour's land (White *et al.*, 1972).

The perception of the government official of the same situation differs mainly in its extension of the range of theoretical choice and in its rating of the alternative sources on quality (Table 7.2(b)). For the government officer, only the borehole and the roof catchment systems are of acceptable quality and the surface water sources fall below. Thus his recommendation would be the borehole (White *et al.*, 1972).

The example provides a model both of the kinds of criteria that are employed in individual choice and the process by which they are linked together. The decision process is seen as an ordered set of bifurcating choices with water quality representing the major watershed on which alternative sources are eliminated or accepted for further consideration. Of those sources that are perceived as acceptable in quality, a judgement regarding cost is made. For those sources meeting minimal levels of cost and quality more refined judgements are made about quality, technique and relationships with other people.

Between the individual user and the water authorities lies another level of choice—that of the community, village or social group. Water authorities are usually dealing directly with a community, or at least its leaders, rather than the individual households, yet so far less attention has been given to alternative supply systems from the point of view of the community as a group.

The frame of reference for communities can be described in terms of a similar perception matrix to those for individual choice. The columns representing criteria for evaluation might be expected to reflect some additional group needs and values; but also, the way the criteria are structured in making a

Table 7.2 Frames of reference for (a) a household user and (b) a government official for evaluating alternative water sources in Ganda territory, Uganda (from White, Bradley and White, *Drawers of Water*, published by the University of Chicago Press; © 1972 The University of Chicago Press)

Table 7.2(a) Perception matrix for a sample household

Theoretical alternatives	Considered as a source	Resource quality	Technology	Economic efficiency	Effect on other people	'Source rating' summary valuation
A_1 Borehole	1	0	×	×	×	0
A_2 Roof	1	1	0	×	×	0
A_3 Spring	1	2	2	2	-2	6
A_4 Spring	1	2	2	2	×	8
A_5 Stream	1	2	2	0	×	0

Table 7.2(b) Perception matrix for one official's view of a sample household

	Perception of alternatives					
Theoretical alternatives	Considered as a source	Resource quality	Technology	Economic efficiency	Effect on other people	'Source Rating' summary valuation
A_1 Borehole	1	2	2	2	1	9
A_2 Roof	1	1	0	0	×	0
A_3 Spring	1	0	×	×	×	0
A_4 Spring	1	0	×	×	×	0
A_5 Stream	1	0	×	×	×	0
A_6 ... 10 (other springs)	1	0	×	×	×	0
A_{11} Possible pipeline	1	1	2	0	×	0

Key ratings: 0—unfavourable; 1—favourable; 2—very favourable; × —not considered or not mentioned.

decision may be different from the model presented by White, Bradley and White for individual choice in East Africa.

An example of community decision making is given by Iwanska (1971) for a Mazahua Indian village in central Mexico, which will be used here to illustrate the community perception of choice. The author is concerned with the process by which the vague aspirations of the villagers and the more articulate Utopian thinking of the village leaders become translated into practical action in a context where tradition and change are both valued.

As has been traditional among Mazahuas from El Nopal, the leaders started to act only when they knew that everybody in the village wanted to get education for children, to get water or to get electricity. Only then did the leaders organize into a group with the help of a friendly outsider (a rural social worker assigned to El Nopal) and begin to contact the proper authorities. In the case of the decision on water and electricity, the 'innovators' had to do a lot of exploring, interpreting and refining of the original ideas. This involved discussions with 'tradition maintaining' leaders and many other people in the village as well.

In the case of water, a great deal of discussion took place as well. Soon after the first negotiations with proper authorities in Las Animas were started, it became clear that people from El Nopal could not possibly gather enough money to bring water to individual houses as they wanted to do. It was suggested by these authorities, and supported by the social worker, Maria Victoria, that at first two or three wells should be installed in places easily accessible to various clusters of huts. However, this idea was soon rejected. Mazahuas from El Nopal decided that everybody would have water at once or they would not have any water in El Nopal at all. They would continue walking to a rather poor and distant well which they had been using so far.

But, still another possibility was discussed: the 'wealthier' families might pay to have the water connected with their houses, while the poorer families would wait until they got enough cash. But this alternative was also quickly rejected by people from El Nopal. In spite of the economic familism, people from El Nopal defined water as communal rather than familial. And as in the case of electricity, the decision not to have any water until everybody would have it in his house, involved both deep, traditional Mazahua values and the commitment to the Progress as well. (Iwanska, 1971).

Table 7.3 illustrates the choice situation in a more prosaic form. The four alternative systems discussed (the theoretical range was probably greater) are evaluated according to the same criteria given in Table 7.2 but economic efficiency is separated into 'effort' and 'cash cost', and the socio-political component is expanded to four additional criteria; social equality, progress, social interaction and village autonomy. In the White, Bradley and White model, social aspects are considered of secondary importance while here they are obviously determining factors, with community values for maintaining social equality and behaving as a 'progressive community' being critical to the outcome.

Table 7.3 differs from Table 7.2 in another important respect; it contains unfavourable (zero) ratings which do not negate the possibility of that alternative being selected. In fact, each of the four alternatives discussed by the Mazahua village would score unfavourably on two criteria; compared to the other possibilities, the old well is antithetical to the idea of progress and unacceptably demanding in terms of effort. As so often occurs in choice situations, each alternative is unacceptable in some respects. Thus the process is one of determining which unacceptability, given the hindsight of realizing no choice will fulfil all criteria, can be upgraded into an 'acceptable pass' on most counts.

The model of community choice we are presenting therefore differs from that of White et al. (1972) for individual choice. In terms of the perception matrices, the community ratings cannot be multiplied together to give a summary valuation because of the tolerance afforded 'unacceptable' alternatives. More fundamentally, it differs in the nature of the choice process that is implied by the models.

The example of individual choice in East Africa is given as one of ordered,

Table 7.3 Community frame of reference for choice between alternative water supply systems for a Mazahua Indian village in central Mexico

Alternatives	Considered as a source	Resource quality	Technology feasibility	Economics		Social equality	Progress	Social inter-action	Village autonomy	'Supply rating' summary valuation
				Effort	Cash cost					(additive)
A_1 old well	1	1	2	0	2	2	0	2	2	12
A_2 2–3 new wells	1	1	1	1	1	0	0	1	2	8
A_3 some house connections	1	2	1	1	1	0	1	1	0	8
A_4 all house connections	1	2	1	2	0	2	2	2	0	12

Key ratings: 0 = unfavourable; 1 = favourable; 2 = very favourable.

binary choices in which some criteria have the power of veto while others merely have a voice. The community choice pattern is more anastomosing with ever-varying subsets of criteria being compared within and between themselves. For example, water quality is considered in a subset with social equality and cash cost. Given that they are incompatible goals, the community adheres to its value for water as a communal good and defers its aspiration for better water until it can pay for it. Thus the community has enlarged the context of decision making in the time dimension. The consideration of alternatives on grounds of technological feasibility is not done in isolation from other criteria, particularly those of cash cost and village autonomy. And the value to be assigned to each alternative on technological feasibility is not the same in the two comparisons:

> technology versus cash cost
> technology versus village autonomy

In El Nopal the decision to reject the advice of the water authorities and the respected village social worker, was an affirmation of the village's autonomy in making its own decisions. The first solution accepted—to continue with the traditional supply—maintained this right. It is likely, however, that the second decision—to have a piped water supply and house connections—would limit village autonomy in the sphere of water resources from that point on. The village would become increasingly dependent on outside bodies for technology and administration and future alternatives.

This comparison of specific examples of individual and community choice leads to more general statements about community decision making:

(1) In community choice there are additional criteria to those of individual choice for evaluating alternatives. These have to do with group (social) values and goals and can be of prime importance,
(2) Community choice is not necessarily, or even generally, a process of ordered, binary choices. The degree to which it approximates such an individual model may well be a measure of the absolute authority of its leader and the individualism of his decisions.

However, the mode of decision-making in most traditional communities is one of seeking out opinion, general discussion and consensus with widespread community participation before the leaders enunciate 'their' decisions. Thus the choices and the trade-offs between conflicting goals become presented as an array rather than an ordered series, and proponents of each particular view actively ensure that their criteria or trade-offs stay within the forms of the debate.

7.3 THE ROLE OF WATER IN THE COMMUNITY

In most cultures and systems of social organization, the way in which water

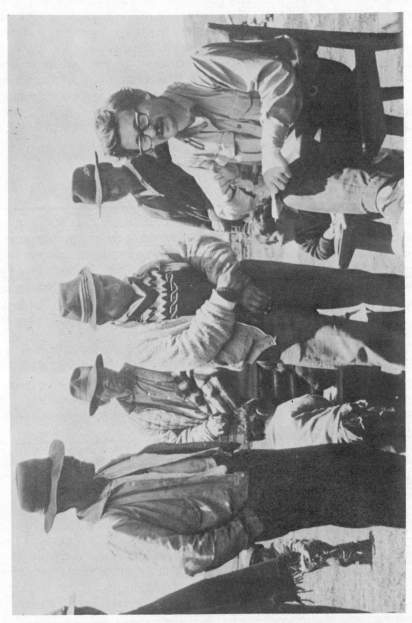

Ecuadorian villagers discuss plans for a water supply improvement scheme with a visiting engineer (photograph: R. G. Feachem)

is distributed serves to band people together and to underwrite their differences. Water is commonly a driving force to keep the community going as an identifiable group—it provides energy for maintaining social relationships as well as economic productivity. Often it is the human health and economic aspects of water that are considered in new water supply schemes and the social aspects are relegated to 'traditional attitudes, values and beliefs' or, in the language of economists, 'intangibles'. The purpose of this section is to provide some indication of the social role of water in traditional rural communities where water is the basis for a system of social relationships within and between communities.

Water distribution systems and related water rights show great variation both culturally and geographically. This is especially so where water is also used for irrigation. The evidence for the social influence of water on society is so widespread that it led Wittfogel to develop his theory of water control as the basis for early civilizations, especially in oriental society (Wittfogel, 1957). His argument was that water, as an agricultural resource, has properties which direct the social organization of people in certain ways—principally in needing to cooperate in order to build and maintain waterworks, and to have an established political hierarchy to command labour and administer group effort.

What Wittfogel was concerned with, and what most societies are concerned with, is the need to establish rules or ways of making decisions, about who takes water, when, and for how long. The necessity for a system of rules reflects the physical nature of water as a resource: if it is a well or qanat it needs cooperation to build and maintain it. If it is a stream or a canal, it flows from a higher to a lower place so that upstream users always have the physical advantage over downstream users. Social rules can either recognize and enforce this advantage (flowage rights) or can try to even it out (riparian rights), or replace it by establishing an alternative rationale for water control (e.g. kinship rights, communal rights). Rules are least necessary where the source is geographically widespread and plentiful, such as a lake or high water table.

For example, among the Kalinga tribe of the Philippines, downstream or upstream users may only use water with the permission of the *first* user on the stream or canal (Barton, 1949). In Moalan Chiefdom society in the Fijian Islands, the upstream users are the 'owners of water' and are responsible for water distribution and the settling of disputes (Sahlins, 1958). Among the Sanjo tribal society of East Africa, control of water is vested in a council of village elders who can take as much water as they like first and are responsible for distributing the rest (Gray, 1963). As we have seen, among Mexican peasant communities, water is considered as a communal resource and is distributed on the basis of adult membership in the community.

Because water is a vital resource, the way water rights are vested can create and maintain almost any hierarchy for social status and political power that a society wishes. Water control can confer power over others on old people, or literate people, or men, or members of a particular family or village, or on the first settler. The very fact that societies differ in where they place the political centre of gravity that water control brings, and that their solutions are not usually economically 'optimizing' solutions, is some measure of the value they assign to their social order. When a new water supply system is introduced, it may bring with it not only new water but also a new social order. The change commonly goes in two directions:

(a) altering the balance of power within communities—often from the traditional leaders to the literate and the politically sophisticated;
(b) altering the external relations of the community—usually towards increased dependency on the national and regional government and a decreased ability to act independently in relation to other communities.

Even where water is used only for domestic purposes, it is a force for both social integration and social differentiation. People from within the community meet at the well, spring or borehole; the women may even spend time there washing clothes and chatting. Strangers are either excluded or may use the source only with permission. The community ownership of the source articulates the boundary between in-group and out-group and reinforces it by providing a meeting place and a reason for cooperation.

Communities nevertheless contain differences in status and power, and these can be daily expressed in the use and distribution of water. One woman goes to the well herself while another sends a servant. One household collects water at the source; another lets it be seen that they buy from a water vendor. Most water carriers are women and children: despite the heaviness of the task, it is not man's work. It is not only a question of time and effort, it is also a matter of dignity, appropriate behaviour and social differences.

In their beliefs about water and its use, people emphasize the symbolic nature of water. Superstitious and traditional practices can often be traced back to roots in both the practical experience of human health and well-being and to the need to establish group rules and social conformity. Thus an important role of water in traditional communities is to enable sets of social relationships to be spelled out and reinforced, often on a daily basis. These relationships can change through time but the changes also *take* time. The effect of new water supply schemes—which by charging for water may change a communal resource into a cash commodity, or by installing house connections may transform the village women into isolated housewives—is to make the changes take place overnight. The failure of villages to maintain the new water systems can often be diagnosed as an adherence to their pattern of social relationships to which the new water scheme was insensitive and disruptive.

7.4 COMMUNITY CHOICE

The principle of self-help as a means of harnessing community energy and involvement with development projects is widely employed to some degree in rural water schemes. Donaldson (1972) has outlined the elements of successful self-help programmes, particularly for Latin America. Partly to reduce cost, but also to reduce the chances of the system falling into disrepair and misuse after the engineers have left, local people are involved in the provision of labour, local materials and/or cash. Local officials may also organize labour and the collection of payments and, less commonly, a local man is trained to maintain the system and do simple repairs. As a minimum, most rural water schemes involve local participation in the contribution of cash or labour. Self-help schemes do not necessarily, or even commonly, allow the community much scope in the making of major decisions about the type of system, or combination of systems, the time scale and manner in which water quality and quantity is to be improved, or the way in which it is to be managed. These are still generally decisions that are delivered to the community on a take-it-or-leave-it basis.

At a first level of analysis, the failure of many self-help schemes can be diagnosed as an organizational incapacity on the part of the community to manage the scheme, and as a lack of understanding and commitment on the part of individuals to properly use the scheme. Miller discusses two examples of this lack of individual commitment to community decisions in a village in Chiapas, southern Mexico. The first decision was to build a medical post which involved the village in the provision of labour and local materials with government support for equipment and personnel. The second decision was to build latrines for each household. In both cases a similar decision-making process to that described for El Nopal in central Mexico took place with the addition that in the case of latrines, each man also signed his personal commitment to build one. Participation in a community decision to provide the facilities did not commit individuals to conform as individuals in using them. Only 59% used the medical post instead of traditional cures and only 65% of those who actually had private latrines used them.

The response of some aid agencies has been to play down the contribution that self-help schemes can make. From the point of view of the 'user-choice' approach argued here, one of the difficulties of self-help schemes is that they are not 'self-help' enough. They are still conceived and implemented within the framework of the 'delivery philosophy' and the choices available to the community are in terms of detail rather than fundamentals.

One of the problems with present self-help schemes is that, despite their spirit of local involvement, at the level of a national or regional programme they tend to be organizationally stereotyped on the pattern of cooperatives and elected committees. This organizational standardization is as unlikely to succeed as inflexibility in the technical design of systems. The texture of community organizational and social differences within an area may be very fine, and no single standardized organizational approach will be everywhere appropriate. Along with a Western imposition of technology there has been a somewhat comparable standardized delivery of management systems.

The principle of community choice is a very important one. We have tried to show that any choice between alternative water supply schemes, or any other development projects, involves the consideration of criteria beyond the direct trade-offs between water quality, cost etc. They involve questions of compatibility with social needs and values, and the degree to which the existing socio-political order will be supported or weakened. A significant element in the last consideration is the question of community autonomy.

When village leaders consider a new water supply, such as a borehole, part of their consideration will be the basic needs and economics of the situation, part will be the effect such an innovation may have upon the social order of the village and their personal positions within it and part will be the effect that decision may have on future decisions. It is a rare, altruistic leader who can willingly make a decision to give up his own decision-making authority. Yet that is often the Hobson's choice that rural water schemes offer communities—to accept a borehole or piped water supply also means an acceptance of an eroded village autonomy—the system will be repaired by external officials and the water controller may well be paid as a government rather than a community official.

Community decision-making styles

In comparing individual and community decision making, the contrast was made between the ordered, binary choice model for the individual, and the multiple-array, discussion-process of the community. Community decision-making styles vary both culturally and geographically—and, as we have argued above, show a considerable range between communities within a local area. In addition to this variation necessitating flexibility in the organizational design of rural water schemes, it also provides for a range of personal commitment to community decisions on the part of individuals and households. Some discussion about community projects among members of the group is common in traditional societies, even where the decisions are 'made' by leaders. The degree of commitment to those decisions by the individuals who will use and maintain the facilities is partly a function of the interaction between

(a) how far the project reflects internally developed aspirations and goals rather than externally generated ones; and
(b) the form the discussion takes and the role played by the leaders.

Group discussions vary in the degree to which they are debated with particular views attached to particular personalities, or a process of anonymous consensus with no individuals explicitly attached to particular opinions. A comparison of tribal nomadic decision-making in Khuzistan, Iran, with the process of peasant decisions in Mexico will illustrate the different discussion styles.

Nomads are making choices in relation to water every few days, that is whenever they move camp (Barth, 1964). All the families in the group are involved in the decision but at no point is there an assembly of people. Indeed it is very important that an assembly does not occur because it would allow each view to be more equal, it would require opinions to be made explicit and associated with particular individuals and it might give rise to a confrontation of views—all of which are carefully avoided. Instead, as soon as the camp has been pitched, individuals will go and consult with one another in pairs and small groups to discuss the probability of water and pasture in various places. Individuals are careful not to commit themselves to a clear alternative; they will always follow one proposal with the opposite point of view. Rather it is a process of feeling out the consensus. Sometimes no clear common view has emerged after hours of discussion and participants retire to bed not knowing if they will strike camp next morning. The discussions are not entirely structureless for although the camp leader has no means of imposing his opinion on the other tent households, he can influence the decision through his family network. If he believes strongly in a particular choice, he will go to the tents of his sons and other close relatives and let them become aware of his view. They in turn will disseminate his opinion in their discussions with their relatives, and so on through the kinship network. If there is lack of agreement anywhere in the camp it will not be revealed by confrontation but by continued discussion until a consensus is reached. Thus each individual is committed to the group choice and will conform as an individual to that choice. This process is vital to the cohesion and viability of the nomad group.

Decision-making in a Mexican peasant village is based on the very acts which Iranian nomads so carefully avoid: an assembly of people; the confrontation of views; explicit, vigorous argument of opinions; and public commitment by individuals to specific choices before consensus is reached. A government project, for example, will first be discussed informally and formally between the village leaders. Individuals will bring what influence they can to bear on the selection of their favoured choice but there is a common attempt to reach an agreed set of recommendations on the issue to be put before the general assembly of the community (usually consisting of all adult males). One of the leaders describes the issue and the alternatives to the community assembly. He then presents the recommendations of the leadership. If the general assembly provides contradictory views the leaders will argue in defence of their opinions. Usually their views hold sway and a consensus is eventually reached. While individuals participating in the consensus agree with the outcome as a community decision, their degree of commitment to it as far as their individual behaviour is concerned may vary considerably, but in any case it is generally less than that of individuals in the nomadic process, of choice by consensus.

7.5 CONCLUSION: THE DESIGN OF USER-CHOICE SCHEMES

The following main observations have been made in this paper.

(1) A new approach in rural water supply is needed which is capable of a

higher survival rate where it is planted and has the ability to spread of its own accord.

(2) A main vector of diffusion and acceptance is community *choice* as well as community participation.

(3) We do not yet have sufficient understanding of the perception and value frameworks in which communities evaluate alternative schemes.

(4) Where a rural water scheme is not in accord with community dynamics (particularly their values, social relationships and organizational capacity), the response is either to (a) abandon or misuse the water scheme or (b) to develop new social forms or habits (such as buying from water vendors) to restore an equilibrium between water and community.

(5) Community choice is partly a question of *which* option to choose and partly a question of how to maintain the capability to choose in the future.

Our area of ignorance in relation to these observations is very large. It is suggested that the question of community autonomy is important, but it is unknown how communities with a strong sense of autonomy differ from those where dependency on the outside world is already well established. Relatively little is known about the organizational resources of communities within the area of most water supply programmes. The recent socio-economic survey of rural Ethiopia (Institute of Development Research, 1975) illustrates the range of traditional and emerging organizational capacities and community institutions which do exist and might be mobilized for rural development.

The immediate needs for developing a more user-choice oriented approach are:

(1) *Technology*. The development of technology and technical packages of components that are within the decision-making compass of small communities. This may include more appropriate, low-cost technology. It also means technology that is understandable, capable of modification at the local level and can be *seen* to be flexible. Thus the community may have to import the materials but they are sufficiently cognizant of the situation and the design to decide for themselves how much to order.

(2) *Design*. The development of methods to evaluate the perceptions and needs of the community and households, and to understand the dynamics of the community, especially in relation to water, as a normal input into the design stage of projects.

(3) *Management*. The development of management systems which can respond to the inputs from the community evaluations at the design stage. The expected needs for much greater flexibility in management systems (in collecting dues, payments, distributing water, handling disputes and breakdowns, co-opting labour) may well imply the development of packages of management components which can be selected and combined to provide a management system fitted to each individual community or group of communities.

These inputs into the development of an innovative, user-oriented approach to rural water supply can best be achieved by providing the encouragement and practical support needed for water authorities to include research, evaluation and experimentation as an integral and priority part of their programmes. At the same time, we should be wary of the delivery of a 'soc-fix' approach to parallel the 'tech-fix' one. User-choice must allow for the rejection of externally promoted choices.

In hindsight, the decision of El Nopal, the village in Mexico, to keep the old well until they could afford a 100% piped water supply, was probably the best one for the overall, long-term physical and *social* 'health' of the community. It was certainly *their* decision, and one taken against 'expert' advice. But in how many water supply programmes would their voice have been heard? And if they had wanted a stone well-head instead, to both protect and beautify the source, would they have been given any support?

7.6 REFERENCES

Barth, F. (1964). *Nomads of South Persia*. London: Allen and Unwin.

Barton, R. F. (1949). *The Kalingas; Their Institutions and Custom Laws*. Chicago: University of Chicago Press.

Donaldson, D. (1972). Rural water supplies in developing countries. *Water Resources Drill*, **2**, 391–298.

Gray, R. F. (1963). *The Sonjo of Tanganyika*. London: O.U.P.

Institute of Development Research (in collaboration with the Development through Co-operation Campaign) (1975). *Survey of Socio-Economic Characteristics of Rural Ethiopia*. Addis Ababa.

Iwanska, A. (1971). *Purgatory and Utopia*. Cambridge, Mass.: Schenkman.

Kirkby, A. V. (1973). The development of a user-choice approach in rural water supply. Working Paper 7, I.D.R.C. *Rural Water Supply and Sanitation Seminar*. Lausanne: I.D.R.C.

Sahlins, M. (1958). *Social Stratification in Polynesia*. Seattle: University of Washington Press.

White, G. F., Bradley, D. J. and White, A. U. (1972). *Drawers of Water*. Chicago: University of Chicago Press.

WHO (1972). Twenty-Fifth Health Assembly. Community Water Supply Programme. *Progress Report of the Director-General*. Document A 25/29. Geneva: World Health Organization.

Wittfogel, K. A. (1957). *Oriental Despotism*. New Haven: Yale University Press.

8

The Economics
of Community Water Supply

IAN CARRUTHERS *and* DAVID BROWNE

8.1 INTRODUCTION

Economics is a body of theory, principles and hypotheses which is concerned with the allocation of scarce resources amongst competing demands for consumption, now and in the future. The economist's role is therefore, to assist and improve the resource allocation processes.

Until relatively recently many investment decisions were based primarily on a financial criterion, on the ability of consumers to pay the total cost of a water supply investment. Nowadays wider social and economic issues are involved in both project selection and design. As a result economists are interested in achieving a proper allocation of resources to the water sector and improving the ways in which these are used within the sector in relation to national objectives. These objectives will influence the criteria by which the allocations are judged.

The key resources are usually *finance* (both capital and recurrent finance, though the distinction is less important in economics than in accountancy), *labour* (skilled and unskilled) and, to a limited extent, *land*. Physical shortages of items such as materials or shipping space also create an opportunity for the application of the principles of economics, e.g. maximizing the return to the most limiting resource.

The objective of this chapter is first to outline a number of simple economic concepts that are basic tools for resource allocation problems. These concepts are central to the work of the professional economist but an awareness of them is also important in engineering, medicine and related areas of water supply and sanitation.

The following sections use the concepts explained in the first section to outline the contribution of economics to water supply planning. Firstly, the question of allocation of resources between water supplies and other sectors is briefly discussed. It is only too easy for those engaged in the water supply sector to see the requirements of their sector in isolation from the needs of the rest of the economy. Secondly, resource allocation within the sector is explored, the key being that programmes must take account of resources as well as needs and objectives so that appropriate projects and standards are adopted.

Economists attempt to improve allocations within the sector by influencing scheme selection and scheme design decisions.

8.2 STATUS OF WATER SUPPLIES

A number of possible views of the status of water supplies are explained below. The status ascribed by decision makers in a particular country will be especially important in determining the resources that are devoted to water and in determining many operational details such as pricing policy.

Social service

Water supplies are generally regarded as an important element of social overhead capital but ambiguity frequently surrounds the status of rural water supplies. Usually there is general agreement that major urban supplies are a public utility but rural supplies are often more akin to a social service; for the most part very poor people are being supplied and the main motive is humanitarian.

The acceptance of rural water supply as a social service requires a change of philosophy because previously water has always been regarded as a public utility which should meet financial criteria. This is a historical result of the fact that water supplies both in the developed and developing world were first constructed in urban centres where their primary role is as a public utility. However, there is a strong case for regarding rural supplies and urban communal supplies as a social service, similar to schools and hospitals, for which only nominal charges are made or which are even free. If water supplies must cover all their costs they will only be received by an urban minority. Therefore, it is recommended that rural water supplies should be regarded as a social service.

Merit want

In an economy where private initiative is encouraged, it is normal for the market mechanism to determine the relative values of goods and services. However, in some circumstances, policy makers may consider that they are better informed than the general public and therefore justified in imposing their own values when making decisions.

The advantages of a good water supply may be more evident to officials of the Ministry of Health and the Water Department than to the average peasant. In this situation, policy makers believe that a good or service is so meritorious that more should be provided than would have been provided by the market mechanism alone, i.e. it is a merit want. As a result Government adjusts individual choice in a situation where the consumers would prefer to spend their money on other things. It decides to elevate the 'merit want' above market criteria to an extent determined by political processes. Many governments

132

consider that water supply development is basic to the health and social well-being of their populations and consequently consider it as a 'merit want'.

However, there are dangers associated with the elevation of any good or service to merit want status, especially in developing countries. In such countries many sectors, such as education, hospitals and roads, could claim this status and any Government decision which in effect gives any service merit want status must be carefully scrutinized, since the resources used may result in a more valuable opportunity foregone elsewhere in the economy. If the real object of a policy is to redistribute income or to create employment the proposal must be appraised on these specific grounds. However, it is suggested that in many developing countries the consumers underestimate the value of good quality water and that there may be justification for granting it merit want status.

Social want

Normally a consumer can be excluded from the enjoyment of a good or service unless he pays for it. However, there is a group of goods and services where this cannot happen; if they are provided they can be enjoyed by all and it is not possible to exclude individual members of society if they refuse to pay (for instance, military protection, or flood protection). Inasmuch as benefits are independent of the level of contribution, most people may not voluntarily contribute. As a consequence the market mechanism fails to satisfy such wants, which are termed social wants. Sometimes they are termed collective goods since they are enjoyed by the group as a whole.

Since consumers cannot reveal their preferences through the market mechanism they must be determined in an alternative way, usually by the political process, so that resources are allocated in a way that is in line with consumer or group preferences. Communal water supplies in developing countries are frequently social wants. For example, it is difficult to enforce payment by users of communal supplies unless charging is practised on a quantity basis.

The provision of public wants

Both social and merit wants are public wants. In the former case the role of the Government is to determine true consumer preferences which are not revealed by the market mechanism and in the latter it is to interfere with the consumer's own preferences. Public wants must be paid for out of public funds but they may be produced by the public or private sector.

Public production

Goods and services produced by the public sector are termed public goods and characteristically, though not necessarily, they satisfy public wants. The inherent characteristic of water supplies suggests that production in the public sector is desirable. There are usually economies of scale in construction and an inelastic demand for water which might prove all-too-tempting to a profit-maximizing monopolist. Furthermore, private costs of supply and public benefits diverge because the market does not recognize the real value of external benefits (externalities), for instance benefits which arise from eliminating foci of epidemic disease or the benefits from tourism which emerge when a country has a high standard of public health. An alternative to public production is public control with subsidies for desirable but unprofitable outlays.

8.3 KEY ECONOMIC CONCEPTS

Economics requires a broad view of investment. Often there are multiple, sometimes conflicting objectives, to be satisfied. Economic analysis helps to ascertain the contribution of alternative courses of action to these various objectives and to make explicit the trade-offs between them. This viewpoint is particularly relevant in determining sector allocations (see Section 8.4). In both sector work and micro-level studies there are a number of relevant, simple concepts, the most important of which are discussed in the next six subsections.

Opportunity cost

This is possibly the concept which the economist is most anxious that other planners should appreciate. The real cost of devoting resources to a particular investment is the value of the best alternative opportunity that is thereby foregone. If resources are devoted to water supplies they cannot be used in another sector of the economy; if funds are invested in urban water supplies these same funds are not available for rural supplies; if resources (e.g. engineering expertise) are devoted to one rural scheme they are not available for another; if extra resources are devoted to rural water schemes that satisfy high design criteria fewer people will be provided with water.

Time preference

The value of a cost or a benefit varies depending upon when it is incurred, the further into the future the lower the present value. This is justified on two grounds. Firstly, the total value of productive resources plus their output will increase over time. Secondly, individuals and society place a higher value on present consumption than on future consumption. Therefore adjustments must be made to the costs and benefits of a project to relate them all to a particular point in time, so that greater weight is given to the present day with the weighting decreasing over time.

Discounting

The means by which all costs and benefits are related to a particular point in time is discounting. The choice of the discount rate is important since the least-cost solution for any given objective may change depending upon the choice of the discount rate. A low discount rate will favour high capital investment projects with low running costs. A higher discount rate will favour projects where the major proportion of costs are incurred in the future.

Basically there are two schools of thought on discount policy. There are those who hold that it is the responsibility of Government not to discount the future too heavily. In fact governments have a unique responsibility to safeguard the future and to adjust the individual's 'defective telescopic faculty'. This requires a 'social time preference' rate which really reflects the politicians' and planners' weighting of present and future consumption. The second school suggests that resources should be diverted to the projects that yield the greatest return. This leads to a high discount rate—a 'social opportunity cost' rate.

Shadow prices

The financial cost of a resource is the cash that has to be paid to acquire its use. The economic cost is equivalent to the opportunity cost. Frequently the economic cost of an input is not equal to the financial cost that has to be paid. The most common examples cited in developing countries are the prices of unskilled labour and foreign exchange. The use of an unemployed unskilled labourer may result in little or no loss of production elsewhere in the economy. The opportunity cost may be very low. (However, increased employment will lead to increased consumption of resources which have a positive opportunity cost. Therefore even if there is no direct loss of output, opportunity cost will be greater than zero.) In contrast the currencies of most developing countries are overvalued by the maintenance of official exchange rates. Similarly, skilled labour is usually scarce and its financial cost does not fully reflect its value.

In an economic analysis the real value of the resources to the economy must be used and, in cases where the financial cost does not reflect the economic value, corrections are made by means of shadow prices. Given the data available in developing countries, no precise calculations can be made of shadow prices, but an estimate in the right direction with an approximate order of magnitude will be a step forward. For example, it is suggested that in many countries with chronic unemployment, unskilled labour should be valued at between 25% and 50% of its wage or financial cost.

Other corrections to financial costs for economic analyses are made when part of the financial cost is merely a transfer payment, e.g. import duties or taxes. These are deducted from the financial cost.

Effective demand for water

Effective demand for water means the quantity of water that people demand and are prepared to pay for at a particular price level. It is determined by a complex interrelationship of a number of factors including the size and nature of the population, the level of education, social and religious philosophy, income, housing conditions, water use habits, climate, available technology and especially the accessibility of the supply. Given a knowledge of the pattern of demand (see Chapter 6) the quantity demanded can then be determined by the price charged. The relationship between the level of water consumption and living conditions suggests that a large increase in water consumption can only be expected with a general improvement in living conditions, which is not likely in many areas in the immediate future. Therefore it can be expected that the effective demand of groups other than the middle and upper class urban consumers will remain low in developing countries for a long time.

In urban areas the demand for water is relatively inelastic, i.e. a small change in the price of water leads to a less than proportionate change in the quantity demanded. This is because: (a) water is a necessity and there is frequently no good feasible alternative source; (b) water expenditure forms an insignificant proportion of many urban consumers expenditure; (c) the poor will carry home a relatively constant amount based on their minimum requirement. Industrial demand is likely to be more elastic owing to the possibility of altering their production techniques, of recycling or providing their own boreholes. However, the overall urban demand curve will be relatively inelastic.

In rural areas, where all consumers have a greater possibility of substitution, the demand will be lower and it may be more elastic when other sources are available. However, this is not always true since many rural people will refuse to pay for good quality water, however low its price, if a natural source is available. In rural areas where there are no alternatives to the improved supply in the dry season, the demand, at low levels of consumption may be as inelastic as urban demand.

Cost concepts and cost structure

The marginal cost of production is the cost of delivering the last (or marginal) unit. The average cost per unit is the total cost of production divided by the number of units produced. Therefore, if marginal cost is less than average cost, average cost will be falling. Conversely if it is greater than average cost, average cost will be rising. Fixed costs are constant as production varies, though the time and range must be specified. However, variable costs alter as production alters.

The major feature of the cost structure of most rural and small urban water supplies is that fixed capital costs are high and that there are significant economies of scale—that is, with increasing capacity, marginal costs are low and average costs are decreasing. For example, if pipe diameters are doubled, the water carrying capacity increases fivefold and the cost may approximately double. There may be high fixed costs for intakes, pumping plant and treatment works. In other words, much of the investment is 'lumpy'.

In addition to high fixed capital costs a large proportion of the recurrent cost does not vary with consumption. Frequently the largest recurrent expenditure item is operation and maintenance staff which is usually independent of the level of water use. It has been estimated (Carruthers, 1973) that only 10% of the total cost of schemes operated by the Kenyan Ministry of Water Development, vary with the level of consumption. This includes pumped and gravity schemes; and the short-run marginal cost of the latter may be practically zero. Longer-run marginal costs will be higher but are likely to be less than those of another new scheme. Hence, over a considerable operational range unit costs fall with an increasing level of utilization.

The marginal costs of large urban schemes will usually be low until existing capacity is utilized. Thus, in the short term, average costs will fall with increasing use. However, it is possible, especially in the largest cities, that the long-run marginal cost is high and increasing, exceeding and thus increasing average cost, owing to the need to use more distant and expensive sources.

The cost of structure of a water supply and the demand for water are especially relevant in examining a number of important issues: the design period, the area to be covered, the quantity of water that should be supplied and, in particular, whether communal points or individual connections should be installed, and pricing policy.

8.4 SECTORAL ALLOCATIONS, OBJECTIVES AND CRITERIA

Sectoral allocations

The current state of water supply facilities in most developing countries is regarded as inadequate and there is a great need for improvement. A modern water supply is a desirable amenity, plays an important role in improving public health and is often perceived as being important for economic development. However, this does not necessarily mean that large quantities of resources should be devoted to high standard water supplies. Disease is not the only constraint on the quality of life in developing countries and water supplies are not the only means of alleviating disease. In addition the current state of many other facilities is inadequate and the need for water supplies cannot be considered in isolation.

The resource endowment situation of poor countries needs little emphasis. Typically there is scarce capital (and even scarcer recurrent finance), plentiful unskilled labour (though there are often seasonal shortages), scarce skilled labour and administrative capacity. Resources which are devoted to water supplies are not available for other urgent requirements, consequently the need for water supplies must not be considered in isolation from the resource availability and the needs of other sectors. Therefore the investment in water supplies should not be taken out of the framework of economic analysis. The perspective for sectoral allocations must be the whole economy so that a balance between sectors is achieved.

Objectives and criteria—national and sectoral

A general goal of supplying water is not sufficient and there should be clear sectoral objectives which will guide the formulation of specific sectoral goals.

These objectives will be derived from, and must be consistent with, national objectives such as national income growth, redistribution of personal and regional income, rural and regional development, increased consumption, improved general welfare, meeting the minimum needs of the population and so on. The major difficulty is that at both national and sectoral levels the objectives are multiple and can and usually do conflict. Redistribution conflicts with maximum growth and consumption now conflicts with consumption in the future.

In order to assess the contribution of a policy or sectoral objectives to national objectives, certain criteria are specified. They are 'tests of preferredness' which enable decision makers to judge the relative merits of alternatives and to see trade-offs that are inherent in selecting options, especially when objectives conflict. Nowadays there are a range of financial, economic and social criteria. In formulating the economic criteria, concepts discussed earlier are relevant. In determining the important rate of discount criterion, time preference and opportunity cost are relevant. When considering income distribution criteria, the central concept is marginal utility. These first order criteria should assist in making sectoral allocations based on the contribution of the sectors to meeting national objectives. In practice trade-offs between sectors are difficult, but planners must be aware of the potential costs of a decision to other sectors.

Second order criteria assist in determining within sector allocations. These planning criteria for the water supply sector are derived from the first order criteria, with which they must be consistent, and from the sectoral objectives. The major sectoral objective may be to generate economic development or to alleviate the worst poverty. This question is discussed in Section 8.8 on water development strategy. However, there will be no single type of water supply suitable for all situations. Good sectoral planning requires diagnosis of the community's development status and provision of the appropriate service. The two major types of planning criteria used to assist planners reach decisions within the water supply sector relate to design and selection of schemes. They are discussed later.

Design criteria are mainly technical criteria which operate at the level of individual design decisions. First order economic criteria have a large role to play in determining these design criteria since, if a specific water supply goal is accepted that meets non-economic criteria, it is important to fulfil that goal in the cheapest way without wasting resources.

8.5 BENEFITS OF RURAL WATER SUPPLIES

A number of impact studies have revealed the gulf that exists between potential and realized benefits of water supplies in developing countries and a number of writers (Saunders, 1975; Warner, 1975) have highlighted the vital differences. The major finding is that very few of the benefits expected from water occur spontaneously, thus supporting the package of inputs strategy for rural development (Carruthers, 1973; see also Chapter 5).

The conclusion of most impact studies is that the provision of water alone, though perhaps necessary, is not sufficient to produce significant benefits. The provision of a safe water supply creates opportunities for extension workers in agriculture, animal husbandry, health, child welfare and home economics. Often these opportunities can be exploited at low cost, sometimes only the cost of conveying information.

Medical authorities often appear to consider the case for health benefits of rural water supplies proven. 'There is no medical need to demonstrate once again the value of a safe domestic water supply in any community. This can be taken for granted and in fact is accepted by the health authorities in this country'. This statement was made by a university professor but could easily have been made by a Ministry of Health official or others whose sincere concern for people's health blinds them to reality. However, health impact studies are often disappointing and surveys show that health education is often a vital missing input.

Although organizations and personnel engaged in rural water supply are either not fully aware of, or unwilling to admit, the limited benefits being achieved at present, they have one reason for overstating the immediate benefits. If governments become convinced of the low level of benefits they may lower the priority of water investment; whereas a long-term perspective should be maintained since the realized benefits are likely to build up over time, especially as people's awareness of how to maximize their value increases. In the longer run complementary facilities will be provided and a start has to be made somewhere.

Water supply organizations should not exaggerate the short-term impact and benefits of rural water supplies but should emphasize the long-term nature of benefit realization. Distortion of the short-term benefits risks governments suddenly becoming aware of the apparently poor return, in the social and economic as well as the financial sense, and diverting resources from the rural water supply sector. Alternatively, if governments are led to overestimate the value of water supplies, they may allocate too many resources to water supply at the expense of other socially necessary activities. Hence it is suggested that as much thought and effort should be given to the realization of benefits as is given to actually installing supplies.

Potential benefits

The provision of a water supply may mean that the quality of water is improved, the reliability is greater, the quantity of water available may have been increased and its distance from the consumers may have been reduced.

The reduced walking distance to the well saves time and energy and releases labour which may be used for productive purposes leading to an economic benefit. Even if the economic value of the saved labour is zero there is a social benefit from the time saved and drudgery eliminated because more time can be spent with the family or on domestic activities and leisure. The improved quality of the water may lead to improved health which can result in (a) lower medical expenditure, (b) an improved sense of wellbeing, (c) increased fitness and hence increased productivity of agricultural workers leading to an increase in crop production and (d) a lessening of the debilitating effects of childhood infections. The reliability of the supply will reduce the risk of epidemics. If water is available for cattle near the homestead the condition of the animals may improve if they do not have to walk so far and are exposed to fewer diseases and the people may then be able and willing to invest in better quality cattle. The potential benefits from a water scheme are illustrated schematically in Figure 8.1.

Which benefits arise, in practice, from rural water supplies? The problem of determining realized benefits is difficult owing to the impracticability of measure-

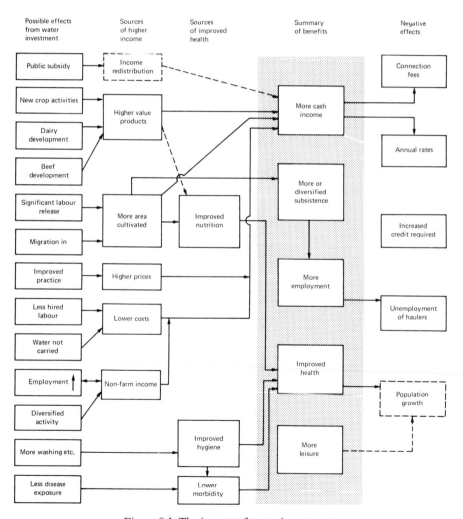

Figure 8.1 The impact of water investment

ment. Firstly, it is impossible to isolate the benefits that are due to water alone. Secondly, the value of the non-marketed benefits cannot be expressed in financial terms. These issues are tackled later.

Health benefits

Chapter 1 shows that several diseases can be reduced or eliminated by improved water supplies. However, the direct relationship between safe water supplies and improved health is not undisputed, largely because of the gap that exists between potential and realized health benefits. Consequently more reliable data is still required and experience must not be transplanted from one environment to another without exercising great care. An unsafe supply is certainly a hazard to health and a safe supply is perhaps necessary for improved health but it is no guarantee. People's exposure to water-based diseases (e.g. schistosomiasis) and water-related insect vector diseases (e.g. malaria) may not be significantly affected, even when accompanied by a health education programme. At the present level of development of many areas it is doubtful if even a very intensive programme would succeed. For example, people may continue to use unhealthy sources for recreation.

Water-borne diseases such as dysentery can be prevented by improving the quality of the water, e.g. by chlorination. Water-washed diseases such as skin infections are associated with the need to wash. They can be significantly decreased by using increased quantities of water. In urban areas water supplies are likely to be an essential health preventive measure, but realized benefits in rural areas will be constrained by the behaviour of rural people.

Firstly it is clear that the potential benefits will only be achieved if people use the water supply rather than their traditional source. Many rural people are only prepared to purchase water if no other water is available. Hence, unless the water is free many people only use the supply when the traditional natural sources are dry. It is not surprising that people who fail to appreciate water quality are not prepared to walk further to obtain a good quality water. Therefore, if consumers are to use an improved supply it must be at least as near to their home as their natural source. Where improved supplies are distant, people only use the supply for part of the year and in other areas some people may not use it at all.

Secondly the potential health benefit from the alleviation of water-borne diseases will only be fully realized if people consume an improved quality water throughout the year. The quality of water from improved supplies is sometimes doubtful, though, as is discussed in Chapter 5, design without treatment may be a rational planning decision. However, even if people obtain good quality water they may contaminate it before consumption. The extent to which people will benefit from an improved supply if they continue to use other water at times is unknown. Unless a large area is provided with water supplies it is unlikely that people will only use water from the improved supply. They will have to use other water when they visit friends. If their supply breaks down they will be forced to use other water. Some experts contend that a very occasional breakdown could be serious, if by using good quality water for a long time people lose some of their present-day immunity to the more common sicknesses.

Thirdly the potential health benefit from the alleviation of water-washed diseases will only be realized if people increase the quantity of water that they use. Low consumption levels of high quality water do not constitute a safe water supply. Increasing the availability of water without improving the quality, even of water generally considered to be unsafe, will greatly reduce the incidence of several unpleasant infections (Chapter 1 and 5). It is possible that increased use of water by rural people presents the greatest immediate opportunity for a significant improvement in their health.

However, it is now apparent that if people have to carry water more than a very short distance that they will only consume 10–15 litres per head per day. The provision of an improved water supply nearer their home, supplying better quality water, will not necessarily mean that they increase their consumption. They will continue to obtain the quantity that they perceive as being their minimum requirement.

The realization of health benefits depends upon the degree of service. A consumer who has a tap on his premises, runs less risk of contaminating the water before consumption; but more important is that he will use considerably more, perhaps up to 10 times more than a consumer who has to carry all the water to his house. Consequently, although health benefits accruing to users of communal points are likely to be slight, significant benefits, especially those related to water-washed diseases, will accrue to owners of individual connections.

Important questions still remain. How much greater will be their sense of wellbeing and their ability to work harder if certain diseases are reduced but they continue to suffer from others? Whatever the answers it is probable that the health benefit for very young children of water supplies is greater than it is for the adult population.

It can be concluded that, until people can be induced to use the water supplies throughout the year and in greater quantities, and health education is more widespread, the potential health benefits supplied will not be fully realized. Often the probability of health benefits is greatest in high-risk epidemic areas, e.g. cholera risk areas, where the benefits should include the value of costs avoided.

Social benefits

Many rural water supplies will significantly reduce the walking distance and will lead to savings of time and energy. One Ethiopian study (Browne, 1974a) which discovered the existence of a 'black market' in which people pay a higher rate for water in order not to queue, showed that many people attach a value to time saving and that it has a real social benefit.

However, savings of time and energy will not necessarily result. As has already been mentioned, people may not use the supply if they must pay for the water. Sometimes the distance that people have to walk to obtain water is not decreased by the provision of an improved supply. Furthermore, time saving may be reduced because people may have to queue at the supply point.

Wherever time and energy savings are achieved the supply will have a genuine amenity value and the mere relief of drudgery is a real social benefit. If the time saved results in extra time being devoted to domestic chores and looking after children, the social benefit of the supply would be important. This was certainly the main direct benefit of the Zania scheme in Kenya (Jakobsen et al., 1971).

In drought risk areas, where the hardships of the inhabitants are increased by inadequate and unreliable water, the provision of an improved supply may occasionally prevent complete social disruption. It is suggested that, in certain very poor rural areas, the benefits arising from the provision of a reliable but poor quality water supply to an area with a scattered or nomadic population, which has very little water or extremely poor quality water, are greater than those resulting from the provision of good quality water to an area which already has plentiful, poor quality natural sources.

Economic benefits

Water supplies may be a necessary input for the realization of economic benefits, but they are clearly not sufficient; other conditions must also be fulfilled. Time saving in collecting water can be devoted to agricultural labour but labour released for agriculture only has an economic value if its marginal product is positive. It is probable during most of the year that labour is not a limiting constraint on agricultural production and the value of extra labour would be very small if not zero, i.e. the opportunity cost of unskilled labour is low. The crucial determinant of the value of the released labour is its contribution during agricultural labour peaks. If at such times other factors are more limiting than labour the economic contribution of the extra labour will be small. However, in many rural situations the marginal product of labour is high at times, e.g. early weeding.

In dry areas where people depend on cattle, water supplies may provide a real benefit in keeping cattle alive if water is more limited than grazing. However, in other areas, the impact of the supplies for cattle may be slight unless individual connections are installed. In Kenya it was found that significant livestock benefits only arose if on-farm connections were provided, so that people did not have to walk their cattle and mix them with other people's animals, and other complementary inputs such as disease control were also introduced. The fact that most facilities, e.g. credit and improved stock, which are complementary to water supplies are missing in rural areas is a major reason why realized agricultural and economic benefits are so limited at present.

One important benefit from a safe reliable communal supply arises when permanent settlement is made possible in fertile areas or grazing areas which are underpopulated owing to lack of dry season water.

Although improved water supplies may be necessary to achieve certain economic benefits, the authors believe that water supplies are not critical to the development process and that the effective use of improved water supplies is more a consequence of development than a cause of development. Evidence from developing countries shows that, at present, benefits from technically adequate water schemes are not occurring in full to the designated consumers. In fact there is very little evidence to show that water supplies by themselves have promoted development.

8.6 COST–BENEFIT AND COST-EFFECTIVENESS ANALYSIS

Cost–benefit analysis is a procedure for determining the value of a project or programme to an economy. The financial costs are shadow priced to calculate their economic values and the economic cost stream is discounted to a particular point in time. Similarly benefits are valued and the stream of benefits is also discounted to the same point in time. If the present value of the benefit stream compares favourably with the present value of the cost stream the project is perceived to be a sound investment.

There are always many problems to be overcome: What are the appropriate shadow prices? What is the appropriate discount rate? What benefits will arise? What is the value of each benefit? Do externalities exist? However, in many sectors, such as irrigated agriculture, these problems can be overcome sufficiently for the answer to be meaningful, though it will always be treated with care and should even then be regarded as a good check and not as a final arbiter of project merit.

Excessive emphasis should not be placed on the outcome of any cost–benefit assessments, even if the project output is readily identified and easily valued, as is the case with most industrial projects and some agricultural schemes. When one is dealing with sectors such as transport and power, there are special appraisal problems associated with identification, enumeration, quantification and valuation of costs and benefits. Those problems are even greater with domestic water supply investments for here the link with the production process and readily valued output is even less distinct. Whilst gains of a productive, health or social nature from water investments may be real and important, the translation of these gains into conventional economic units presents both conceptual and empirical problems. Furthermore, an improved domestic water system supplies only potential gains and often a joint input is necessary for this gain to be realized. For example, accessible and plentiful water supply undoubtedly creates opportunities for improved dairy husbandry; but dairy cows have to be available and credit is often required before the opportunity can be realized. It is, therefore, reasonable to question the feasibility and utility of attempting to attribute benefits to such joint inputs.

Some authorities (for example the World Bank) consider that it is possible to apply cost–benefit analysis to urban water supplies. Costs are easily determined and revenue forecasts are used as a measure of benefits. The logic for this is that consumers will not be willing to pay more for water than the benefit they derive and that revenue therefore indicates the minimum benefit. This is true but the actual benefits may greatly exceed this minimum, for three reasons. Firstly, water rates are often kept low for political or social policy reasons. Secondly, consumers receive considerable benefit from the priority uses (such as drinking, cooking and washing) and would be willing to pay very high prices for water for these uses, rather than do without it. However, because they pay much less than they would be willing to pay, they enjoy what is termed a 'consumers' surplus'. Consumers' surplus is exluded from revenue but it is, nevertheless, a real benefit from the service. The characteristics of the demand for urban water mean that consumer surplus is likely to be large in relation to revenue. The third reason for revenue underestimating benefits, is that external benefits (for instance improved health of one's neighbours), though important, are excluded. Therefore revenue is considered to be an inadequate proxy measure for benefits in urban areas. In rural areas the situation is further complicated in that inhabitants, through ignorance, will greatly underestimate the value to them of good quality water. Hence revenue is likely to be a totally worthless measure of the value of benefits in rural environments.

There is no satisfactory method of evaluating the benefits of urban or rural water supplies in developing countries at present. To attempt such an evaluation would mean making heroic, if not absurd, assumptions and result in a meaningless answer. It is not unusual for cost–benefit analysis, although basically very simple, to be used as a means of impressing the decision maker or layman of the validity of a particular investment, without making clear the rather spurious assumptions on which the values are based. Nevertheless, though the task is difficult, some judgement is necessary on the value of water investments. Cost-effectiveness analysis is the process for finding the least cost means of achieving a particular goal—say 2000 houses with 500 litres of water per day. In this process economic concepts such as shadow prices, discounting and effective demand are very relevant.

Decisions will always be taken in the field of water supplies on the basis of intution and judgement, but cost-effectiveness analysis should help to improve or sharpen judgement.

8.7 APPROPRIATE STANDARDS AND DESIGN CRITERIA

Appropriate standard of service

There is little merit in providing water supply and related facilities if it is beyond the capacity of the community to use and sustain them properly. This statement needs elaboration and emphasis because a number of organizations involved with water supply investment, especially rural supplies, do not appear to be fully conscious of limitations upon otherwise desirable courses of action.

Over-supply of water is a misuse of resources whatever the potential public health value of an ample supply of water. Public policy should aim at obtaining a fit between the peoples' needs, attitudes, capacities and resources, at a particular stage of development, and the standard of water service and the administration and institutional methods used to supply this service.

The attitude of people to water supplies will depend on education, religion, ability to accept innovation etc. The capacity of people to make effective use of water improvements is reflected by their commercial awareness, their ability to cope with cash transactions, the other resources which they possess and their knowledge of good health practices. Describing the needs of the people is extremely difficult because it necessarily involves value judgements and political decisions.

If the demand for improved water supply is the result rather than a cause of development, it follows that the more developed areas and communities should be provided with a higher degree of service to coincide with their effective demand and greater ability to use the water effectively. The provision of a safe chlorinated supply to every house in a country may be a desirable objective but in most developing countries it would not only be unrealistic but positively damaging to overall national development.

It is suggested that the appropriate service for poor and scattered communities should be a guaranteed source within reasonable walking distance with comparatively little emphasis on quality. Whereas, in semi-commercial farming areas, on-farm connections should be encouraged. Thus in areas with reasonable natural sources it may only be appropriate to invest in water supplies if the area is 'ready' for individual connections.

Individual connections and communal water points

It is generally recognized that benefits from individual connections are always much greater than benefits from communal water points. The cost of a scheme based on individual connections will be greater than the cost of a communal point scheme, the cost ratio depending on the type of supply, local topography and other factors.

In urban areas a communal point system demands a dense distribution network and the marginal cost of taking the water to an individual's premises is relatively low. The benefits of individual connections in urban areas are high and thus wherever the individual can afford his own connection they are clearly desirable. (Where there is risk of epidemic disease there is also an economic case for subsidized individual connections based on the notion of externalities.) However, communal points must be provided for those who are unable to attain to their own connection.

However, in rural areas the issue is not so clear. Firstly, the effective demand may not exist owing to lack of cash, insufficient appreciation of the benefits and lack of complementary resources to maximize the benefits. Secondly, many rural water supplies are single-point supplies, such as a hand-pump at

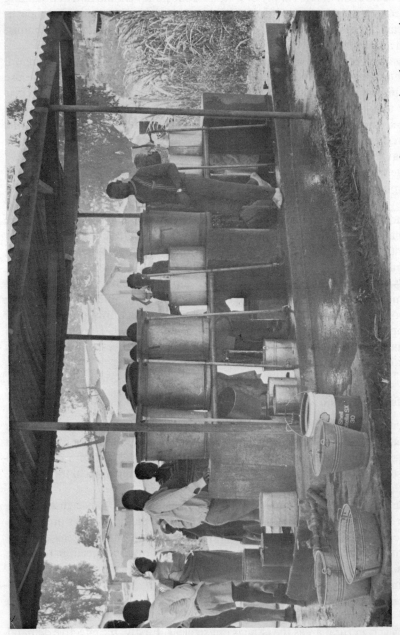

A government-owned water selling point in a suburb of Blantyre, Malawi. A government employee supervises the operation and collects the money. His receipts may be checked by reading the water meter (visible at ground level on the left of the photograph) which records the volume of water sold (photograph: M. G. McGarry).

the head of a borehole. A distribution system to provide on-farm supplies would increase the cost of the supply many times over. In certain countries, for example Ethiopia, it would be inconceivable that rural water schemes would be anything other than point supplies. Even in the worst drought-affected areas, people and cattle rarely die of thirst. However, the amenity value of a safe assured water supply would be a great social benefit.

The situation where the choice is most difficult is in well-endowed rural areas which are to be provided with a gravity scheme. A communal point network will necessitate an expensive distribution system. The marginal cost of a scheme designed for individual connections will be the cost of the small-dimension pipes to individual farms, and the marginal cost of larger pipes in the main network required for the greater quantity of water that will be demanded. The latter, however, will be able to take advantage of the economy of scale characteristic of distribution pipes. It has been estimated by the Ministry of Water Development in Kenya that the cost of an individual connection scheme is typically double that of the same scheme catering only for communal points.

In these areas, on-farm supplies would give opportunities for keeping grade cattle, crop spraying and minor irrigation (of vegetable gardens, for example). They would maximize savings of time and energy and would ensure that all those connected actually used the water. They would minimize the risk of contamination and the health benefit potential would be maximized. Finally, they enable a high level of rate collection to be achieved and the net financial cost of the more expensive scheme to Government could be lower in the long run.

It is suggested that, in areas such as the densely populated area of Central Kenya, the marginal benefits of a communal point supply over the abundant natural sources is small, but that the marginal benefit of individual connections over the communal point is very large. Therefore, in such areas, resources should be concentrated upon individual connections, even though costs may be at least double.

Design criteria

If schemes are underdesigned, demand will not be satisfied; if they are over-designed, scarce resources will be wasted. Of course there are many purely technical aspects of design, but nevertheless the economist has a role to play in predicting demands and helping to set design criteria appropriate to the resource base of the country.

There is a wide spectrum of opinion on the merit of design criteria. Some engineers maintain that design criteria are of very limited use. Because of wide variations in local conditions they claim to need maximum flexibility. Others argue that, in order to maximize the use of very limited skilled man-power, fairly rigid standard designs should be adhered to. In practice a middle course, with design criteria laid down only as guidelines, is probably best. In the following sections some typical design issues are discussed.

Design consumption figure

The design consumption figure should be based on estimated demand which in turn will depend on factors such as cash income, education, climate, complementary facilities and, above all, on accessibility. In particular, consumption is dependent upon whether or not individual connections will be provided and on the likely rate of take-up.

In rural areas water for cattle and for human consumption should not be considered as separate goods and the design figure must include water for both. It is possible to find examples of schemes where the designers have provided water for people alone, much to the puzzlement of herdsmen, with predictable unsatisfactory results.

Sometimes developing countries tend to adopt very high and inappropriate standards. Numerous empirical studies have shown that if people have to walk more than a few hundred metres they are unlikely to carry more water than 10–15 litres per head. Therefore water supplies based on communal points should be designed for low consumption figures unless there is evidence of a future effective demand for individual connections.

The fact that quantity demanded is related to general living conditions means that low levels of supply must be accepted until general welfare increases. In urban and rural schemes with individual connections the design figures should be based on the best estimates of future demand and not on experience from the developed world nor on levels that planners believe are 'desirable'.

Within urban areas there will be regional differences based on income, household facilities etc. and the design of the distribution system must take these into consideration. An interesting example of proposed design is cited by Lee (1969). The Master Plan for Water Supply, Sewerage and Drainage for Calcutta adopted two levels of demand but this could be traced to supply rather than demand considerations. In areas of the city supplied by groundwater the design figure was nearly 100 litres per head but in areas using surface sources the design figure was 180 litres.

Design period

Water supplies are designed to meet the demand for water. If they are designed to meet present demand they will obviously fail to meet increasing demand. If they are designed to meet demand in the distant future expensive investments will be under-utilized for many years. The objective of designers may be to meet demand at all times at minimum cost. If, for example, a decision is being made between a 10- and 20-year design period, the marginal present cost of the 20-year design must be compared with the cost of scheme augmentation in year 10. Economies of scale will favour a longer design period but costs incurred in year 10 will be discounted to the present day. Therefore longer design periods will be favoured in situations where economies of scale are very significant (for instance, in distribution pipes) and where the appropriate discount rate is low. The decision will not only depend on these calculations because certain practical considerations will favour the longer design period; aid funds are often only available for capital investment and many governments are more liberal to increases in development (capital) budgets than recurrent budgets. Another practical factor is that often the greatest constraint is design capacity, the marginal cost of designers time for extra installed capacity may be close to zero.

Technology

In developing countries it is desirable that the technology utilized should be as simple as possible. In a situation where skilled labour may be the greatest constraint to water development, the scheme must not be so complicated that it is impossible to maintain properly; and the simpler the scheme the less training is required by the operators.

The use of cheaper materials, such as plastic rather than steel piping, should be encouraged. In labour surplus economies the use of labour-intensive construction methods and local materials may mean that the real economic (shadow priced) cost is lower.

Storage

In order to ensure supply at times when demand exceeds the capacity of a water source, storage is required. This may be provided at various points in the system; from a major reservoir receiving water from a distant source to individual storage tanks on consumers' premises and at communal water points. The greater the storage provision the more reliable but expensive is the supply. Thus there is a trade-off decision between increasing cost and decreased risk of shortage. The conventional wisdom of engineers probably results in reasonable storage decisions in capital cities of developing countries, but in small towns and rural areas this may lead to overdesign. Inhabitants of small towns and rural areas can adjust with little hardship to peak periods either by avoiding use at this time or by queueing. One study has shown that at a major rural supply in Kenya storage absorbed more than 10% of the capital cost but was less than 10% utilized in the early years (Carruthers 1973). In addition to covering peak demand, consumption point storage is supposed to cover breakdowns but in rural schemes it is unlikely that breakdowns will be discovered until the storage is empty. In any event, breakdowns are less important than in urban areas because alternative sources usually exist. Therefore it is suggested that storage on rural water schemes may often not be worth the extra investment except in cases where storage is required as a form of water treatment (Chapter 5 and 9).

However, storage at boreholes may enable very significant capital savings on pump and engine. Storage may allow longer pumping hours and therefore the installation of equipment with a smaller capacity. Similarly there may be pumped surface schemes where night storage allows investment savings or gravity schemes where the streamflow is so low that night storage must be provided.

There is in some schemes the possibility of a trade-off between the cost of storage and of pipes. It may be worthwhile, taking advantage of the economies of scale of piping, to design the system, without storage, so that the main distribution system is capable of supplying peak requirements in the early years. As demand builds up, storage can be added in phases at a lower present value cost. The saving of storage costs will contribute to the extra pipe costs. The overall cost may or may not be greater but the system has the possibility of greater eventual capacity and this flexibility is important since the final demand in rural areas is still not well defined.

Standby capacity

Standby pumping capacity, despite the engineer's instinct to cover all contingencies, is basically an economic decision. There is a trade-off between risk of failure and the cost of the standby capacity. The cost of an urban failure may be high and therefore the cost of covering very unlikely situations may be acceptable. In rural areas the cost of failure is lower and consequently standby capacity should only cover more likely situations.

Standby capacity is also linked with economies of scale, which could mean that the greater the economies of scale, the greater the standby that should be provided. It may also be acceptable to have significant standby in the early years of a scheme since that capacity will later be required as base capacity and will be available when the early snags are being sorted out.

Optimal scheme size

The optimal size of a rural scheme is frequently determined by technical considerations such as the topography. The economy of scale characteristic of schemes can lead to an interesting design problem. The economies have to be balanced against the increasing cost of carrying water over longer distances. Alternatively two smaller schemes, with separate intakes, but a higher proportion of smaller diameter pipes, might be considered.

Water treatment

The question of water quality and treatment is not just a technical matter. Improved water quality is only achieved at a cost of resource utilization and may mean fewer schemes. Again the cost quality trade-off may be based on different criteria in urban and rural areas, i.e. a higher minimum standard is required in urban areas. Furthermore there is little point in constructing treatment works in rural areas if their maintenance is unlikely to be satisfactory. Also the marginal benefit of improved water quality in rural areas may be zero if health education is absent and people are subject to many other sources of illness. These matters are discussed at length in Chapter 5.

Gravity supply or pumped supply

An economic approach is required when there are alternative gravity and pump solutions for a scheme. The higher initial costs of the gravity scheme may have to be balanced against greater operation and maintenance costs of the pumped alternative. The latter will be incurred in the future and must therefore be discounted to achieve a true comparison.

Communal water point design

Communal water points should be as simple as is consistent with being strong enough to be capable of resisting 'reasonable' misuse, because extra benefits are unlikely to result from more luxurious points. The spacing of the points should take into consideration the fact that closer spacing by reducing the average distance that the consumer has to walk will, at least, result in a social benefit of time and drudgery saving.

Metering

There is little economic merit in metering in rural areas. Meters involve capital, administrative and maintenance costs on which there is little return other than to minimize waste. Restricted flow can be used instead. In rural areas with low marginal costs waste is not necessarily a crucial matter.

Optimal design of an individual scheme versus the optimal programme

The optimal size of an individual scheme may be very large, owing to economies of scale, when that scheme is considered in isolation. However, political and social criteria determining the overall programme may require a spread of investment and may conflict with the concentration of resources on a few large schemes. A few large schemes results in less people being served in other parts of the country.

Similarly the use of higher standard design criteria, e.g. through emphasis on individual connection schemes, may mean that fewer people will be supplied elsewhere. If, however, administrative capability and professional staff rather than finance is the major constraint, e.g. if foreign aid donors are willing to provide as much aid as they believe can be effectively used, larger schemes and design criteria may not deprive other people of water.

The optimal design period for any scheme may well be 20 years or more, but the result of using this long-term optimal figure will be that fewer people are served in the immediate future. The provision of treatment on a particular scheme may also mean that fewer people elsewhere receive water supplies. This illustrates that there is often a basic conflict between optimum scheme and programme design. This is one area where designers would benefit from planning guidelines.

Merit of the second best

This section commenced by raising the question of the appropriate standard of water service, and pointed out that in certain rural areas individual connections may be more appropriate than a communal system. However, owing to the higher costs involved, a consideration of the design issues discussed above may result in the appropriate standard of service appearing to be a sub-standard supply. For example, it may not be worthwhile chlorinating a particular supply, borehole water may be chemically contaminated, and even an improved water service may be irregular. However, if the new supply is an improvement over the previous supply in quality, quantity, reliability or proximity, at a cost considered to be less than the (broadly conceived) benefits, then an investment might be considered worthwhile. These matters are also discussed at length in Chapter 5.

Even when technicians can be persuaded of the need for appropriate, rather than high, standard supplies politicians may object with cries of 'second class supplies for second class citizens'. In these circumstances the idea has to be conveyed that increasing the standard of supply may greatly increase the costs but that the benefits may not increase sufficiently to justify the cost increase, given the country's resource endowment situation. Concentrating resources into a few high standard schemes will make the majority worse off than they need be. The key to obtaining appropriate supplies is to subordinate technical criteria and see merit in second best solutions.

8.8 SELECTION CRITERIA

Only a small proportion of the population of most developing countries have access to a water supply other than their unimproved natural source. Governments cannot provide all of the population with water supplies immediately and the function of selection criteria is to decide in which order different areas should be provided with water, i.e. the priorities of timing.

The urban–rural choice

The first choice facing Government is the distribution of funds between urban and rural water supplies. In most countries the supply of the capital and other large towns receive priority. It is suggested that this is a rational choice for the following reasons. Firstly there will be a more immediate public health impact, the risk of a serious epidemic is much greater in urban areas without an adequate water supply. The alternative sources in the urban areas are frequently very polluted, whereas the rural people have the source which they have been using since time immemorial. The economic and social benefits from a supply in an urban area are likely to be greater because of the existence of complementary inputs and because of the more probable effective demand (demand backed by willingness to pay) for individual connections. The latter will also mean that there is a greater probability of a high level of rate collection and it is much more likely that financial criteria can be satisfied.

One argument sometimes advanced for the provision of facilities in the rural areas is that by making the rural areas more attractive it may be possible to slow down the rural–urban migration that is creating difficulties in most developing countries. It can, however, be argued that experiencing urban facilities in the form of piped water is likely to whet the rural inhabitant's appetite for a full range of such facilities and thus to accelerate the urban drift. The important point is that vital aspects of public policy, such as whether to concentrate upon urban or rural areas, are determined by untested hypotheses. Economic research can help determine the empirical evidence to support or refute such assertions.

However, rural water development must proceed simultaneously with urban water supply development, and an equitable balance should be maintained in allocating funds between urban and rural areas. The decision as to what constitutes an equitable balance will be an important political decision.

The second level of choice is between individual schemes. Scheme selection will always remain subjective to a certain extent, and subject to political considerations. However, the official introduction of comprehensive planning criteria should assist in achieving greater objectivity.

Rural development strategy

The need for water in different regions in different developing countries generally varies greatly. In the drought-stricken areas of the Sahel it may be needed to keep the people and their animals alive, whereas in the high potential regions of Kenya it may be needed to boost an already relatively high standard of living.

The major strategic choice is between a 'worst first' and a 'growth point' strategy. The policy of concentrating water supply investments in 'growth points' which possess complementary facilities will increase the probable economic and health impact but is in direct conflict with a policy of priority to the poorest areas. This is likely to be a high cost (no economies of scale) policy with a low probable pay-off. There may be greater operation and maintenance difficulties and little likelihood of a significant proportion of total cost being raised by rates. Although most rural water schemes at present are bad risks for economic development and improved health, this policy increases the risk.

However, on humanitarian and political grounds governments will not be able to ignore the poorest areas, and the strategy that is adopted will depend on the national objectives and their relative importance. The water development policy should be determined by these objectives, subject to the resource constraints. It is likely that the policy followed in practice will be a mix of the alternative 'worst first' and 'growth point' strategies.

Proposed criteria for selecting rural schemes

It is suggested that rural supplies should be divided into two categories: those which are provided to assist development and which lead to economic as well as health and social benefits, and those which are provided on humanitarian grounds and which will result primarily in health and social benefits. It is appreciated that the distinction will not always be clear-cut and is only made to assist decision making.

Empirical evidence shows that an improved water supply, though perhaps necessary for improved health, welfare and economic progress, is not by itself sufficient. Hence the most important criterion for schemes which are designed to assist development is the presence of complementary inputs. This in effect means either giving more facilities to those areas which already have some facilities or providing a comprehensive package of inputs. This must be accepted if the criterion is whether or not economic benefits, are likely to result.

The economic scheme should assume high priority if it is going to support another development programme such as a Government Agricultural Package Programme. It is preferable that the scheme includes a rural centre that can provide the focus of development. If there are institutions such as schools, hospitals, wealthy merchants, etc. who could afford individual or household connections this would provide the most promising source of revenue to finance the operation and maintenance of the scheme. Even in schemes where the probability of installing individual connections is low, the likelihood of high revenue collection could be an important practical criterion. The expected health benefits of water schemes will be an important consideration. In areas with complementary facilities health improvement may in time lead to economic benefits stemming from an increase in the quality of agricultural labour inputs and improved livestock. These would be in addition to social benefits such as an increased sense of wellbeing and time and energy savings.

For schemes which are provided for humanitarian reasons the main criteria should relate to the distance, reliability and quality of existing supplies. The worse those characteristics are, the higher the priority. Inasmuch as the availability of water is more important than quality to most rural people, it is suggested that distance to a reliable source should be the main criterion. This has the practical advantage of being easily applied.

If one is considering two alternative areas for an improved supply, it is easier to discover which is further from an existing reliable source than it is to apply other criteria. Initially the objective may be that nobody should have to walk more than a certain distance to a reliable dry season source.

In principle it would be desirable to include a criterion concerning individual social and health benefits, including improved health and time and energy savings, but in practice this is difficult and the distance criterion may be a reasonable proxy in many cases. In areas with a high risk of epidemic disease this factor alone should give the area high priority. At any time special priority areas will probably exist, e.g. drought-affected areas will have high social and political priority.

In both economic and humanitarian based schemes the choice will be tempered by practical technical considerations such as accessibility of construction machinery. In addition there are a number of criteria which are very important for all rural supplies. If a new water supply will allow settlement in an area that is underpopulated with respect to other resources it may influence migration and lead to both economic and social benefits. In all cases there should be evidence of local involvement and desire for a water supply. This evidence may take different forms but it is inadvisable for Government to provide water supply to an area unless there is evidence of local involvement. It is suggested that a simple request from the local people does not constitute sufficient evidence because everybody would like to have a supply within easy reach. Another important criterion would be cost per head. At present most developing countries are spending a very limited sum of money on water supplies each year. If those funds are used for low-cost schemes more people will be supplied in the near future than if higher-cost schemes were built.

8.9 QUESTIONS RAISED BY SELF-HELP

In many countries planners believe that water schemes will be more likely to be successful if the local people are able to participate. This participation may take a number of forms ranging from cash contributions and providing labour to complete planning and construction. If the initiative for a water supply originates outside the community there is a risk of lack of communication with the local people and that the supply may be regarded as 'the Government water supply'. Consequently there is the possibility of the benefits not being fully realized or even early abandonment due to inadequate operation and maintenance.

Self-help movements for water improvement are emerging in a number of countries, a good example being Kenya. Here there is a current wave of interest in using the self-help movement to promote water schemes in the rural areas. It is a reflection of the genuine desire of the people for water and of their impatience with the speed of the government's programme strengthened by leadership of local politicians who realize that water supplies will benefit all their constituents. The cynics would add that they see water schemes as a means of self-promotion or re-election.

However, there are a number of characteristics which are common to most self-help water supplies: the projects proceed with inadequate planning; they are technically unsound; they are more expensive than is necessary; self-help labour is often disorganized and makes an insignificant contribution to lowering the cost of the project; the finance collected is often insufficient but people feel that they have made a once-and-for-all payment and are reluctant to make contributions to operation and maintenance. These weaknesses are recognized by the professional staff in the water supply sector and efforts are being made to overcome some of the problems, e.g. by making technical advice available to self-help groups.

In addition there is another less well recognized but equally important danger that self-help schemes may interfere with national planning efforts. Although the people may be dissatisfied with the government's water supply programme, that programme may well be realistic in relation to the complexity of the problem and the limited resources available. If planners have devised a logical water supply investment programme, which they perceive as being in the national interest, self-help pressure leading to programme alterations or expansion may be undesirable.

This pressure could have two effects. Firstly, additional funds may be allocated to water supply and this enlarged programme may even be a better reflection of the political will than the planners original programme. However, it will mean that other vital sectors of the economy may be deprived of resources. Unless the most constraining resources, such as skilled engineering manpower, are increased in proportion, it is likely that the additional available funds would not be properly utilized.

Secondly, it will frequently be difficult if not impossible to increase implementation capacity quickly and self-help proposals will simply be a means of political lobbying and queue-jumping over other schemes. This will mean that other areas of possibly greater priority are relegated in the queue. This is particularly serious in a country such as Kenya where increasing size of some self-help projects means that individual schemes absorb a significant proportion of funds available for national water supplies. This puts serious limitations on development in priority areas which are less successful in their political lobbying.

Therefore although an economic planner would not wish to discourage local participation, a large number of self-help schemes, and in particular large schemes, could create problems and distort the national allocation of resources.

8.10 FINANCE OF WATER SUPPLIES

Water supplies can be financed by a variety of means ranging from free water with a 100% government subsidy to the consumers paying the whole of the capital and recurrent costs. It is especially important to resolve the means of financing water supplies in developing countries where the lack of finance has often led to deterioration of existing supplies and a curb on development of new supplies.

One major problem in selecting a rating policy is that there are several functions of the rating procedure, some of which conflict. The main functions are economic, financial and social. The economic function is to ensure that resources are used efficiently and that price equals marginal cost. If price exceeds marginal cost the resources will be underutilized; if marginal cost exceeds price, capacity may quickly become a constraint. The short-run marginal cost of many rural schemes may be negligible when they are operating below full capacity, and even in the longer-run marginal cost may be low because of the economies of scale that exist (see Section 8.2). However, the long-run marginal cost of large urban supplies may be high and increasing and exceed average cost because more distant and expensive sources must be used for new augmentations.

Therefore the economic criterion may suggest a very low price for rural supplies but a very high price for large urban supplies. The social function of rating is subjective but would generally be considered to include the attempt to relieve abject poverty, redistribute income and develop backward areas. Therefore the social and economic functions may coincide for rural water supplies and suggest a very low rate; but they are likely to conflict in large urban areas.

The financial function of rates is to cover all the costs of the supply, capital, operation and maintenance and collection. Thus a financial criterion requires a rate based on average cost. In rural schemes with their significant economies of scale this will be much higher than marginal cost and would preclude economic use of the facility. In addition, it would clash with the low rate demanded by social criteria and, since the complete demand schedules are often entirely below the average cost curve, it would be a practical impossibility to adopt financially sound tariffs successfully. Thus, in rural areas, a financial deficit is probable.

In large urban areas with increasing long-run marginal cost, a rate based on average cost may be below the rate suggested by marginal cost and would thus lead swiftly to capacity crises. On the other hand, a long-run marginal cost rate would generate a large financial surplus.

Governments in developing countries, with a narrow tax base, and where many necessary infrastructural investments preclude the raising of revenue have been anxious to use any opportunity to raise finance and have often given greater weight to the financial rather than economic criteria.

Reconciling the conflicting rating functions

One possible way to attempt to reconcile the conflicting objectives of water rates is to practise price discrimination. To achieve this consumers must be separated. In the rural areas this can be achieved by discriminating between those with their own connection and those walking to a communal point. The social objective of a very low price for the poorest consumers can be met and those with connections should pay at least marginal cost. It is very unlikely that the financial criterion could also be met and a subsidy is the best solution. The need for subsidizing rural water supplies must be faced by governments who wish to pursue a rural programme.

The social objective demands that poor urban consumers are charged a low rate but the economic objective may demand a high rate to coincide with the increasing long-run marginal cost. A degree of reconciliation can be achieved by having a two-part tariff with a low rate for minimal use but increasing the rate for use above a certain low level to that demanded by the economic criterion, subject to political constraints. In addition communal point users could be charged at or below the minimal individual connection rate. Even if the long-run marginal cost is above average cost the financial criterion should be met since the low level users will only account for a small proportion of the total water used. In Addis Ababa although a significant proportion of the city's population uses communal points a 10% increase in the rate for individual connection owners would more than cover the cost of free water from communal points.

A two-part tariff can also be used in the situation where marginal cost is low and a flat rate is imposed irrespective of quantity combined with marginal cost rate for quantity. The flat fee contributes towards meeting the financial criterion and the low rate encourages economic use. This is a reasonable policy in small towns with spare capacity but a low rate for large quantities is often applied in large cities which have increasing long-run marginal costs. It means that capacity will become a constraint sooner and brings forward the time for future water investments.

However, whatever policy is adopted must be practicable. For example, in Kenya, communal point schemes' rates are often based on a low flat fee irrespective of use. However, it has been found impossible to effectively enforce payment since unsupervised points are in effect collective goods.

Rural rating policy

Rating policy should distinguish between individual connections and communal water points. The former provide a high level of service to the higher income groups whilst the latter provides a minimal level of service to the poor.

It is suggested that there is a strong case for free water from communal points and that governments should give greater consideration to such a policy than in the past. It would involve a loss of revenue but frequently this will be small. The major reasons for a free policy are:

(1) In the rural areas the short-run marginal cost of water is frequently close to zero and, over the longer-run, marginal cost is often low. Thus a free policy may accord with an economic efficiency criterion.
(2) Rural water supplies should, as was discussed above, be regarded as a social service and the financial criterion should play a secondary role.
(3) Governments which consider social criteria as important determinants of rural policy may elevate certain goods above the market place and there is a strong case for regarding water as such a merit want. However, owing to their lack of education, people may not immediately appreciate the full value of improved rural water supplies. Therefore, unless the supplies are free they

are unlikely to realize the potential benefits. For example, people may only use the supply in the dry season and use polluted sources in the wet season resulting in little or no health improvement. In addition the large capital investments will be heavily underutilized.

(4) Income redistribution is often a major objective of developing countries, the redistributive effect of providing rural water supplies is unclear. One approximate measure of the redistributive effect of a free water policy is the amount of cash that the rural people would have spent had it not been free, plus the value of the extra resources (fuel for a pump) that their increased consumption due to free water requires. The former being a direct personal cash saving is clearly an efficient means of income redistribution. It has been estimated (Browne, 1974b) that in rural Ethiopia cash savings are four times the value of the extra Government resources that would be required.

(5) Rural communal point users receive a low degree of service, they use small quantities, often walk a considerable distance to the supply and sometimes have to queue.

(6) The ability of rural people to pay is usually low. They will only purchase water when no alternative is available. It is often the case that the poorer the area the greater the period of the year when no alternative exists. Therefore poorer people may have to pay over a longer period, and thus pay more than people who live in better-off areas which have higher rainfall.

(7) Finally the revenue lost by a free policy will usually represent only a small part of the total cost; and a free policy would mean that the cost of collection would be saved.

The major argument against free water is that the water authority must meet financial targets. In urban areas free communal water will often be covered by a small increase for other users but in the rural areas there may be few if any individual connections. It has been stated that: 'The idea that water for drinking and hygiene should be free or heavily subsidized tends to inhibit financing and is a major cause of the shortage in less developed countries which already is critical and is growing worse' (Ripman, 1967). However, a proper subsidy scheme will not inevitably lead to poor service, although when embarking on such a policy governments must appreciate their future liabilities. The average cost of providing rural water supplies is often so high that it would be impossible to meet strict financial criteria and therefore the alternative to Government subsidy is no water supply. The effective demand for water is low and the demand schedules lies entirely below the average cost curve, if not below the marginal cost curve. If Government has limited funds for rural water supplies, it may be better to have fewer supplies which are free but which are being properly utilized than a slightly greater number, provided out of the small revenue collection, but which are being underutilized with the consequent waste of national resources. Advocates of strict financial criteria tend to ignore the low level of rural incomes, the amenity value and the indivisibilities and economies of scale of water supplies.

There are many countries where poor scattered communities render individual connections in rural areas inconceivable. But in areas where the population density is high, the topography is favourable and an effective demand exists, as for example in the Central Province of Kenya, individual connections should be positively encouraged owing to their greater effectiveness. Although one of the objectives of the policy would be to generate revenue the adoption of the connections may be encouraged by a low initial connection fee but combined with realistic rates, possibly based on an area ability to pay criterion.

Urban rating policy

As in the rural areas there is a strong case for free communal supplies in large urban areas. In this way the poorest inhabitants who receive a low degree of service would be provided with free water as a social service. This would mean a desirable redistribution of income. There are external benefits from this policy because there is a general public health risk if these people use alternative polluted sources.

The policy for individual connections, which are normally metered, should depend upon the long-run marginal cost structure. If long-run marginal cost is high and increasing, rates for industrial and other larger users should be in line with marginal cost, though a lower rate should be charged for domestic users. This policy would generate a financial surplus for the operating authority and would dampen demand so that expensive augmentations could be delayed.

In urban areas where marginal cost is decreasing or where there is much excess capacity no policy will be entirely satisfactory. A low rate for all users would have both economic and social merit but the authority would incur a large deficit. A two-part tariff might meet financial criteria by means of a flat minimum charge and satisfy economic criteria by a low rate reflecting marginal cost; but it would penalize low-income consumers. This could be modified by a low flat rate for a limited quantity of water.

It is concluded that, if effective demand for and effective use of water supplies are a consequence rather than a cause of development, either (a) income growth must be awaited before investing in water supplies or (b) inefficient use of the facilities must be endured for some time and heavy and continuing Government subsidies must be provided for most supplies. Social criteria support the latter policy since widespread availability and use of improved water is considered desirable. The alternative means that only an urban minority would receive the service.

8.11 REFERENCES

Bradley, D. J. (1971). *Infective Disease and Domestic Water Supplies.* (Water Supply Research Paper No. 20 BRALUP.) University of Dar es Salaam.

Browne, D. G. (1974a). *Dongore Water Supply—A Study of a NWRC Rural Well.* Addis Ababa: National Water Resources Commission.

Browne, D. G. (1974b). *Rural Water Pricing Policy.* Addis Ababa: National Water Resources Commission.

Carruthers, I. D. (1971). Cost–benefit analysis and agricultural development. *Farm Economist*, **12**, 107–112.

Carruthers, I. D. (1973). *Impact and Economics of Community Water Supply*. Ashford: Wye College.

Donaldson, D. (1974). Progress in the rural water programs of Latin America. *Bulletin of the Pan American Health Organization*, **8**, 37–53.

Jakobsen, B. Ascroft, J. and Padfield, H. (1971). The case for rural water in Kenya. In: *Strategies for Improving Rural Welfare*. (Occasional Paper No. 4; Ed. M. Kempe and L. Smith.) Nairobi Institute of Development Studies.

Lee, T. R. (1969). *Residential Water Demand and Economic Development*. (Department of Geography Research Publication No. 2.) University of Toronto.

Musgrave, R. (1959). *The Theory of Public Finance*. New York: McGraw-Hill.

Ripman, H. (1967). Water use and economic development. In: *Proceedings of International Conference on Water for Peace*. Washington, D. C.

Saunders, R. J. (1975). Economic benefits of public water supplies in developing countries. *Journal of American Water Works Association*, **67**, 314–317.

Warner, D. (1975). Evaluation of the benefits of rural water supply projects in Tanzanian villages. *Journal of American Water Works Association*, **67**, 318–321.

WHO (1972). *Kenya Sectorial Study and National Programming for Community and Rural Water Supply, Sewerage and Pollution*. (Report Nos. 2 and 4.) Brazzaville: World Health Organization.

9

Water Treatment in Developing Countries

JOHN PICKFORD

9.1 WHY TREAT WATER?

The minimum possible

Whenever water is provided for low-income people in developing countries there should be the minimum possible treatment, and the best supply is one which needs no treatment at all. The trouble with treatment is that it needs looking after. If the treatment process, however simple it may be, does not receive adequate attention, it will not function properly. Inadequate attention may, in fact, lead to a positive danger to public health. If the raw water is contaminated with disease-causing organisms which are not properly removed, then a large number of people can be infected at the same time. Wagner and Lanoix (1959) claim that there is plenty of evidence of outbreaks of typhoid fever, cholera and epidemic jaundice due to breakdown of treatment, and even in the United States 20% of water-borne disease cases have been attributed to deficiencies in the operation of treatment plants (Craun and McCabe, 1973).

A survey carried out by the National Environmental Engineering Research Institute, Nagpur, showed that in India 80% of the water treatment plants studied were not receiving proper attention (Arceivala, 1971). This survey covered municipal plants and it is reasonable to assume that a higher proportion of small rural works are not maintained efficiently, and the situation is likely to be worse still in countries without India's vast resources of technical ability. Even if reliable staff are available for a treatment plant and they have access to reliable technical advice when they need it, their salaries have to be paid throughout the life of the scheme. For some forms of treatment chemicals have to be provided and paid for.

It is therefore important that all possible sources of water should be considered when a water supply scheme is devised. A distant reliable source involving a long pipeline but needing no treatment may well be cheaper in the long run than a nearby source whose waters require a great deal of treatment to make them suitable. The full total cost of all sources, allowing for all capital and running costs, should be calculated. In addition, requirements for imported equipment or chemicals to treat water should weigh heavily against a particular process. Chapter 5 deals at length with the problem of deciding whether or not it is feasible and necessary to provide treatment for a particular water supply.

Treatment involves aspects of quality other than those like removal of pathogens which directly affect health. If treated water is not acceptable for other reasons, the users will continue to draw water from traditional sources and so will not benefit the disease-reduction of the treated water. For example, if treated water has an unpleasant taste, polluted but better-tasting water will be preferred; if the treated water discolours clothes during washing, women may continue to use an infected stream or pond. Provision of sufficient water for all needs is particularly important in areas where schistosomiasis is endemic. There is little point in providing a treated water supply if people go to polluted water for uses with greater bodily contact such as washing clothes or bathing in a stream (WHO Expert Committee, 1973).

Sources of water

Rainwater, highland stream water and some groundwater is generally good and little or no treatement is required. Water from village ponds, lowland streams and some underground sources may contain a variety of impurities which must be removed to make the water acceptable. The water in ponds and streams, which has passed through other inhabited places, is often contaminated by human waste and so may contain disease-causing organisms. For climatic reasons the flow in many hot-country streams and rivers is very variable. At times there is low discharge or the flow may stop altogether. After high-intensity tropical rainfall, the water level rises rapidly and the water contains a great deal of soil. Heavy rain can cause pollution of groundwater by pesticides and by animal and human waste, and groundwater may vary seasonally in quality and quantity.

Treatment largely consists of preparing *good water* by removal of *undesirable substances* by various *processes*, and we will consider these three aspects in turn.

9.2 WATER FIT FOR USE

The *International Standards for Drinking Water* (WHO, 1971) states that 'water intended for human consumption must be free from organisms and from concentrations of chemical substances that may be a hazard to health. In addition, supplies of drinking water should be as pleasant to drink as circumstances permit'.

Good water is sometimes described as 'wholesome and palatable', a term which is described as follows by Fair, Geyer and Okun (1966): 'To be wholesome, water must be free from disease organisms, poisonous substances, and excessive amounts of mineral and organic matter. To be palatable, it must be significantly free from colour, turbidity, taste and odour . . . and well aerated'.

Temperature is also important, and coolness is regarded by New Guinea Highlanders to be the most desirable characteristic of good water (Feachem, 1973). The desired temperature is around 10 °C and water at 25 °C is considered unpleasant. High temperature also stimulates the growth of plankton and water can become oversaturated with dissolved gases. However, in hot climates it is not usually possible to reduce the temperature of water by any form of treatment except on a household scale where water may be contained in porous vessels.

Bacteriological quality

From the health point of view the most important characteristic of good water is obviously an absence of pathogenic organisms. Most micro-organisms are actually harmless. However, some of the people who pollute a water source may have diseases and therefore all faecal organisms should ideally be absent. Faeces of healthy as well as ill people contain millions of *Escherichia coli* and these are generally taken as a measure of faecal pollution, although faecal streptococci and *Klostridium perfringens* are also used (Chapter 3).

The WHO *International Standards* lay down that in piped supplies there should be no *E. coli*. This high level of purity is attainable; for example, there were no *E. coli* in 13 000 samples taken in London in 1964–65 (Southgate, 1969). For small household supplies such as wells the WHO suggests that a zero *E. coli* count and not more than 10 coliforms per 100 ml are appropriate standards. However, it has already been stressed (Chapter 5), that these standards are too high for general applicability in developing countries.

Toxic substances

Chemical or poisonous substances are often the result of industrial pollution, and so are unlikely to affect rural water supplies. Maximum levels of arsenic, lead, mercury and other toxic substances are given in the *International Standards*. Pesticide-residuals are not normally present in dangerous concentrations.

Fluorides

The concentration of fluorides is critical for dental health in children. Too high a concentration can result in dental fluorosis in some children, but a small amount is essential for the prevention of dental caries. The desirable concentration varies with average ambient temperature; it should be 0·9–1·7 mg/l at 10 °C, 0·7–1·2 mg/l at 20 °C, and 0·6–0·8 mg/l at 30 °C, all concentrations expressed as F (Miller, 1962).

Mineral matter

Water should not contain any settleable suspended solids and should be clear, although clear water is not necessarily fit for human consumption. Turbidity, which is measured by looking at a candle through a vertical column of water, should if possible be less than 5 units, with a maximum desirable level of 25 units.

Salinity

The main effect of salinity is on taste, discussed below. Excessive salinity, especially if present as magnesium sulphate, can have a laxative effect. Local people can become accustomed to water with more than 4000 mg/l total solids, but the effects are often distressing for visitors.

Hardness

Carbonates and bicarbonates of calcium and magnesium cause hardness. Expressed in terms of calcium carbonate, water with less than 50 mg/l total hardness is 'soft', and water with more than 100 mg/l is 'hard'. Hard water requires more soap to form a lather than 'soft' water, although this advantage is less important as detergents replace soap for clothes-washing. Hardness also causes scale formation in pipes and fittings.

Organic matter

If organic matter is of vegetable origin it may be quite harmless. After all, tea may contain 2000 mg/l of organic matter; wine and soup may have higher concentrations.

Taste and odour

Objection to taste and smell is to some extent subjective; for example the concentration of iron which makes water unacceptable varies from 0·04 mg/l to over 200 mg/l. Water with chlorides in excess of 250 mg/l is sometimes considered as unpalatable although a concentration of sodium chloride of 1400 mg/l is provided for public supply in parts of Essex, England (Overman, 1968). Odours are stronger at higher temperatures. They may be due to the release of dissolved gases such as hydrogen sulphide, to the growth of micro-organisms which release taste-and-odour-producing substances, or to the decomposition of dead micro-organisms, leaves, grass and aquatic vegetation. Even if tastes and odours are harmless in themselves consumers often interpret them as evidence of pollution and consequently use other sources which are inferior from a health point of view.

Colour

Iron and magnesium are the main causes of colour, although organic material may discolour some water. Strong colour makes water unsatisfactory for washing clothes and is especially objectionable when textile-processing is carried out.

Oxygen

Dissolved oxygen is needed in water to give a pleasant taste and to prevent corrosion. It may be absent from underground water even when it is not polluted.

Incrustation and corrosion

If water is to be passed through pipes, as when it is distributed after treatment, it is necessary to consider the effect of the quality on the pipework. Very hard water can result in incrustation of pipes and fittings. Corrosion, on the other hand, is less with hard than with soft water. The rate of corrosion is also less with increased alkalinity, but is proportional to the content of dissolved oxygen and carbon dioxide, and to the temperature and velocity (Cox, 1964). Corrosion of galvanized tanks used to store rainwater is common as the water is soft and well-aerated. Corrosion by sulphate-reducing bacteria, which occurs particularly in anaerobic soils such as waterlogged clays, can be very serious and can result in perforation of cast-iron pipes within a few years. Iron bacteria may produce tubercles which reduce the flow in pipes. Protection can be provided by coatings of coal tar or other material, and trenches may be back-filled with limestone (Mara, 1974).

9.3 IMPURITIES IN RAW WATER

Water at the source of supply may require treatment because of naturally-occurring impurities or because of pollution. Water is polluted when it 'is altered in composition or condition, directly or indirectly as a result of the activities of man, so that it becomes less suitable for any or all of the uses for which it would be suitable in its natural state' (Key, 1967). Unpolluted surface water may not be suitable for water supply without treatment because of soil content following heavy rain, and because of weeds and algae. Impurities may be concentrated in groundwater giving so high a content of iron, manganese or salts that the water is unsuitable for use.

Impurities resulting from man's activities may be divided into five groups

(1) Wastes of animal or human origin, which contain bacteria and sometimes viruses. Such wastes may be carried in streams and rivers, are common in village tanks and may occur in unprotected wells and springs.

(2) Run-off from farms, where cultivation may increase erosion; fertilizers and pesticides may be included.

(3) Domestic sullage—wastewater which has been used for bathing, washing

clothes and cooking utensils. This may contain a high content of food waste.
(4) Industrial wastes, which are very variable in quantity and composition.
Mine drainage and mineral-processing water may be included in this category.
Wastes from food-processing industries are often heavily contaminated with
organic matter.
(5) Accidental pollution, such as that resulting from discarding engine oil.

In order to ascertain the nature and quantity of impurities, samples of the
water should be taken which are truly representative of the water. When there
is a seasonal variation, samples should be taken in all seasons.

Suspended matter

The silt content of many tropical rivers is very high. The mean content of
the Kosi river at Chatra in India is 2860 mg/l (United Nations, 1953) and the
maximum suspended solids contents of some other tropical rivers is reported
(Reid, 1956) as:

    10 000 mg/l in the Irrawaddy at Prome
     4000 mg/l in the Nile at Cairo
     4000 mg/l in the Jamuna at Delhi
     3600 mg/l in the Hooghly at Calcutta

In addition to silt, rivers may carry a load of grit and gross solids such as
floating debris.

Dissolved inorganic matter

Most inorganics are of natural origin. For example, groundwater in Ghana,
Burma and parts of northern India has a very high iron content (Reid, 1956).
This gives a characteristic red colour to the water. Water with a high manganese
content is blackish. Water which is colourless underground may become dis-
coloured when it comes into contact with air. Groundwater in Zambia is very
hard, some groundwater in Ghana has a great deal of nitrate, and groundwater
in parts of Kenya has high concentrations of fluorides. Sulphates abound in
groundwater under the deserts of North Africa and the Middle East.
    A high chloride concentration may be due to seawater intrusion. When
associated with ammonia, chlorides may give an indication of pollution. If
ammonia is high and chlorides low the source is likely to be vegetable, but
if both ammonia and chlorides are high the pollution may be of animal origin.
In disinfection of water supplies, any ammonia in the raw water requires
extra chlorine, which combines with the ammonia to form chloramines. These
are poor disinfectants compared with free chlorine and sometimes additional
chlorine amounting to ten times the ammonia concentration is required to give
effective disinfection.

The effects of metals and salts have already been mentioned in relation to the quality of good water. Apart from the removal of iron and manganese, normal treatment suitable for rural areas has no effect on these substances. Phosphorus and nitrates can contribute to eutrophication, the biological enrichment of an aquatic environment as a result of high nutrient input. Eutrophication is characterized by excessive plant growth, particularly of algae.

Organic matter

Water rich in organic matter may be suspected of bacterial or chemical contamination. Their stabilization by aerobic bacteria exerts an oxygen demand and measurement of oxygen demand is often used as a measure of pollution. The simplest test is to oxidize the organic material chemically with potassium permanganate to give the permanganate value (PV). The test may be carried out by boiling for ten minutes, or at room temperature for a longer period such as four hours. Other commonly used tests are the 5-day biochemical oxygen demand test (BOD_5) and the chemical oxygen demand (COD) using dichromate.

Some forms of organic matter give rise to colour and bad taste as they favour the development of algae, fungi and bacteria, which become attached to pipe walls in distribution systems where they secrete substances with an unpleasant smell. Some organics produce malodorous compounds with chlorine. Pollution of groundwater by hydrocarbons, for example by accidental spillage of oil, can result in pollution lasting for many years owing to their slow biodegradability in the absence of oxygen.

Micro-organisms and macro-organisms

By far the majority of micro-organisms in water have a beneficial effect, breaking down organic matter and effecting self-purification of streams and rivers. However, even a few pathogens can be disastrous and whenever possible all sources of water should be checked for evidence of faecal pollution. As with treated water this is done by selectively cultivating cultures of *E. coli*, faecal streptococci or *clostridium perfringens*. The bacteriological examination of water, although simple, has to be carried out very carefully (Mara, 1974). Micro-organisms which are present in raw water include bacteria, virus, protozoa and metazoa. The largest bacteria are about 50 μm long and the smallest only 1 μm long. In many developing countries the water consumed from untreated sources is heavily contaminated by faecal bacteria. A survey of the water from 300 open dug wells in Delhi and its surroundings (Arceivala, undated) revealed that over 90% of the samples had a MPN (most probable number) exceeding 20 per 100 ml for both coliforms and enterococci.

Macro-organisms are also important in assessing the quality of polluted water; the invertebrate animals of the stream bed are the most popular group of indicator organisms. Trouble in treatment works and pipes is often caused by the growth of plankton. *Phytoplankton* are of vegetable origin and *zooplankton* are animal. Zooplankton infestation in water mains is difficult to eliminate and can be unpleasant in delivered water. Some micro-organisms release taste-and-odour-producing substances, and the decomposition of dead micro-organisms can lead to tastes and smells.

9.4 PROTECTION AND TREATMENT AT SOURCE AND INTAKE

If impurities can be prevented from polluting the water in a source, its quality will be improved. For example, the use of vegetable cover in rainwater collection areas can reduce erosion and hence reduce the suspended solids at the intake. Public health education may lead to more sanitary disposal of excreta by encouraging the use of properly constructed latrines to replace indiscriminate defecation in or near surface water, but it is virtually impossible to observe complete sanitary control over the entire watershed (Wagner and Lanoix, 1959).

River intakes

An intake should be sited to prevent the entry of suspended matter under all regimes. In order to reduce the abstraction of sediment with water the intake should not be close to the river bed and the pipe should be large enough to keep the velocity below 0·15 m/s. The intake should be protected from large floating objects, for example by a wooden crib as shown in Figure 9·1. A small diversion dam placed across the river can be used to maintain a sufficient depth of water when the river is low. The basin so formed reduces turbidity by slowing down the flow. Where water is pumped from a river with considerable variation of level, a floating intake can be used. This may be supported on oil drums. In order to protect the treatment plant from large objects, including fish, a coarse bar screen is sometimes provided. Bars are commonly about 20 mm diameter spaced 60–100 mm apart. If it is impossible to avoid the entrance of

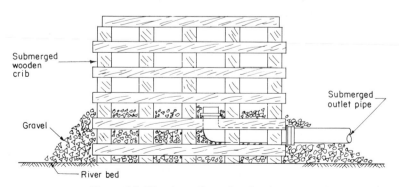

Figure 9.1 Wooden crib at river intake

sand and grit, a separate grit trap may be provided. The velocity should be about 800 mm/s to prevent the deposition of organic matter.

Infiltration galleries and wells

With suitable bed conditions water can be abstracted from a river by digging tunnels parallel to the river or wells alongside the river. To some extent water is filtered in passing through the bed material. At Aurungabad in India an infiltration gallery nearly three thousand metres long with a brick arch was built during the sixteenth century. The gallery was nearly four metres below the bed of the river and in 1886 yielded 7700 m³ of water in 24 hours (Wallace, 1893).

Protection of wells

In many places water is withdrawn from shallow hand-dug wells by going down to the water (step wells), and elsewhere the top of the well is open in such a way that the water becomes polluted. Improvements to hand-dug wells should include the following:

(1) The sides of the well should be lined with impervious material to a depth of about 3 m to prevent the entry of water flowing near the ground.

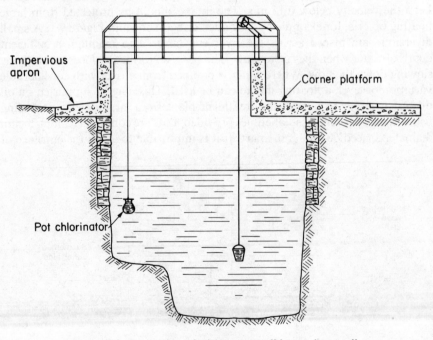

Figure 9.2 Conversion of a large step well into a draw well

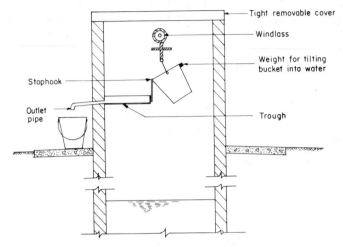

Figure 9.3 Draw well with windlass

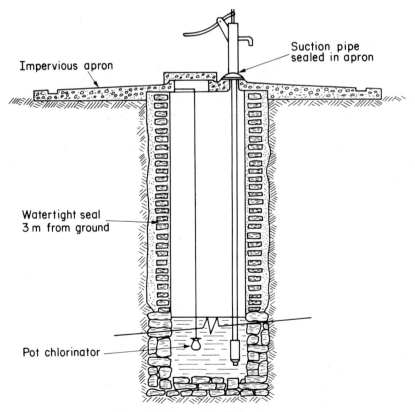

Figure 9.4 Dug well with hand-pump

(2) An impervious aprun should be constructed round the well mouth to prevent surface water from entering the well, to divert spilled water away from the well-mouth to a soakaway and to provide a comparatively dry floor for well-users.

(3) An area within about 15 m of the well should be kept free from pollution. In this area there should be no dumping of refuse and any pit latrines, soakaways or cesspits should be relocated.

(4) The method of abstraction should be improved. Figure 9·2 shows a structure for converting a large step well into a draw well. This includes a parapet wall to prevent users entering the well. A further improvement is to avoid all contact with the bucket and rope so that water in the well cannot be contaminated by dirty hands. The windlass shown in Figure 9·3 achieves this and the roof prevents dirt entering the well. Figure 9·4 shows a dug well fitted with a hand-pump.

It will be noted that in Figures 9·2 and 9·4 a pot chlorinator is included. Improvements (2) and (3) above also apply to shallow tube wells used with a hand-pump. There should be no perforations for the ingress of water in the top 3 m of the tube.

Protection of springs

Spring water is usually of good quality but may easily be contaminated by people collecting water and by polluted surface water. Protection can be provided by digging a ditch at least fifteen metres from the spring to divert surface water and providing a covered cistern to collect the spring water (see Figure 9.5). The supply may be drawn from a tap near the spring or piped to buildings. An overflow and a drain for cleaning ditritus should be provided and all pipes should be screened. Wastewater from any tap, from the overflow and from the drainage pipe should be led well away from the spring by adequate drains. A further precaution is to exclude any animals from the area around the spring by erecting a fence.

Abstraction from ponds or tanks

For a newly constructed pond, or a pond where a portion can be dammed temporarily, a trench can be dug from the side under the pond. A collector pipe is laid in the trench and is surrounded by a layer of large stones around which are piled two or three layers of gravel of gradually decreasing size and the trench is finally filled with sand. The collector pipe leads to a well built of impervious material or to a sand filter. Water can be lifted from the well by installing a hand-pump. For existing ponds which must remain in use, a 40 mm diameter plastic pipe can be pushed from a well and a floating intake provided as shown in Figure 9·6.

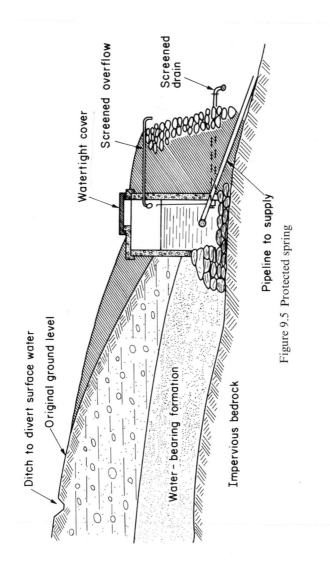

Figure 9.5 Protected spring

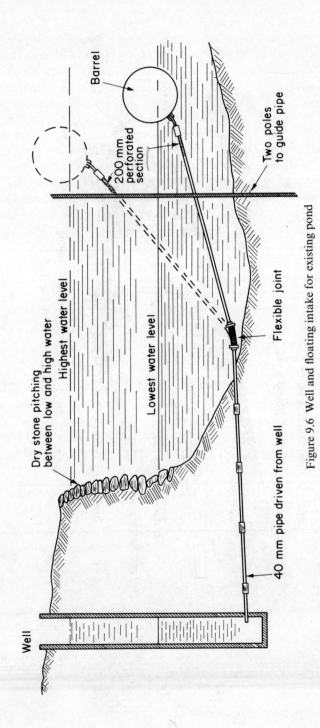

Figure 9.6 Well and floating intake for existing pond

Barrel

200 mm perforated section

Two poles to guide pipe

Dry stone pitching between low and high water

Highest water level

Lowest water level

Flexible joint

40 mm pipe driven from well

Well

9.5 STORAGE AND SEDIMENTATION

Tanks, reservoirs or ponds through which water passes slowly are often provided for the settlement, or sedimentation, or suspended matter and reduction of turbidity. The rate of settlement of solids depends on the particle size and may only amount to a few millimetres an hour for fine clays and colloids unless coagulation is aided by chemicals such as alum. Occasionally concrete sedimentation tanks of conventional design are constructed. The retention time should be based on jar-tests on samples typical of all regimes of the river. Twort, Hoather and Law (1974) advise that sedimentation tanks should be three times the theoretical size, but point out that with tropical temperatures 50% less detention time is possible owing to faster settling of solids. Reservoirs or storage basins reduce turbidity by sedimentation but their primary purpose is to enable water to be drawn throughout the year when the streamflow is variable. They also balance the quality by mixing highly turbid floodwaters with clear settled water.

Storage basins and underground cisterns have been used for thousands of years to retain seasonal rainfall or streamflow through dry weather. An unusual tank still employed in Kordofan in western Sudan is the bulbous baobab or *tebeldi* tree *(Adansonia digitata)*. Homar tribesmen cut a 400 mm hole leading to a large cavern hollowed out inside the trunk. Some of these 'reservoirs' are large enough to hold fourteen cubic metres of water which is poured in by hand during the short rainy season (Davies, 1957). A large number of *tebeldi* cisterns are still in use.

A storage basin may be formed by building a simple earth dam up to nine metres high, and small basins can be made from stabilized soil. They may be lined with concrete, masonry or polythene sheeting. The minimum depth of water should be 1·8 metres, and allowance should be made for losses by evaporation and seepage. Evaporation may be up to 2 metres a year. In the first year of impoundment of the *hafir* at Baggara for the supply of El Obeid in western Sudan losses by seepage and evaporation were 25 mm/d during the dry season. In the second year the losses were 15 mm/d. The capacity should be sufficient for deposited silt which may amount to 7% of the total capacity in dry areas where the catchment has little vegetation. Waste drains can be provided to get rid of bottom deposits during flood-flow; it is important to keep the valves of these drains lubricated. When first constructed the area to be flooded should be cleared of vegetation, and routine maintenance should include the control of weeds, especially when the water level is low.

During storage there is a substantial reduction of bacteria and especially of pathogens which are sensitive to changes of food supply, temperature and other environmental conditions. Removal of bacteria is partly due to sedimentation and chemical changes. In addition ultraviolet rays in sunlight have a germicidal effect which may penetrate to a depth of three metres in water of low turbidity, and bacteria are consumed by protozoa and other predatory

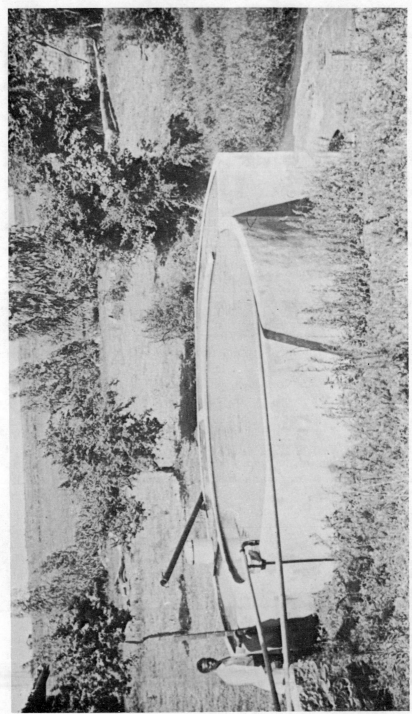

A farm water supply in Kenya. The water is pumped from a stream into the sedimentation tank. This young sanitary engineer is experimenting with various alum doses to overcome severe seasonal turbidity problems (photograph : D. D. Mara)

organisms. About 90% of bacteria are removed in a week and there may be higher mortality depending on local conditions—for example, the reduction of bacteria is greater in alkaline water. Provided there is no added pollution during storage, water should be held for as long as possible to reduce the number of human faecal bacteria.

Storage can be valuable in the control of schistosomiasis. In the life-cycle of the schistosome, free-swimming *miracidia* excreted by an infected person die within 24 hours if they do not reach the intermediate host, the fresh water snail. *Cercariae* from infected snails can only live for 48 hours if they do not reach a human or animal host. So two day's storage capacity provides an effective barrier to transmission of the disease as long as cercariae-shedding snails do not enter the tank. However, storage basins can act as breeding grounds for host snails which are usually established in shallows along the shoreline. Deepening and straightening the banks of the basin is helpful and galvanized screens with a 3 mm mesh can be provided to trap snails from upstream flow. Planned variation in water level has been successfully used to reduce the snail population; snails are stranded as the water drops and become desiccated or are eaten by land birds or animals (McJunkin, 1970).

In all tanks and reservoirs the inlets and outlets require careful siting. In a small tank incoming flow should be distributed evenly to prevent currents and the outlet usually consists of a weir extending across the whole width. Short-circuiting should be reduced as much as possible although this is difficult as the flow through tanks depends upon a number of variable factors including any temperature difference between incoming water and the contents of the tank. For large tanks and reservoirs the outlet is often sited some distance below the surface layer where there may be a high concentration of algae. Deeper water is usually cooler, but in certain areas may have a higher content of iron and manganese.

Algae help in the purification of water by symbiosis with aerobic bacteria, but excessive algal growth causes great problems in many areas. Eutrophication, or biological enrichment, depends on a supply of nutrients like phosphorus and nitrogen, and run-off from fertilized agricultural land has led to eutrophication problems including the blockage by algae of intakes and other parts of the treatment plant. Copper sulphate in concentrations of about 0·50 mg/l can be used to eliminate algae, but such doses can be lethal to some fish. Fish have been deliberately introduced to some tanks as a means of algal control. Wagner and Lanoix (1959) advise designers to look at other local ponds and reservoirs to see the extent of algal growth. Since sunlight is essential for photosynthesis, some small tanks are covered, and this also reduces the chances of contamination.

Access to sedimentation or storage tanks should, of course, be restricted as much as possible to limit pollution. In large reservoirs where it is impracticable to control pollution over the whole area, it should at least be prevented within three hundred metres of intakes.

9.6 AERATION

Water may be aerated to remove excess gases or to cure an oxygen deficiency. Cox (1964) states that the primary purpose is to improve taste by removing hydrogen sulphide and the volatile taste-and-odour-producing waste of algae or decomposition of organic matter. Aerated water is more palatable, as unaerated water has a 'flat' taste. Aeration may make water less corrosive by removing carbon dioxide, although it rarely reduces the carbon dioxide level below 4·5 mg/l, and corrosion is then prevented only if the alkalinity of the water exceeds 100 mg/l.

In water which is supersaturated with oxygen, aeration causes excess oxygen to be released, thus avoiding possible lifting of the surface in filters. On the other hand, increasing the oxygen content of oxygen-deficient water results in the oxidation of ferrous and manganese ions. Where the iron and manganese content of natural water is high this may be the greatest benefit of aeration. When water is alkaline (pH greater than 7) ferrous bicarbonate or sulphate is reduced in the presence of oxygen to ferric oxide which is insoluble. If the iron content is less than 5 mg/l it can be removed by aeration and filtration; with a higher iron content other means may be employed to remove the ferric precipitate to prevent filters becoming overloaded.

For rural plants there are four methods of aeration—spray nozzles, cascades, inclined aprons and tray aerators.

Spray aeration

When water is already under a pressure head of 7 m or more, as when discharged from boreholes, it can be sprayed into basins through nozzles of special design. The nozzles are usually 25–40 mm in diameter and each will deliver at least 18 m^3/h. The basin should be large enough to catch wind-blown spray, or the aerator may be surrounded by louvers. Up to 75% of carbon dioxide can be removed in a spray aerator. If the total flow is low, efficiency can be maintained by closing the supply to some of the nozzles.

Cascades

Water is allowed to fall as a thin sheet over one or more concrete steps, as shown in Figure 9.7(a). Overman (1968) states that a single cascade with a 400 mm supply can aerate 9000 cubic metres of water a day with 50%–60% carbon dioxide removal.

Inclined aprons

Water passes down as inclined channel (Figure 9.7(b)) fitted with studs or plates so that the flow is turbulent with a zigzag movement. 25–50 per cent of carbon dioxide may be removed.

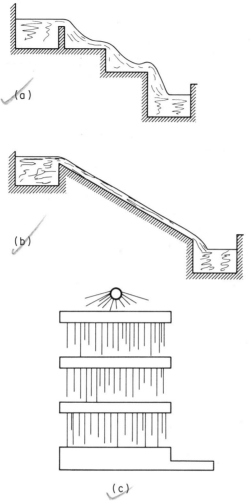

Figure 9.7 Cascade, inclined apron and tray aerators

Tray aerators

In these water falls through a series of trays perforated with small holes (Figure 9.7(c)). These should be 5–12 mm in diameter at 25–75 mm centres (Ministry of Health, India, 1962). The area of the trays required varies between 0·015 and 0·045 square metres per cubic metre of water passing through each hour. Tray aerators are often built in stacks of four to six trays giving a total height of 1·2–3 m. The trays may be filled with layers of coke or gravel of about 50 mm size. Tray aerators give 30%–60% removal of carbon dioxide and sufficient oxygen for iron removal.

A hand-operated unit for iron and manganese treatment has been developed by NEERI in India (Arceivala, undated). The unit consists of four cylinders

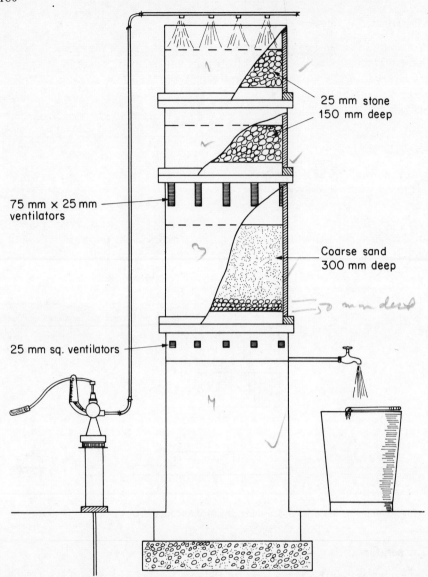

25 mm stone
150 mm deep

75 mm × 25 mm
ventilators

Coarse sand
300 mm deep

25 mm sq. ventilators

Figure 9.8 Hand-operated unit for iron and manganese removal

placed on top of each other as shown in Figure 9.8. A 150 mm layer of assorted 20–50 mm stones is placed in each of the top two cylinders. In the third layer a 50 mm deep layer of 10–20 mm stones supports a 300 mm layer of coarse sand. The gravel becomes coated with oxides of iron which help in the further oxidation of iron and manganese. Water is collected in the bottom cylinder and is withdrawn through a 12 mm tap into a bucket.

Maintenance of aerators

Protection of water during aeration is advisable to prevent the access of insects that might breed on slime. Slime and algal growth in basins, cascades and aprons can be controlled by applying a solution of copper sulphate or copper sulphate and lime with a whitewash brush. The solution should be mixed in a plastic bucket.

9.7 FILTRATION

Filtration is the most important treatment process. Slow sand filters have great advantages for developing countries, although other types are also widely used.

Household filters, such as the Berkefeld shown in Figure 9.9, will completely remove bacteria if the diatomaceous filter candle is fine-grained. The candle should be thoroughly cleaned and then boiled every few days. Some candles are impregnated with a silver catalyst which kills bacteria. The candle only has to be cleaned when it becomes clogged (WHO–IRCCWS, 1973).

Rapid sand filters, in which water passes through a bed of sand under gravity or pressure, are commonly used for the treatment of urban supplies. When the filter sand becomes clogged it is cleaned by backwashing, often assisted by compressed air. Clogging can be reduced by using two or more layers of filtering media, such as anthracite and sand, so that the water first passes through coarse material which retains larger solids. On back-washing the lighter anthracite, with larger pore size, stays on top.

Upflow filters enable small particles to pass through the lower, larger-sized grains of media and to be retained on the higher, smaller grains. The stratification of the media is preserved during backwashing.

Intermediate and series filtration have received a great deal of attention in India and elsewhere. Patwardhan (1975) proposed a number of standard

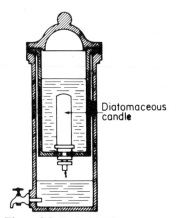

Figure 9.9 Berkefeld filter

filter types depending upon the turbidity of the raw water and NEERI recommended a roughing filter operated at a very high rate followed by slow sand filtration or an upflow filter (Arceivala, undated). Agarwal and Agrawal (1975) have successfully used intermediate rates following alum dosing.

Local media have been used successfully in Thailand. Following experiments at AIT, Bangkok, Frankel and Sevilla (1972) proposed that for turbid waters a roughing filter of coconut husk fibre should be followed by passage through a burnt rice filter. Field trials were later carried out in villages using locally-made earthenware pots of one cubic metre capacity to contain the filter media (Frankel, 1974).

Slow sand filter

Huisman and Wood (1974) claim that 'no other single process can effect such an improvement in the physical, chemical, and bacteriological quality of normal surface water'.

Advantage of slow sand filters

'Biological' filters, or slow sand filters, are used for the water in some of the world's largest cities, such as London and Amsterdam. The quality of the treated water is very good and micro-organisms are removed to such an extent that there is no aftergrowth in distribution pipes. No chemicals are used and no unpleasant taste is added.

For developing countries there are a number of special advantages:

(1) The cost of construction is low, especially where manual labour is used.

(2) Simplicity of design and operation means that filters can be built and used with limited technical supervision. No special pipework, equipment or instrumentation is needed.

(3) The labour required for maintenance can be unskilled as the major job is cleaning the beds, which can be done by hand.

(4) Imports of material and equipment can be negligible and no chemicals are required.

(5) Power is not required if a fall is available on site, as there are no moving parts or requirements for compressed air or high-pressure water.

(6) Variations in raw water quality and temperature can be accommodated provided turbidity does not become excessive; and overloading for short periods does no harm.

(7) Water is saved—an important matter in many areas—because large quantities of washwater are not required.

(8) Sludge, which is often a major problem with water treatment by more sophisticated methods, is less troublesome. There is less of it and it is easily dewatered.

Purification in slow sand filters

Figure 9.10 shows the essential parts of a small filter. In a mature bed a thin layer called the *schmutzdecke* forms on the surface of the bed. This *schmutzdecke* consists of algae, plankton, bacteria and other forms of life and is very active. The processes causing purification of the water as it passes through the filter are as follows

(1) Water is stored in the reservoir for anything up to 12 hours during which it is improved in the same way as in any storage basin. Heavy solids settle and light solids coagulate; bacteria are reduced: algae increase during daylight, producing oxygen; and there is some chemical oxidation of organic matter.

(2) In the *schmutzdecke* micro-organisms break down organic matter and a great deal of inorganic suspended matter is retained by straining.

(3) In the sand bed there are complex processes at work. As Shah (1971) has pointed out, a filter in no way resembles a tea-strainer, which only retains solids which are larger than the size of the holes. In a biological filter, minute particles are acted upon by a variety of forces. The space between sand grains is gradually reduced as the grains become covered with a sticky layer formed of material attracted to the grains by adsorption. As water goes through the bed it is constantly changing direction so that particles come into contact with the grains by centrifugal and intertial forces. Between the grain there are pockets which act as tiny sedimentation basins. At the same time the active microscopic life in the sticky layers around the grain, consisting of bacteria, protozoa, and other micro-organisms, feed on impurities and each other. This life-filled zone extends about half a metre down from the surface, but gradually decreases in activity downwards as the water is purified and contains less food. In the bottom layers of the bed the compounds formed by biological activity are further reduced by chemical action.

Organic matter and micro-organisms in the raw water (including bacteria and viruses of faecal origin) have been converted to simple and harmless inorganic salts in solution. During this conversion oxygen in the water has been used up and carbon dioxide has been evolved and absorbed. The final process is therefore aeration. As the filter effluent passes over the weir oxygen is taken up and surplus carbon dioxide is rejected. At the same time the weir, in conjunction with the regulating valve, controls the flow through the filter and the water level in the reservoir over the bed.

A new filter takes some time to 'mature'—to build up the *schmutzdecke* and the sticky layers round the sand grains. During this time effluent water will not be satisfactory. For several weeks the filter will operate well with the regulating valve almost fully closed. Then as the *schmutzdecke* becomes clogged the valve is gradually opened, a little each day, to maintain the required rate of flow. When the valve is fully opened and the flow again decreases, the filter must be cleaned. This is done by lowering the water level to a couple of hundred

184

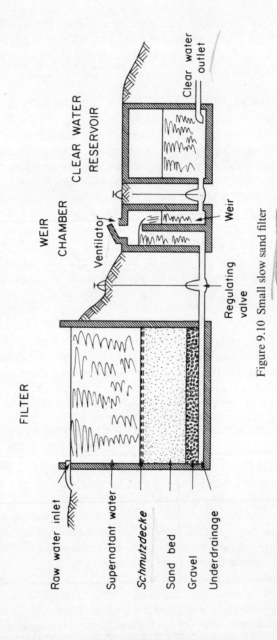

Figure 9.10 Small slow sand filter

millimetres below the surface of the bed and then carefully removing the *schmutzdecke* using flat-nosed shovels. The *schmutzdecke* and the sand dug up with it may be tipped, or the sand may be washed for re-use.

Sand beds are usually made with depths of about half a metre over what is required for purification so that 10–20 mm may be removed every two months or so. After four or five years, when the sand surface is at its lowest limit, new or washed sand is brought in to bring up the bed to its original depth. New sand should be placed under old by 'throwing over' the old sand. In this way the top layer which is richest in microbiological life can be kept at the top.

Performance of slow sand filters

Although raw water turbidities of 100–200 mg/l can be tolerated for two or three days, biological filters work best with fairly clear raw water—an upper limit of 50 mg/l is sometimes taken as a guide. If river water turbidity is often higher than 50 mg/l some preliminary treatment such as storage or 'roughing filters' should be used. Biological filters produce a clear effluent free from organic matter and nutrient. This limits the formation of slime and bacteria in distribution systems. Between 99·0% and 99·99% of bacteria may be removed, and biological filters remove all cercariae of schistosomiasis if properly designed, constructed and maintained (McJunkin, 1970). They can be used following aeration to remove iron and manganese, and reduce colour in raw water.

9.8 DISINFECTION

In many small water supply schemes where the physical and chemical quality of water is satisfactory, disinfection is the only treatment provided. Since the prime object of water treatment is health-protection, it follows that the destruction of pathogens is of major importance. Ozone is a disinfectant widely used in some industrial countries but it required a degree of technical supervision beyond the means of rural areas in most developing countries.

Chlorination

Chlorine, in one form or other, is the most common disinfectant. Its action is to destroy the enzymes essential for the existence of micro-organisms. In addition to its germicidal ability, chlorine oxidizes iron, manganese and hydrogen sulphide; it destroys taste-and-colour-producing constituents; it controls algae and slime; and it aids coagulation (Rajagopalan and Shiffman, 1974). Because it is an oxidizing agent, part of any chlorine applied is used by organic matter, forming chloramines. Enough chlorine must therefore be applied for reaction with organic matter and micro-organisms (the 'chlorine demand'), and to leave a surplus to deal with further infection by pathogens. This surplus is called the 'residual chlorine'. The chlorine takes some time to act on the organic matter and micro-organisms, a period which is called the 'contact

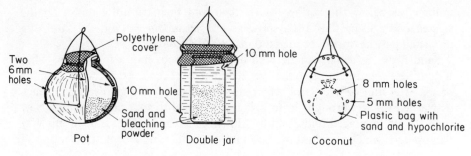

Figure 9.11 Simple chlorination pots

time'. The effectiveness of disinfectant potential is therefore expressed as residual chlorine after a certain contact time.

For distribution systems carrying treated water, a residual chlorine concentration of 0·2 mg/l after 20 minutes contact is usually sufficient. In general for rural supplies, with or without treatment, 0·5 mg/l after 30 minutes is recommended. Chlorine residual of 1 mg/l after 30 minutes will kill schistosomiasis cercariae (WHO, 1965), and amoebic cysts may require 2 mg/l after 30 minutes. At these higher concentrations the taste of the water is unpleasant. The amount of residual chlorine is measured by tests using orthotolidine, which are simple and require little equipment. The orthotolidine–arsenite (OTA) test gives by calculation the chlorine demand, the residual chlorine and the total chlorine.

Bleaching powder

For urban water supply chlorine is often applied as a gas, but for rural schemes a solution made from a powder is more convenient. The most common material is bleaching powder, which is a mixture of calcium hydroxide, calcium chloride and calcium hypochlorite. It has 20%–35% available chlorine, is easy to handle although it is bulky and comparatively unstable. If opened only once a day for ten minutes, 5% of its strength is lost in 40 days: if left open all the time it will lose 18%. Bleaching powder has been used for the disinfection of wells in India for a long time (Turner, 1914), and recently simple chlorination pots have been developed in India (CPHERI, undated and 1972) and elsewhere. These are charged with an equal-weight mixture of bleaching powder and sand. As can be seen from Figure 9.11, the containers have small holes so that water passes slowly through.

Solutions should be kept in the dark as there is a serious loss of strength if they are exposed to light. Containers should be of wood, plastic, ceramic or cement which are resistant to corrosion. The maximum chlorine concentration is 5%, made for example by mixing 4 kg of powder having 25% available chlorine with 20 litres of water. Bleaching powder contains an excess of lime which can block feed pipes and so a solution should be decanted from the mixing tank into a feed tank.

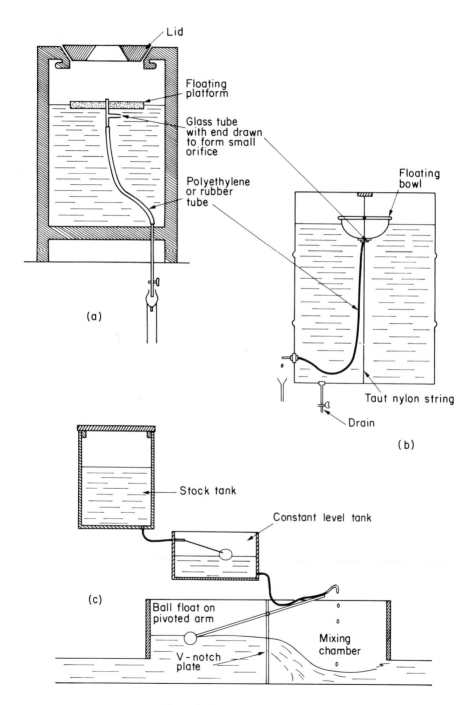

Figure 9.12 Apparatus for drip-feed

High-test hypochlorite

This is a granular material with higher available chlorine (60%–70%). It is more stable than bleaching powder, especially in tropical conditions, but containers have been known to burst if left in the hot sun (WHO–IRCCWS, 1973). It is completely soluble in water.

Drip-feed apparatus

Several devices have been introduced to enable chlorine solution to be applied at a uniform rate as the level in the container drops. Some of these are shown in Figure 9.12. A simple arrangement to meter the solution feed so that it is approximately proportional to the flow of water in a channel is shown in Figure 9.12(c).

Disinfection of tanks and wells

Before using new storage tanks, wells, pipes or surfaces which will come into contact with water (such as trays of aerators), they should be thoroughly disinfected. There are two ways of doing this. One is to put sufficient bleaching powder or high test hydrochlorite in the water to give 50 mg/l available chlorine and leave it for twelve hours, adding more chlorine if there is a continuous flow of water, as in the storage tank for a protected spring. The solution is then removed or allowed to flow out, and is replaced by fresh water. The second method is to clean walls and other surfaces and then apply a strong solution, such as one which gives 200 mg/l available chlorine. A whitewash brush can be used to apply the solution.

Household disinfection

Chlorine or iodine tablets can be used to treat drinking water. Iodine is a good disinfectant but is too expensive for community use. Some iodine compound tablets are effective against bacteria, cysts, cercariae and some viruses. Boiling is an effective method of disinfection. It is essential to bring the water to a 'rolling boil' and Nnochiri (1975) recommends that it should be boiled for 30 minutes to destory protozoal cysts and ova. To prevent recontamination the water should be cooled in the container in which it was boiled.

9.9 PLANS AND PROGRAMMES

Having considered the various ways in which water can be treated, we return to our first thesis: the ideal rural water supply scheme in most developing countries is that which requires no treatment at all.

Field studies

If maximum value is to be obtained from any resources of money, material and time which can be made available, it is absolutely essential that plans for water supply should be based on full and correct information. This can usually only be obtained on site and the importance of field investigations cannot be emphasized too strongly. Plans for water treatment based on the situation during dry weather may be completely inappropriate in the rainy season, and vice versa. Apart from alterations in the quantity and quality of available water, the habits of local people may change depending on whether farm work can be carried on or not. The field study must ensure that plans for all but the simplest water treatment are based on properly-measured analysis of water quality—physical, chemical and bacteriological.

Simplicity

All schemes should be as simple as possible, even where semi-trained personnel and adequate supervision are available. It should not be necessary for the operator to make complicated calculations and simple 'yes or no' decisions should be the most that are required in most cases: 'if the water level drops below the painted mark, rotate the valve one turn in the direction of the arrow'. If, exceptionally, a range of choices is inevitable as in applying a dose of bleaching powder, it is often wise to use nomograms rather than tables of figures or graphs (Dunn, 1949).

Maximum use of resources

The availability of land, labour, equipment and funds is completely different in industrialized and developing nations. Commenting on this, a WHO Scientific Group (1967) concluded that there is a 'need for the development of engineering programmes that take into account the general availability of land and labour in developing countries'.

Planning land use

Because land is often plentiful, simple treatment methods which require a substantial area can be used; simple storage basins and slow sand filters are examples. Land may be available 'anywhere around' and advantage should be taken of this by placing any works at the best possible place in relation to the fall required to carry water through. Allowance should always be made for extension in the future. Sufficient space should be left for additional capacity and any structures, pipework or valves should be planned so that they can be incorporated in a future enlarged scheme.

Labour and incentive

In most developing countries there are plenty of people who are not fully employed throughout the year even if there are seasons of intense agricultural activity. This valuable resource can be utilized if the community is anxious to improve its water supply. The importance of community participation is stressed throughout this book. At a conference in South-East Asia, Unakul (1970) reported that when village community development committees were involved in the management of water supply in Thailand the systems were better managed. A WHO Expert Committee (1969) stated that 'promotion of community interest and participation is essential for the initial and continuing success of any community water supply programme', and Pineo and Subrahmanyam (1975) wrote that 'it is hard to find a successful rural community water supply programme that did not involve active community participation'.

The crux of the success of any water treatment programme is therefore likely to be the concern of the people. If they know the value of good water and are aware of the importance of avoiding pollution and carrying out the required maintenance, then the scheme will have a chance of success. Although technical skill is required, especially in relating the treatment process to the raw water, the most important factor in the treatment of water is consumer education.

9.10 REFERENCES

Agarwal, I. C. and Agrawal, G. D. (1975). Intermediate rate filtration for hot and developing countries. Paper presented at the Conference on *Water, Waste and Health in Hot Countries* (Ed. John Pickford). Loughborough: University of Technology.

Arceivala, S. J. (undated). *Rural Sanitation*. Nagpur, India: Central Public Health Engineering Research Institute.

Arceivala, S. J. (1971). In: *Proceedings of the Seminar on water supply and sanitary problems in urban areas below one lakh population, Roorkee, 1971*.

Cox, D. R. (1964). *Operation and Control of Water Treatment Processes*. (Monograph Series no. 49). Geneva: WHO.

CPHERI (undated). *Disinfection Techniques for Small Community Water Supplies*. Nagpur: Central Public Health Engineering Research Institute.

CPHERI (1972). *Disinfection of Well Waters*. (Technical Digest no. 26). Nagpur: Central Public Health Engineering Research Institute.

Craun, G. and McCabe, L. J. (1973). Review of the causes of waterborne-disease outbreaks *Journal of the American Water Works Association*, **65**, 74–84.

Davies, R. (1957). *The Camel's Back—service in the Rural Sudan*. London: Murray.

Dunn, J. S. (1949). *The application of nomograms to the purification by chemical treatment of tropical waters*. Accra: Government Printing Department.

Fair, G. M., Geyer, J. C. and Okun, D. A. (1966). *Water and Wastewater Engineering*. New York: Wiley.

Feachem, R. (1973). *Domestic Water use in the New Guinea Highlands: the case of the Raiapu Enga*. (Report no. 132.) Sydney: University of New South Wales, School of Civil Engineering.

Frankel, R. J. (1974). *Evaluation of low cost water filters in rural communities of the lower Mekong Basin*. Bangkok: Asian Institute of Technology.

Frankel, R. J. and Sevilla, A. S. (1972). *An Asian technological approach to water reuse: series filtration using local filter media*. Paper presented at the 6th Conference of the International Association of Water Pollution Research, Jerusalem.

Huisman, L. and Wood, W. E. (1974). *Slow Sand Filtration*. Geneva: World Health Organization.

Key, A. (1967). Water pollution: a world-wide problem. In: *Report on the Water Pollution Seminar*. Dublin: Institution of Civil Engineers, Ireland.

McJunkin, F. E. (1970). *Engineering Measures for Control of Schistosomiasis*. Washington: Office of Health, Agency for International Development.

Mara, D. D. (1974). *Bacteriology for Sanitary Engineers*. Edinburgh: Churchill Livingstone.

Miller, A. D. (1962). *Water and man's health*. (AID Community Water Supply Technical Series No. 5.) Washington: Agency for International Development.

Ministry of Health, India (1962). *Public Health Engineering manual and code of practice: Section 1-A, Manual on water supply*. New Delhi: Government of India.

Nnochiri, E. (1975). *Medical microbiology in the tropics*. London: Oxford University Press.

Overman, M. (1968). *Water: solutions of a problem of supply and demand*. London: Aldus Books.

Patwardhan, S. V. (1975). Low cost water treatment for developing countries. Paper presented at the Conference on: *Water, Waste and Health in Hot Countries* (Ed. John Pickford). Loughborough: University of Technology.

Pineo, S. C. and Subrahmanyam, D. V. (1975). *Community water supply and excreta disposal situation in the developing countries*. (Offset Publication No. 15.) Geneva: World Health Organization.

Rajagopalan, S. and Shiffman, M. A. (1974). *Guide to simple sanitary measures for the control of enteric diseases*. Geneva: World Health Organization.

Reid, E. F. (1956). Water treatment in the tropics. *Journal of the Institution of Water Engineers*, **10**, 515–530.

Saunders, R. J., and Warford, J. J. (1974). *Village water supply and sanitation in less developed countries*. (Public Utilities Report No. RES2.) Washington D. C.: International Bank for Reconstruction and Development.

Shah, N. A. (1971). *Water-supply engineering*. London: Asia Publishing House.

Southgate, B. A. (1969). *Water: pollution and conservation*. London: Thunderbird Enterprises.

Turner, J. A. (1914). *Sanitation in India*. Bombay: The Times of India.

Twort, A. C., Hoather, R. C. and Law, F. M. (1974). *Water Supply*. London: Edward Arnold.

Unakul, S. (1970). Thailand's rural community water supply program. In: *Water supply and wastewater disposal in developing countries* (Ed. M. B. Pescod and D. A. Okun). Bangkok: Asian Institute of Technology.

United Nations (1953). *The sediment problem*. Bangkok: UN Economic Commission for Asia and the Far East.

Wagner, E. G. and Lanoix, J. N. (1959). *Water supply for rural areas and small communities*. (Monograph Series no. 42.) Geneva: WHO.

Wallace, J. (1893). *Sanitary Engineering in India*. Bombay: Education Society's Steam Press.

WHO (1965). *Snail Control in the Prevention of Bilharziasis*. (Monograph Series no. 50.) Geneva: World Health Organization.

WHO (1969). *WHO Chronicle*, **25**, 70.

WHO (1971). *International Standards for Drinking Water*, 3rd ed. Geneva: World Health Organization.

WHO (1969). *Community Water Supply*. (Technical Report Series No. 420.) Geneva: World Halth Organization.

WHO (1973). *Schistosomiasis Control*. (Technical Report Series No. 515.) Geneva: World Health Organization.

WHO–IRCCWS (1973). *The purification of water on a small scale*. (Technical Paper No. 3.) The Hague: World Health Organization International Reference Centre for Community Water Supply.

WHO Scientific Group (1967). *Treatment and Disposal of Water*. (Technical Report Series No. 367.) Geneva: World Health Organization.

III

Institutional Development

10

Institutional Development
for Sanitation and Water Supply

MICHAEL G. MCGARRY

10.1 BACKGROUND

In recognition of the fact that the provision of water supply and sanitation services to low-income populations is pitifully inadequate and that the rate of providing these services is insufficient even to catch up with population growth, several international agencies including the World Health Organization, the International Development Research Centre, OECD, UNICEF, IBRD, UNEP and UNDP undertook collective action to promote and assist the improvement of water supply and sanitation in the rural and squatter settlement populations of developing countries. In a background document the Ad Hoc Working Group (1975), comprising representatives of these organizations, stated that:

The lot of people living in rural areas and on the fringes of cities is becoming a matter of increasing concern to governments. From the standpoint of sanitation and public health, the conditions in which these people live usually are extremely bad. About four-fifths of the world's rural population, or well over 1000 million men, women and children, do not have safe water available to them in adequate quantities. Basic sanitary services are largely absent.

The prospects for 1980 are unfortunately worse. At the present pace of installing needed facilities, it would be optimistic to hope to reach even 25% of the people in the rural or fringe areas by that year. With the expected growth of the world's population, moreover, by 1980 some 60 million more people will be without safe water than in 1970. At the same time, the volume of human waste will have increased, further aggravating environmental pollution and leading to preventable illness, debility and death because of poor water supply and inadequate facilities for the disposal of human excreta.

Stripped of the statistical evidence, the stark global facts are that: people need and want water; the pace of providing it is miserably slow; the existing prospect of speeding up the pace over the next 5 or 10 years is not promising; and where installations have been provided, they have been left with distressing frequency to fall into disrepair and disuse through faulty operation and maintenance.

In 1974, a technical panel of the Ad Hoc Working Group met to consider the factors constraining development of this sector. It concluded that in the main technology *per se* could not be considered either a weighty or controlling constraint. Rather, the slow pace is caused primarily by lack of appropriate national and local institutional infrastructures. Less dominant problems were considered to be internal and external financing. In order to meet the needs of water supply and sanitation, many institutions have responded on an individual basis. This has led to the spontaneous growth and interest in this sector within several agencies. In recognition of the technical nature of many solutions to water supply problems, jurisdiction has drifted away from medical personnel in ministries of health to sanitary engineers in water authorities and departments of sanitary engineering. Seldom are these activities coordinated. In some cases, 10 or more separate agencies are involved in supplying water within one country. As a consequence, interdepartmental and professional jealousies have arisen and misunderstandings and conflicts prevail.

There can be no single institutional infrastructure which all countries can adopt as an optimal model. Undoubtedly, several agencies within any one country will need to be involved in this sector. However, efforts must be coordinated to maximize benefits to the low-income populations. The most effective institutional infrastructure will need to reflect political and economic realities. Thus, at the present time, the most appropriate infrastructure to, say, Tanzania, will by no means simulate that of Bolivia.

Historically, efforts to expand water supplies were first made in the larger cities which, being assisted by UNDP, WHO, the World Bank and the Interamerican Development Bank, have in many cases succeeded in reaching the majority of the urban population. Only more recently have the national and international agencies begun to focus their attention on low-income populations in rural areas and the slums. Whereas the cities are normally able to form their own autonomous water and sewerage authorities or to work within the municipal government, responsibility for providing small town and dispersed populations with health infrastructure falls on the shoulders of the ministries of health, community development agencies and non-government organizations. At the present time, however, the main thrust of activity is still centred on medium-sized cities.

10.2 URBAN SANITATION AND WATER SUPPLIES

Out of necessity the larger urban centres have developed institutional infrastructures to cope, in one way or the other, with urgent demands of their rapidly growing populations. In contrast to rural villagers who may have several alternative sources of water supplies and locations for excreta disposal, those in urban areas, and particularly those in densely populated slum areas, are faced with having to draw water from centrally distributed supplies or purchase water by the pail-full usually at exorbitant prices from local vendors.

Only the largest city centres can claim financial viability in both water and sewerage. Financial efficiency is, however, at the heart of any successful programme. In many areas, water has traditionally been a natural right. With increasing costs of resource development, treatment and distribution, a point is reached where the government can no longer continue to provide free or nearly free supplies. This is particularly true of the urban centre where the majority is able and willing to pay for its water. On the other hand, the smaller rural communities invariably need some form of subsidy. Water supply and sanitation development programmes provide an opportunity for the government to put wealth redistribution policies into effect. It is somewhat surprising that, in countries purporting to follow such policies, city water supply and sewerage projects are subsidized by national funds which include revenues acquired from the rural areas.

Putting urban water supplies and sewerage on a sound financial footing begins in convincing the politician and householder of the necessity to pay for the services provided. Tariff rates and charges have in the past commonly been too low to meet even the costs of operation and maintenance, let alone those of amortization of loans, depreciation and establishment of reserves for future expansion. Most urban projects have been supported by straight non-return grants which are frequently spread too thinly and are inadequate to cover project and programme requirements. Many have been left incomplete and inoperative as a result. Grant programmes tend to be fragmented and badly coordinated, which only exacerbates poor financial management.

In recognition of the political difficulties in raising tariff rates to realistic levels the Brazilian government encourages municipalities to establish special water agencies to handle all aspects of water supply. These are either public authorities or 'mixed' companies—the board of directors of which comprises public officials and representatives of the commercial sector. This latter type of authority has the advantage of being as far away from the political arena and bureaucratic red tape as possible. Donaldson (Chapter 11) describes the system of revolving funds used to great advantage in financing municipal water services in several Latin American countries.

Professional personnel and technical manpower is more readily available in the urban centres than in the rural areas. Once trained at university level the young engineer is loath to lose himself in the rural hinterland. His career prospects are far brighter in the city. It is therefore easier for the municipal water and sewerage authority to attract engineers and technical personnel. As described later there are still difficulties in keeping the engineer in local government employment. Governments are commonly unable to compete with the commercial sector for qualified personnel. Likewise, there is a constant debilitating brain-drain of scarce manpower to the developed countries.

The provincial towns and, what Donaldson terms the 'rurban' centres, the smaller rural towns, are faced with a similar set of problems. Manpower shortages are even more severe and financing, whether derived from external sources or from within the country, is never sufficient to satisfy demand. During the past two decades it has become clear that the ministries of health and departments of community or rural development have neither the resources, administrative infrastructure nor the experience to cope with the problem alone. Central governments have been transferring authority for this sector to departments of public works or newly-formed national water authorities. Although a step in the right direction, this transfer of authority coupled with a lack of motivation on the part of the urban centred central government has often resulted in conflict, duplication and a political scramble for jurisdiction. The *modus operandi* behind such programmes is the same. The conventional approach to improving water supply and sanitation in the primate city is extended down to the smaller towns. Technologies, administration and even tariff mechanisms are similar. Provided that resources are not limiting, this approach is successful and have been widely supported by the international banks in reaching an ever-increasing number of households. As the government successfully completes its programmes in the larger cities, it turns to the smaller and less wealthy towns where this approach is less applicable. It is unfortunate that the cut-off point is reached at village-sized communities where communication between the community and central government is infrequent and inefficient, trained personnel are not available, and where the import of a technology and installation of equipment alone is wholly inadequate. In many countries, and in Latin America in particular, emphasis has been given to the major cities and provincial towns, largely on the basis that they are amenable to purely technical solutions, give greater return on investment and are more accessible. By taking the easiest path first, the way ahead has become more difficult.

In many ways this emphasis can be interpreted as subsidizing the wealthy at the opportunity cost of the poor who are greater in number and need. The theory that by supporting the wealthy sectors development benefits will trickle down to the poor, has not universally proved valid. Urban services projects have not had a multiplier effect as was once hoped. Rural development is not a natural consequence of urban prosperity. It is not until there is a conscious effort and a real shift in orientation towards rural development by governments that any real progress can be made in this sector.

10.3 MANPOWER DEVELOPMENT

Reacting to a deterioration in the urban environment, conscious of national prestige and with an eye towards tourism, many governments have made application for aid to develop master plans for water supply and sewerage for their largest cities from international aid and UN agencies. Most such studies, normally utilizing the services of foreign personnel at key managerial and technical levels, have all pointed to shortages in trained manpower—sanitary engineers, administrators, accountants and operating and maintenance staff. Wallpapering the crack is a relatively inexpensive exercise: promising young individuals are sent overseas or trained on-site during the final design stages of the project. Unfortunately, the national demand for this trained manpower is often far greater than can be met by these means. The commercial sector is able to offer higher salaries than the government and such personnel frequently leave government employment for higher salaries elsewhere. This approach to manpower development is very common. Unfortunately it is piecemeal, project-oriented and largely ineffective in attempting to solve a much larger, more complicated and longer-term problem. Manpower development is a dynamic, time-consuming process which cannot be taken lightly. Only through a carefully planned programme extending over a number of years can the required number of personnel, with sufficient education and experience, be acquired for efficient programme planning, implementation, management and operation.

With a view to medium-term manpower requirements, developing countries also look to international technical assistance which is not specifically tied to projects for the training of its professional sanitary engineers. This practice is a direct result of the lack of local facilities available and does not give adequate recognition to the long-term national demand in both the public service and the commercial sectors. Superficially, it may appear to be a valid approach; in theory, the better students are trained abroad in the donor countries' more advanced institutions at the donor's expense and return home to contribute to the recipient's national economy. To the chagrin of the developing country its better-educated students often fail to return but remain in the donor country to enjoy the relatively higher salaries while contributing to an already-developed economy. Efforts to curb this brain drain include 'bonding' the student to his former government department for a period of 2 to 5 years. This often fails as the returned student becomes discontented with his situation at home and ineffectual in his work.

Apart from draining the more educated manpower from the developing countries at substantial opportunity cost, the practice of sending students abroad for training has the additional drawback of not supporting local educational programmes. Although a number of students may return to be gainfully employed within the economy, no provision is made for local post-graduate programme development. The developing country thus becomes more and more dependent upon overseas aid. Particular mention is given here to the curricula of overseas postgraduate sanitary engineering programmes as not meeting the needs of developing countries. Major differences in climate, cultural and economic circumstances and the specific research objectives of the donor country institutions often result in inappropriate education being given to overseas students. Thus, a student who should be acquiring training in overall wastes management systems design ends up studying such obscure topics as the production of polysaccharides by microbes involved in the activated sludge process!

Again, there is a strong and natural tendency to respond to the needs of the largest city which are most obvious to the view of the elite. There are, however, much greater demands in the rural areas and smaller towns which often make up 90% of the population. Bangladesh, Burma, India, Indonesia and Thailand have a combined rural population of over 600 million without reasonable access to adequate water supplies. The estimated 1000-odd graduate sanitary engineers of the region who should ostensibly be responding to these demands are located in the larger cities with orientation towards urban problems. There has not been any serious attempt at conducting manpower surveys for environmental health requirements in any part of South-East Asia (WHO, 1974).

Most of the educational institutions of tropical countries which do offer courses in this sector have curricula patterned after those of the industrialized countries and do not respond to local needs. In regions other than Latin America, the sanitary engineering profession has suffered from having little prestige in terms of social acceptance. Thus, few good students are willing to enter programmes in this profession. In general, there is seldom any priority attached to education in environmental health engineering. No real emphasis is given to it in undergraduate programmes so that most students wishing to undertake such courses must go through an additional two years of study. Lack of sufficient priority given to this sector results in inadequate levels of funds to support the required number and quality of institutions undertaking educational activities.

Likewise, there is a severe shortage of training personnel, with the high demand of the environmental engineers in the private sector offering some two to three times government salaries, most graduates gravitate towards that sector thereby reducing the capacity to generate more environmental engineers. There is also an unmet demand for personnel to be trained at the sub-professional level, particularly in the rural areas. This demand is acutely felt in Latin America where water supply and sanitation programmes have developed more rapidly than in other regions. It is not even entirely clear what kind of sub-professional training is required. In the urban centres, the need is for more, and better trained, operating and maintenance personnel. However, at the village level, not only is maintenance of pumping and treatment equipment required, but also the technician or village health worker must be responsible for the promotion of the proper use of water supply, excreta disposal facilities and improvements in hygiene in the home at the basic preventative level.

There should be a relationship between demand and supply of trained personnel. As things now stand, with no quantitative data to hand, the priorities and funding of educational programmes to produce the required number of graduates is largely a matter of guesswork. Manpower planning programmes need to be initiated with a clear outcome-oriented approach, with well defined objectives and a commitment by the government to its implementation.

10.4 HEALTH AND CONDITIONS OF THE RURAL POOR

There are now about 550 million people living in absolute poverty, that is, with incomes of less than the equivalent of $ US 50 or less than one-third the national average income (World Bank, 1975a). Approximately 85% of these live in the rural areas of developing countries; most subsist in Asia while only 4% are to be found in Latin America. Within each country there are further disparities as exemplified by comparisons between rural and urban areas. The absolute poor of the rural areas are interspersed with the relatively wealthy, primarily providing a source of cheap labour. Vested interests militate against them, subjecting them to inequalities by means of unequal distribution of benefits from production. They are therefore denied access to the support and services necessary to raise the quality of their lives. In many countries the socio-economic system is firmly entrenched to their disadvantage. As an example, in some parts of Central America 90% of the land is owned by 1% of the population. As may be expected that 90% of land is the most productive; the worker being relegated to less valuable land is drawn into debilitating credit arrangements with the landlord and merchant. Without adequate land tenure the poor are unable to escape from the feudal web and so are forced to remain in a state of undernourishment, ignorance, disease and passive submission.

Emphasis in most developing countries has been on high rates of economic growth without adequate control over the distribution of wealth. As a result the industrial and urban sectors have prospered in many cases and have in effect established new and enlarged classes of wealthy, educated urban elite. The theory was that high rates of growth in the more receptive sectors of the economy would spread the benefits thereby accrued to the poorer sectors. Such growth however has taken place almost to the exclusion of the absolute poor who have been exploited by way of remaining an unorganized source of cheap labour. The gap between the urban elite and the rural poor continues to widen in most developing countries.

The positive correlation between socio-economic level and ill-health has been well documented. The core health problem of developing countries are infectious and parasitic diseases and malnutrition. These take their greatest toll amongst the poor. The inequitable distribution of ill-health according to socio-economic status places further debilitating burdens on the rural poor and slum peoples. Further distortion is introduced by means of the parasitic infections and diarrhoeal diseases which have their greatest impact on children that are between weaning and five years of age. Once weaned from the breast the child's food intake deteriorates in quality; he becomes more susceptible to the greatly increased number and variety of disease-causing agents. At least half of all deaths in developing countries are those of children under five (World Bank, 1975b).

Relative to the industrialized states most developing countries are characterized by a high proportion of children in the total population. High rates of population growth, ill-health and malnutrition are combined in a complex set of interactions which drive the peasant in a vicious circle towards poverty. Children are valuable assets to the household and provide security in old age; where poverty and high rates of child mortality persist families tend to be large and fertility rates high. It is understandable that under such conditions parents respond to a child's death with a desire to replace it. Population pressure on the land may lead to reduced per capita food availability, overcropping, soil degradation and malnutrition. Population pressure in the home lowers the quality of housing, induces crowding, insanitary conditions in the home and leads to ill-health which interacts with malnutrition to reduce productivity and drives the family further into the web of poverty.

Reduced fertility, morbidity and mortality rates are associated with raised socio-economic status. The high fertility/mortality cycle is difficult to break because the response to reduced mortality in the form of reduction in birth rates is slow. Improved health is one way of enabling the peasant to control his environment better. The net result of change in the complex balance of interrelated factors depends critically on the magnitude, nature and timing of responses. Health improvements, for example, reduce mortality rates, can increase fecundity and increase maternal survival—factors all fostering higher population growth rates. Thus when effected in isolation health benefits can be counterproductive by encouraging more rapid population growth and thereby undermining health gains. Improvements in health need to be integrated with other changes aimed at raising life's quality and thereby maintain that delicate but complex balance of factors leading to overall socio-economic advance.

10.5 VILLAGE SANITATION AND WATER SUPPLY

In addressing the difficulties of improving sanitation and water supply in villages and the more dispersed populations which are both geographically and culturally inaccessible one must first establish the basic objectives of such activity. The primary objective is, of course, to raise health levels although major secondary benefits related to overall development can be accrued through water supply in terms of improved village organizational structure, agriculture, communications with government and reductions in time and energy spent in fetching water. However, the question must be asked: Is the gift of a water pump in the village centre the most cost-effective way to achieve such objectives? The answer is, unfortunately, almost universally—no.

Even in purely technical terms it has been amply demonstrated (Saunders and Warford, 1974; McGarry, 1975) that the installation of water supply mechanisms in the community can go only part of the way towards improving health levels. If full benefits are to be realized, sanitation, hygiene in the home, changes in attitude and levels of health education must be implemented in conjunction with water supply. Despite this well demonstrated fact, national and international agencies continue to propagate water without any significant concurrent effort to improve basic sanitation levels. Reasons for this are relatively clear; firstly, technology is a means of communication and often the only medium through which central governments can interact with remote communities. Indeed, it is often used as a means of promoting government policy whereby the promise to provide water supply is made to the rural community behaving in some manner in line with government wishes. Water is a felt need of the peasant; a demand based largely on the wish to increase the availability and accessibility of water but rarely one connected to the wish to improve health. The concept of improving health by means of sanitation and water supply is an abstract one and difficult to communicate. It is only natural then that government agencies short-circuit educational requirements and social needs out of their programmes and rely solely on providing technology. Worse still, the almost universal failure in applying the technical approach to sanitation (for example, by providing water-seal slabs) has resulted in the deletion of excreta disposal improvements from nearly all such projects.

In trying to achieve our basic objectives a series of questions *must* be raised before we rush off in a charitable frame of mind to distribute tubewells, pumps and latrines. These relate to the very nature of central governments' interaction with the rural peoples, the stated and *de facto* politico-economic philosophies propounded, the basic motivational forces behind rural development policy and the means of communication used to project this policy.

Obviously such questions cannot be elaborated in a short paper on institutional development. I will, however, attempt to draw attention to their relevance to the manner in which government agencies implement water and sanitation programmes in the village and dispersed populations.

Viewpoint of the villager

For decades, even centuries, the villager and his forefathers have been engaged in making a living from the land. Government participation in his affairs is, more often than not, a recent phenomenon. His economic and social life qualities may have deteriorated or be in jeopardy in modern times and there may well be valid reasons for government interference in his life. He can appreciate the need for a more accessible plentiful supply of water and when offered it, is eager to accept—other things being equal. In many instances the officials are able to convince him that it is even worthwhile to provide labour at no cost to the project. The equipment arrives and the facilities are installed. The engineer and administrator are able to report another successfully completed task, one of perhaps thousands. Unfortunately, there is a real possibility, even a likelihood, that the installed equipment will breakdown in a relatively short time and, despairing of any alternative, the villager will return to his old source for water. The net benefit is thus zero, perhaps actually negative when measured in terms of opportunity costs and the subsequent deterioration in the villager's respect for his government.

The peasant is normally characterized by his humility, being both submissive and receptive to outside suggestions where past experience with officialdom has not been to his disadvantage. He tends to let the outside experts decide for him and to remain passive and lack self-confidence in the face of external pressures. His experience so far has indicated that the government wishes to assist him by providing material and technical assistance and has in fact assumed that responsibility. Little wonder then that upon mechanical breakdown he is willing to wait patiently over a period of perhaps six months or more for assistance in its repair. In the meantime he returns to the former, unimproved source of water.

Government attitudes and approaches to the village

The peasant is the nub of rural development. The rather typical case described above may have been a well-meaning attempt by the government to introduce a change in the village environment in order to improve the well-being and thus productive capacity of its inhabitants. But the reverse sequence should have prevailed. Recognition should be given to the fact that raised village organization, motivation levels and productive capacities will lead to improvements in its environment and well-being. The common approach of first 'providing' water, apart from its being purely technical and therefore unbalanced, results in no greater degree of motivation or self-confidence, the villager acquires no new productive skills and becomes sceptical of solutions proposed by the government. If any advancement occurs at all it can only be described as dependent development. The prospects of the equipment being maintained and used in absence of the promoter are very slim indeed.

There are many references in the literature to self-help and the need for local participation in construction. Care must be taken to distinguish between the different kinds of participation. In the case described above the villager may have provided his labour as part of the bargain but he did not participate in the planning and decision-making process, and he had no control over its outcome. As described by Tschannerl (1973) his participation came strictly as an alienated component of the project; from the outset the government authority look the decisions, installed the unit and by implication accepted the responsibility for its maintenance.

There has, in the past, been a strong tendency to attend to those communities which show greatest potential for growth, are wealthiest and best educated, have the greatest capacity to repay capital loans, have the strongest political influence and are most vocal in their demands. In contrast Tanzania's current development plan places the highest priority on villages of the greatest need. In fostering its cooperative programme, water supplies are being supported first in Ujamaa cooperative villages, in areas of acute scarcity of water, areas of population concentration and where productive activities may be promoted. There is an increasing awareness that financial return and economic development are only components of the overall development process. In parallel with economic development (which, indeed, may not in itself be measurable) must come advancement of the individual as the focal point of the development process. Technical performance and economic efficiency, currently the primary measures of success, need to be complemented by such parameters as social development, community organization, individual participation, development of skills and the advancement of self-confidence on the part of the individual and his community.

Although technical efficiency should not be discounted, the technology selected and the way it is chosen must be suited to the physical and social conditions in which it is placed. Technology is not neutral; it can be, and often is, badly selected, with the result that the village becomes totally dependent upon the government for its installation and maintenance. Introducing improvements to the village involves a process of technology adaptation and transfer; it is an extremely delicate one and all-too-often underestimated in terms of its importance and complexity. We hear of the culture gap between the foreign expert or consultant and the developing country he attempts to advise, less recognized but far more important is the cultural, economic and even geographic separations between the indigenous urban civil servant and the rural villager. Coming from a completely different background and educated towards a Western style of life, the national faces the same problem as the foreign consultant. Segre (1974) describes the frustration which this gap engenders:

Thinkers, planners, advisers and administrators have all fallen into one or another of two errors concerning the import of modern techniques and techniques of modernization. They have not tried to obtain the legitimization of these by the accepted traditional leadership, assuming that it must be impossible to receive legitimization by an inferior society for superior techniques of foreign origin. They have usually either tried to impose these imported ideas and techniques on the natives, without paying much attention to local traditions or mentality, or they have appealed to local innovators who, though indigenous by birth, are equally foreign in outlook.

Whyte and Burton (Chapter 7) have emphasized the need to involve the community in the decision-making process, to react to its demands in fundamental terms and to respect its reasoning which may not be easily accepted by the technocrat but may be fundamental to the success of the project in terms of its accounting for social constraints in technology selection. Each ethnic group will have its own method of coping with external pressures; thus when a technology is proposed, to be successful it will have to go through a process of becoming accepted both by the community at large and by the individual. Legitimization of the proposed technology is an absolute necessity. Segre emphasizes the role of the community's elite in accepting and adopting the technology. This is the most common mode of village acceptance but not the only one. In their frustration, impatience and misunderstanding the engineer and administrator often ignore this necessary legitimization process, bypass the village hierarchy and install the equipment. To their chagrin the innovation, which has not been freely internalized and accepted, is sooner or later rejected as an imposition. It is emphasized that the 'social design' of the technology is just as important to its continued use and maintenance as the technical. Incorporation of this fact into design procedure will require profound changes in attitudes and approaches by the engineers if they are to succeed in the rural areas. It also requires the addition of the social scientist to the conventional team of engineer, physician and administrator.

The word 'motivation' has been mentioned several times. It is perhaps instructive to examine this aspect of rural development *vis-à-vis* water supply and sanitation. Often as not the principal reason behind lack of progress in this sector is that the central government and its functionaries are not adequately motivated to assist the low-income groups. This is reflected implicitly or explicitly by those who are involved in rural development work but who live in, and are oriented towards, the city. National water authorities most often measure success in terms of numbers of facilities installed instead of social development and health improvements effected. It becomes more important that the physical structure is technically sound than that it is socially acceptable, assured of continued use and maintenance and effective in improving public health. The primary motivation of the engineer is too often job security and his own legitimization within the administrative superstructure. As illustrated by Tschannerl (1973):

The progress reports on water supply talk about so many boreholes drilled, so many people supplied with water, so many kilometers of pipes laid, so many projects designed, etc. No mention is made of the process of how this was accomplished or other results aside from the structure. One never reads, for example, that the engineers have decided to spend more time with the peasants so that they would get better acquainted with their problems, or that so many plumbers in the village were trained in the course of construction, or that as a result of suggestions from the villagers a different, cheaper design for a particular item was adopted.

By maintaining a social distance from the villager and by emphasizing the complexity of technical design the engineer becomes assured of a place in the bureaucracy and establishes himself firmly in a monopolistic position and thereby forces the village to accept the technological 'black box' he offers, to become dependent upon his expertise and reliant on his services.

Development aid for water supply in rural areas

Much of what has just been said of the central government's relationship with the rural community also applies to that between the international technical assistance donor and the government itself. Aid has been available for economically productive projects for two decades but only recently has it become available for rural water supply. Just as it has often had a net negative impact on development of other sectors so it has limitations in assisting health infrastructure which the developing country should be fully aware of.

Aid has the habit of making the recipient reliant upon the donor in several ways. By its very nature aid makes a desired goal attainable with something less than the total input normally required. Whereas the initial project may appear successful its failure becomes apparent when, upon contemplating the next project, more aid is required. This form of dependent development fosters a reliance upon technical assistance and a lack of self-confidence in the recipient. Accordingly, most technical decisions are made by the overseas consultant, or where a choice is offered it is the foreigner who designs the alternatives. The aid donor agency operates under a series of self-imposed constraints. Normally, with due respect to the taxpayer, the donor requires a large part of development aid funds to be spent on donor-country equipment and personnel. The funds are used for the project's overseas exchange component but freedom to select equipment from other countries or their own manufacture is commonly not given to the recipient country. This is particularly dangerous where numerous items such as pumps are purchased for installation in rural areas. Insistence on donor country pumps as a condition of the loan imposes a kind of technological fix on the recipient. Inevitably the pumps will require repair at which time spare parts will need to be purchased from the donor country. In keeping with a policy to standardize government equipment the recipient may well be forced into the position of having to choose the given pump as standard. It is then at the mercy of the manufacturer or will require more aid from the original donor without any freedom to select alternatives, thereby becoming more reliant on aid funds and less in control if its own development, so allowing the technological fix to set in more deeply. Unknowingly, crucial decisions were taken at the point of accepting the first parcel of aid when the 'golden carrot' was brightest. Typically, at the time of the initial decision there were few national professionals with adequate training and experience to foresee its long-term implications. Consequently, short-term benefits were achieved at the expense of longer termed goals.

The relevance of the foreign consultant's basic motivations to the development process is in question. True, professional ethics stipulate that the consultant is to act on behalf of his client, but the question may be raised: Who is his client, the donor or recipient? The decisive powers as to which consultant should be used are invariably held by the donor country; the consultant's next contract will probably come from the donor not the recipient. Unfortunately the objectives and motivations of donor and recipient are not always synonymous. Whatever else, the consultant's firm is a profit-making concern, constrained to narrow terms of reference. Its goal is all-too-often oriented to producing a well-bound thick report which is seldom written in the recipient country's first language and is well furnished with technical jargon. The profit motive is likely to minimize professional man-hours spent on the project. Inherent in overseas projects is the fact that the foreign consultant does not have to live with the final outcome of his design. He is not part of the national government and thus may have different motivations, objectives and priorities. In many cases these may be in conflict with those of the developing country he purports to serve.

10.6 PRIMARY HEALTH CARE AND THE IMPROVEMENT OF RURAL SANITATION

As described above, national water authorities, departments of public works and Ministries of the interior have, in general, been unable to deal effectively with the problem of water supply and sanitation in the dispersed and village populations. They have stressed the installation of water supply infrastructure and not changes in attitudes, hygiene and improvements in sanitation in the household. Their technique has been one of extending approaches normally used in the city to the smaller towns. This has been widely successful in the more advanced and wealthier urban centres. Unfortunately, success has stopped short of the more dispersed rural peoples who often comprise the majority of the rural poor and indeed the majority of the national population.

In like fashion, where ministries of health have held responsibility for development of rural sanitation and water supply, difficulties have also been encountered in reaching out to the hinterland. Health services have been concentrated in the urban centres and available for the most part only to the relatively privileged classes. This distortion is underpinned by the inadequate level of expenditures on health which averages 87 US cents per year per capita in those countries with annual income per capita of less than $ US 100 and seldom rises to above $ US 4 in others (World Bank, 1975b). Comparable expenditure in the United Kingdom is over $ US 100/capita/year. It is unfortunate that most of the funds which are allocated for health expenditure in developing countries are spent without due consideration of their cost-effectiveness. Instead of their being invested in preventative and environmental measures, the emphasis has been on creating sophisticated centralized health services, the training of highly competent qualified medical personnel and an orientation towards curative medicine practices. A large part has been spent on hospitals in urban centres, providing them with modern equipment and staffing them with expensively trained doctors and nurses. These personnel are trained in 'Western' fashion and have a natural inclination to remain in the larger cities. Thus they are qualified and committed to meet the medical requirements of those that can afford their services. Their training and function are more suited to the needs of the industrialized state than those of their own country. These practices are underpinned by a lack of clearly defined objectives and priorities. The outcome is a rigid and over-centralized, urban-oriented administrative superstructure which, although purporting to serve the rural poor, lacks the necessary ability to reach out to them. The distribution of resources is inequitable; the over-concentration of personnel, institutions and facilities in the towns causes the central authorities to be too far removed from, and out of touch with, the rural population's needs and expectations. The frustration of working through such an organization is typified by one Central American health official's complaint, 'How can we be expected to service villages when they aren't even on the map and can't speak our language?' The cultural, geographic, even linguistic separations make this approach to improving rural health levels entirely inappropriate. Unfortunately, the modern medical profession in most countries is entrenched and resistant to change, so much so that the attitude that only physicians are qualified to conduct medical practice has become legalized. The medical faculty has become protective in outlook and monopolistic in practice. Unfortunately, the very high cost of producing physicians, their inherent desire to remain in the city and their 'brain-drain' to developed states are not compatible with the objective of raising the health status of the population—the majority of which resides in the rural areas.

In attempting to meet such a challenge a few countries have undertaken real commitment to the rural poor and have given high priority to rural health programmes. These include China, Cuba, Tanzania and, to a certain extent, Venezuela (UNICEF–WHO, 1975). Others encouraging localized endeavours, some on a trial basis, include Bangladesh, India, Nigeria, Columbia, Iran, Nepal, Malawi and Guatemala. There is considerable concern being expressed at the international level over the inadequacies of the urban-oriented curative approach and a reorientation is being effected towards the strengthening of health services through primary health care in rural developing areas. With the exception of the larger national programmes in China and Cuba, most primary health care efforts have not made full use of their potential to improve water supply and excreta disposal practices. Likewise, there is still a dominant tendency towards the treatment of illnesses, albeit at the village level. Just as simplified medicine can make major inroads into ill-health without use of the accredited physician, so too can simplified technological improvements be accomplished without the use of the graduate engineer.

Each system of primary health care differs according to the needs and conditions in the country and community. There are, however, some common characteristics. As mentioned above, the first is motivation and real commitment to the social betterment of the rural peoples. Primary health care employs low-cost effective organizational structures and technologies which include preventative, promotive, curative and rehabilitative health measures and community development activities which are accessible to those in need. Primary health care is normally integrated into the national health scheme and centrally coordinated, *but locally controlled*. The 'reformed' health service as described by the World Bank (1975b) should enjoy the full confidence of the community it serves. The key functionaries are the village health worker and local midwife who, preferably, come from the community they serve and are responsible to it. Normally the health worker has some degree of primary school education and 2–3 months training in basic principles of preventative and curative medicine periodically returns to the training centre for further education and retraining. He is responsible in the village for organizing community efforts in environmental health, sanitation and water supply, and health education. He is also responsible for identifying and treating the more important diseases. Curative skills are, however, quite limited; most effort is being directed towards preventative measures. The village health worker may be supervised by medical auxiliaries who have had up to two years of health training with substantial background in the technical aspects of disease prevention, including sanitation and water supply. Emphasis here is again on the promotion of community health rather than the cure of disease on an individual basis. The auxiliary is responsible in turn to the primary care managerial physician who has had full training as a physician. Unlike the typical doctor, however, the managerial physician has had a stronger background in epidemiology and community health promotion. He has also received elementary training in traditional medicine, agronomy, nutrition and rural development.

The promotion of sanitation and water supply in the dispersed and village population could advantageously be made through primary health care systems. It is obvious that at the current rate of expenditure by national and international authorities this, the most difficult sector of the population, will not be adequately covered by the technology-oriented approach common to national water authorities.

The primary health care system is designed to reflect needs of the community, both technically and socially. It relies to the greatest extent possible on local resources—materials, manpower and finance. It also fosters use of low-cost simple technologies in a stepwise approach to village development and does not require such improvements to meet standards set by urban-oriented engineers. While suggesting the primary health care system as a means of meeting the rural challenge in sanitation and water supply, it must be emphasized that— apart from successes in China—primary health care is in its infancy and has had an insignificant impact on overall global needs to date. It is, however, appropriately oriented and holds a very great potential for this sector.

10.7 CONCLUSIONS

Ill-health and poverty are inequitably distributed between and within nations. The positive correlation between health and socio-economic status has been well documented; yet those in greatest need of improvements in their sanitation and water supply, the rural poor, are also those least able to afford and maintain them.

The initial conjecture that benefits to be accrued by means of rapid industrial and urban growth would spread out to the rural areas has not proved valid. In particular, urban water supply programme development has not had its supposed multiplier effect on the rural community and village.

In most tropical regions the present rate of institutional, manpower and budgetary allocation to rural sanitation and water supply improvement is wholly insufficient to meet current demand or even to keep up with population growth.

The development of new and improved technologies can only be a partial solution. Major institutional changes are required. Fundamental shifts in orientation and approaches need to be made if the very limited available resources are going to be made cost-effective. In order that effective, long-lasting improvements be made at the village level, the peasant will have to be brought into the decision-making process and the technology legitimized by his community as a whole. Otherwise the technologies being introduced will continue to be regarded as externally derived and as the responsibility of the government to keep and maintain in working order.

Comprehensive manpower planning is badly needed in nearly all developing countries. The current practice of appending training components to individual projects or of providing for postgraduate education at overseas universities through aid programmes is proving to be inadequate in meeting the demand for environmental engineers and sub-professional technicians. National, or at least regional, facilities need to be established to provide training through curricula which are more relevant to local problems.

Emphasis has been placed on potable water schemes for urban centres.

Comparable improvements have not been made in urban excreta disposal facilities. Insufficient recognition is being given to other components of the sanitation 'package' which are requisite if full health benefits are to be realized. In the rural areas sanitation facilities are wholly inadequate and insanitary, if indeed not entirely absent.

The purely technical approach to urban water supply has illustrated its relevance to that sector. However, attempts to extend it to the village have almost universally failed, as evidenced by the notoriously high rate of well-pump failure in rural areas. In most countries, financial and manpower resources of the central government are not sufficient to meet the demands of the rural areas if anything approaching urban standards of water supply are to be met. There is a wealth of manpower resources available at the village level which has remained largely untapped. Ministries of health have emphasized the curative approach in combating disease and have suffered heavy losses of manpower through training physicians more suited to meet the needs of industrialized states than those of their own country. There are, however, encouraging examples of primary health care delivery programmes in which the village health worker is given a limited training that emphasizes prevention rather than cure of the more important diseases.

With few exceptions these examples of primary health care programmes have not adequately stressed water supply and sanitation; training has tended to be more medically than engineering oriented. However, where sanitation and water supply can be emphasized, this approach is seen to offer real potential in terms of its cost-effectiveness. Although integrated into the national health care scheme and centrally coordinated, it should be locally controlled. Improvements thereby made in the village are viewed as its own; the technologies introduced are likely to be more appropriate to local conditions, and the villagers more capable and more willing to maintain and use them effectively.

10.8 REFERENCES

Ad Hoc Working Group (1975). *An international programme for the improvement of water Supply and sanitation in rural areas of developing countries.* WHO, UNDP, IBRD, UNICEF, IDRC, UNEP and OECD, Washington.

McGarry, M. G. (1975). *Developing country sanitation.* A report to the International Development Research Centre, Ottawa.

Saunders, R. J. and Warford, J. J. (1974). Village water supply and sanitation in less developed countries, *Public Utilities Report No. RES 2.* Washington: World Bank.

Segre, D. V. (1974). *The High Road and the Low.* London. Allen Lane.

Tschannerl, G. (1973). Rural water supply in Tanzania: is 'Politics' or 'technique' in command. Paper No. 52, *Annual Social Science Conference of the East African Universities,* Dar-es-Salaam.

UNICEF–WHO (1975). *Joint study on alternative approaches to meeting basic health needs of populations in developing countries.* (Paper JC20/UNICEF-WHO/75.2.) Geneva: World Health Organization.

World Bank (1975a). *Rural development sector policy paper.* Washington.

World Bank (1975b). *Health sector policy paper.* Washington.

WHO (1974). *Education and training in sanitary engineering.* Report on a seminar held in Bangkok, November 22–29. New Delhi: World Health Organization Regional Office for South East Asia.

WHO (1975). *Promotion of national health services.* World Health Organization. Paper A28/9, 28th World Health Assembly Provisional agenda item 2.6, April.

11

Progress in the Rural Water Programmes of Latin America

DAVID DONALDSON

11.1 INTRODUCTION

A challenge accepted

By signing the Charter of Punta del Este in 1961, the Governments of the Americas adopted the goal of supplying water and sewerage to at least 50% of their rural population by the end of that decade. At the time they were set, these goals represented an unparalleled challenge, for only about 8 million rural dwellers (7% of the total rural population) had adequate water supplies (PAHO, 1969). To meet this challenge it was obvious that numerous rural water programmes would have to be created and many tens of thousands of projects would have to be planned, designed and built in order to bring water to the target population of 64 million people.

Furthermore, it soon became evident that existing organizational concepts would have to be revised and that new skills would have to be sought for the revised programmes. Thus the stage was set. Dostoevsky might say of a similar moment, 'taking a new step, uttering a new word is what people fear most'. But the step was taken.

Achievements to date

Examining the progress that rural water programmes of the Americas have made in the last ten years, one is struck first by the magnitude of the accomplishments and the promise they hold for the future; secondly, by the deep and growing concern for rural areas and a parallel intensification of efforts to promote modernization of rural life; and, third, by the vastness of the unfinished portion of the task.

This paper was originally presented at the Seminar on Rural Water Supply and Sanitation in Developing Countries sponsored by the International Development Research Centre and held in Lausanne Switzerland in May–June 1973. It was originally published in *Bulletin of the Pan American Health Organization*, **8** (1), 37–53 (1974). It is reproduced here in a slightly shortened form by permission of the Pan American Sanitary Bureau. © Pan American Sanitary Bureau, 1974.

Considering the progress made, the past decade should be viewed as one of solid achievement. The best data available (PAHO, 1969; 1972) show that by the end of 1972 the countries of the region had raised the proportion of rural dwellers having a potable water supply from about 7% to 27%—thus increasing the population served by a factor of about 4·7. This means that about 33 million rural inhabitants are now being served by approximately 30000 systems that they themselves helped national programmes to build.

For several years now there has been an organized rural water programme in every country of the region, largely because during the 1960s the Pan American Health Organization helped the countries to experiment and develop new concepts and solutions. While some of these programmes achieved less than the desired results, each served to refine existing techniques and to increase understanding of existing problems.

It is also worth noting that those involved have had the experience of obtaining and disbursing $ US 73·5 million from the 24 loans that international credit agencies made in this field between January 1961 and December 1972. Realizing that for each loan there are national matching funds in the amount of 40% to 60% of the loan, and that the Government often contributes 20% to 30% more in construction grants and an additional amount for operational funds, it has been estimated that about $ 400 million was invested in rural water programmes between 1961 and the end of 1972. About 80% of this has come from national sources.

While much remains to be done, a solid base has been laid. As in most development programmes, the effort to date—that of building the foundations for future efforts—is not readily apparent to the casual observer. But those who know where to look can see that many of the programmes can be traced from national/PAHO/UNICEF demonstration efforts, through PAHO-assisted pilot programmes, to full-scale national rural water programmes.

The success achieved should not be measured only by the numbers of new consumers. Concepts and approaches changed; consciousness of the need to speed modernization of rural life developed; and a new awareness of what could be accomplished in the rural sector emerged. Many of the first programmes had very limited goals—often seeking to develop little more than a series of individual community systems serving water from standpipes. But very quickly the success of these individual projects caused formation of national or regional programmes in which the people served demanded more complex solutions (such as water piped to the patios of private dwellings) and showed a willingness to pay the cost. The time needed for this transformation has varied from country to country but, in nearly every case, once the initial projects were installed the improvements inexorably evolved.

Hand-pumps v. piped connections

Here it is interesting to note a major difference between programmes in this hemisphere and those in other parts of the world. In many programmes outside the Americas it is argued that water delivered from a house connection—which implies developing a programme for collecting and distributing the water and for administering the resulting system—should be considered one of the advanced steps in the rural water supply process. Therefore, in many of these programmes hand-pumps are the immediate goal, with any type of piped water being a long-term objective.

While hand-pumps have their place in our programmes, and many thousands have been installed in the Americas, our assessment of the problem indicates that the best approach is that of piped water systems developed, built and operated with strong local participation. We believe that, even with the very limited human and financial resources available, this approach is the quickest way to give the most water to the most people at the lowest cost.

'Rural water'—a dynamic process

While most programmes in the Americas started by building systems that would supply safe water from public fountains, experience has shown that this was only the beginning of a process—and that it was generally only a prelude to the next stage, i.e. systems that pipe water into users' homes.

The time it takes to evolve from one stage to the next depends on many factors—local economic conditions, the type and intensity of promotional efforts, awareness of health benefits, etc. But the limited data available indicate that within about eight to ten years after their inauguration many of the early public fountain systems became 'patio connection' systems—i.e. systems delivering piped water to single taps in the patios of about 80% of the houses served.

11.2 CURRENT GOALS AND APPROACHES

Rural water goals

In October 1972 the Ministers of Health of the Americas held their Third Special Meeting in Santiago, Chile. There, after reviewing progress to date, they developed the 'Ten-Year Health Plan for the Americas', which contained the goals for the 1970s (PAHO, 1973). With regard to rural water they set the following targets:

Provide water for 50% of the rural population, or, as a minimum, reduce that population without service by 30%.

They also indicated that the countries should

Utilize [the] techniques of 'mass approach' and concepts of community self-help to provide water in rural areas and use ... revolving funds to finance rural water supply programs.

It was pointed out that

... there still are many, especially in the rural areas, who lack these essential services [water and sewerage] and who are equally entitled to have them. Our priority task is undoubtedly to devote special attention to those most in need, those who usually live in villages and on the outskirts of major cities. With this in view, we have established goals which we hope to achieve through the application of modern techniques, those which make it possible to speed up installations through improved use of domestic resources, foreign capital, and, what is most essential, active community participation.

'Rural' and 'Rurban' programmes

In reading about the rural water supply programmes of Latin America, one often finds the statement that '27% of the rural population had a safe source of water at the end of 1972'. To understand this properly, one must be aware of several concepts and definitions. Among other things, one needs to identify the types of 'rural' programmes in Latin America.

There has been a tendency in the past to lump several different programmes under this single heading. In reality, however, there has been at least three separate and distinct types of 'rural' programmes, consisting of (1) community well programmes for dispersed populations; (2) rudimentary aqueduct programmes for semi-concentrated populations; and (3) more advanced aqueduct programmes for villages and other concentrated populations.

Usually, in referring to a 'rural water programme' the writer is talking about the third category, together with some rudimentary aqueducts, but one can never be sure. Furthermore, the official estimates of 'rural' (hereafter called 'rurban') water coverage are often based on arbitrary numbers or definitions. (In fact, even the definitions of 'rural' vary from country to country, though the most common one used in referring to water supply in Latin America is any population concentrations of 2500 persons or less (Donaldson, 1972).

The three basic 'rural' programmes

The most basic programme—an individual source programme—involves developing a protected spring or providing a well with a hand-pump to serve a number of scattered families. Little or no formal community structure is associated with its operation, and it is usually maintained and paid for by a national programme or a ministry at no cost to the user.

The second programme, that of rudimentary aqueducts, utilizes a well or spring, a small storage tank, and a limited distribution system for delivery of water to public fountains and perhaps a few patio connections in order to serve a semi-concentrated population. The users of such a system pay a small sum, but depend heavily on the national programme to assist them in maintenance, operation and future expansion.

The third programme (i.e. the 'rurban' programme) is the one most people are referring to when they talk about 'rural water programmes of the Americas'. It is usually designed to serve a community with a 'central core' of at least 100 houses and the immediate surrounding area. The system normally utilizes a protected spring, a pumped well or a treatment plant, and delivers water to

Table 11.1 Characteristics of different rural programmes

Type of Programme	Population served	Source	Distribution systems	Water delivery	Local organiza-tion	Financial recovery
Individual source	Dispersed	Well or protected spring	None	At well only	None	None
Rudimen-tary aque-duct	Semicon-centrated	Pumped well or protected spring	Simple	At public fountains plus a few patio con-nections	Minor, mainly for operation and mainte-nance of system	Little or none
Rurban	Concen-trated around a 500-person core	Well, spring, or treatment plant	Complex, serving core area plus nearby con-centrated areas	At patio connections and a few public fountains	Major, for operation, maintenan-ce, and administra-tion of system and collection of rates	Enough to pay for operation, maintenance and local administra-tion of system and to set up a reserve fund

a storage tank. Its distribution system is designed to supply water through 'house' or 'patio' connections, making minimal use of public fountains. A local water board—with the assistance of the national programme—operates, maintains and administers the system and collects water rates. Characteristics of the three programmes are summarized in Table 11.1.

Clearly, each of the three programmes is part of an interrelated process. The community wells serve to attract the surrounding people and, with time, the nearby population density grows. When the density gets high enough, a rudimentary aqueduct can be considered. In the past the changeover from well to rudimentary aqueduct took an average of 12–15 years, while the next step—from public fountains to about 80% patio connections—took an average of eight to ten years.

At this point a logical question is: Why did the programmes start with the concentrated instead of the dispersed population? The answer is that dealing with more concentrated groups produces the greatest public benefits and the quickest financial returns. Thus the countries of this region have elected to concentrate their efforts in the 'rurban' area while carrying out the 'individual source' programmes at a slower rate.

The work in this second area has been slow for many reasons. Among them are: complexity of the problem; high unit cost of benefits received; and lack of human and technical resources. But as the problem of the concentrated

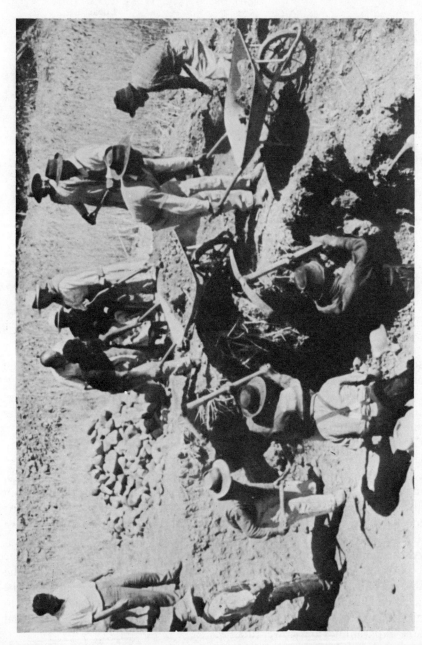

Self-help labour working on a rural water supply scheme in Latin America (photograph : D. Donaldson)

population approaches a solution (in some rurban programmes coverage is now up to 50% of the target population) more attention must be given to solving the problems of the dispersed areas.

The rurban water programme

Despite differences of scale and technique, the various rurban programmes of the Americas have much in common. For instance, they have all been based on three fundamental concepts. These are: (1) strong and active community participation in the development, construction, administration and financing of the local systems; (2) focusing of resources on the problems of concentrated instead of dispersed populations; and (3) extensive use of technicians to assist a limited number of professional personnel. Other common features include the criteria used to select target communities, the methods used to finance projects, the widespread use of 'mass approach' techniques and the use of local boards which administer and operate the systems.

Community selection criteria

The criteria for selecting target communities and scheduling the construction of systems are determined at the national or regional level after a review of existing manpower and financial constraints.

Table 11.2 shows the criteria used by one of the more successful programmes to choose those communities that would be included in its construction programme. In practice, the criteria were not applied in a rigid manner but were used as guidelines. It was later found that selections made in the 'project identification' phase were adhered to about 70% of the time. Failure to meet the third and fifth criteria was found to be the main reason for removing communities from the list.

Table 11.2 Criteria for selection of target communities

No. 1—Communities with largest number of inhabitants (not more than 2000)
No. 2—Communities with access by road for trucks
No. 3—Communities that have expressed interest, have requested the system and have offered financial or other assistance for construction and operation of the proposed system
No.4 —Communities located within one of the zones of influence of the national or local development plan
No. 5—Communities where the project can avoid unusual or expensive solutions

Programme financing

The construction cost of the system has usually been broken down as follows: (1) about 50% is covered by a loan from an international agency, which is often repaid by the central government; (2) about 30% is granted by the national and state programmes; and (3) the remaining 20% is obtained from the community in the form of cash, materials and labour during construction.

In general, the operating and administrative costs are paid by the community, together with an additional amount which can serve as a reserve or help amortize loan costs. These revenues are obtained through water rates collected by the local water board under the direction of the national programme. The basic financial responsibility is thus a local one, but it is carefully watched, supervised and coordinated by the national programme, which carries out financial planning for the programme as a whole.

Programme structure

Table 11.3 shows a typical programme structure and the major areas of responsibility at each level. Regional programmes, which exist in a few countries, are usually organized as separate operations, but are tied together under the 'umbrella' of the national programme through common criteria, design and techniques.

Tatle 11.3 Functions of various levels of a typical rural water programme

National	Provide a financing channel for national counterpart funds, international loans, national grants and local contributions Develop norms and policies (technical and administrative) Supervise execution of national plan Conduct long-range planning Coordinate construction efforts Supervise regional programmes Exercise overall financial control Provide technical and administrative assistance Provide training
Regional	Supervise programme execution Carry out design (in case of larger countries only) Supervise construction, operation and administration of projects Undertake community promotion and supervision of projects
Local	Administration of system Operation of system Maintenance of system Collection of water rates

The revolving fund

In order to implement techniques which will permit low-cost solutions, it is necessary to establish sound *long-range* financing for rural water programmes. The revolving fund appears to offer the best possibilities in this regard, because of its flexibility and its adaptability to local conditions. However, it should be noted that the term 'revolving fund' has often been misused. A formal definition would be: A fund that is continually replenished as it is used, either

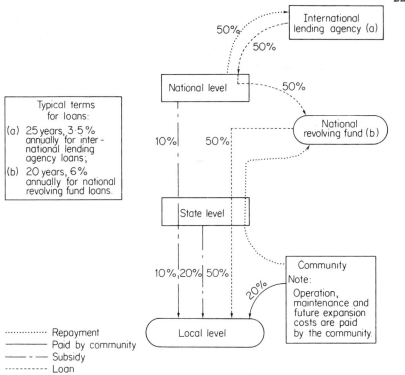

Figure 11.1 A typical revolving fund plan

through further appropriation or by income generated by the activity that it finances.

In terms of rural water programmes, a revolving fund implies establishment of a fund on a regional or national level to finance construction of individual community projects. The loaned funds are recovered by having the benefited community repay the revolving fund. As the repayments come in they are reloaned to finance additional projects (see Figure 11.1). An advantage of the technique is that methods for obtaining the original financing, terms of the loans and terms of the repayments can be adapted to local conditions.

While the style of the revolving funds used has varied from place to place in Latin America, the fact that they require a repayment scheme has tended to promote effective organization at the local level. The communities (as well as local and national officials) thus become accustomed to community financing of services received. This community involvement is one of the major benefits that result from establishment of a revolving fund.

In practice, the establishment of these funds has followed three general patterns:

(1) A grant is used to obtain the initial financing; the fund is then kept in operation by relending repayments as they are collected.

(2) The fund is created in conjunction with a national or international loan and is then maintained by relending those community repayments that exceed the amounts needed to pay off both the loan and the loan amortization. (3) The fund is created in conjunction with a loan and is maintained partly by national government servicing of the loan and partly by income from community repayments over and above the amounts needed to pay off the loan.

A recent study of conditions in Latin America (Davia, 1968) indicates that it is feasible for a rural family with an income of between $250 and $500 to pay for operation and maintenance of a typical rurban water system *and* for capitalization of at least half of the total investment.

Whether or not this is done, development of new revolving funds requires the highest possible degree of local community participation. Without it such funds often become little more than construction funds that 'revolve' only once.

Future financing

The Inter-American Development Bank has been highly instrumental in the growth of the hemisphere's rural water programmes to date. But there is a need to develop additional or alternate financing sources and to explore new schemes. The question of self-financed projects or subsidized ones must be faced and the monetary recovery from each type of project must be realistically determined. We also need to find ways of interesting more official agencies (such as central banks and social security institutes) in making long-term, low-interest loans.

Up to now about 50% of the initial funding has been covered by international loans, about 30% by government grants, and about 20% by local contributions. However, the international agencies are beginning to require more matching money, a development which will require the programmes to revise their financing sources and techniques.

In May 1972 the 25th World Health Assembly considered the special needs of the rural sector and recommended that WHO Member States 'take such steps as would lead to increased allocation of resources to rural water supplies' (WHO, 1972). The task will not be easy. For example, the World Health Organization technical assistance budget for the water supply area is only $26 million, a tiny fraction of the roughly $13 thousand million needed for the countries to achieve the WHO goals for 1980.

Therefore, while the work of the 1960s can serve as a guide, we must be prepared to finance new solutions. For instance, it might be desirable for lending agencies to make loans for administrative development just as they now do for project construction.

The mass approach to 'rural' water supply

When one compares the need for 'rural' water systems against what has been achieved to date, the need to increase the output of the various programmes is readily apparent. To meet this challenge a technique called the mass or 'systems' approach has become widely used in Latin America. Its objective has been to develop a coordinated and integrated 'packaging' of those concepts that permit more rapid promotion, design, installation, operation, maintenance and administration of the various projects. Because a rural programme must repeat the same tasks for hundreds of villages—in some countries thousands— the development of such 'standardized' techniques is essential in order to multiply the impact of limited resources.

Regarding technical standardization, existing maps or aerial photographs are often used to plan the project, while modular design criteria, predesigned elements and standardized equipment lists are used in the speedy development of both project equipment lists and project plans. The materials are brought together in a central yard and sent to the community as a package, along with all necessary tools and other items not readily available at the site.

With regard to standardized personnel practices, technicians train and supervise volunteer workers at the local level. These workers carry out developmental and promotional activities in accord with the carefully designed and coordinated guidelines of the package programme. Naturally the design and timing of a particular project must be closely coordinated with the needs, resources and goals of the overall programme.

Experience in Latin America has shown that these 'modules' and this standardization can be a powerful and practical tool when the solutions developed are constantly reviewed to see that they produce maximum benefit at minimum cost.

11.3 CURRENT AND FUTURE PROBLEMS

Administrative v. technical needs

A rurban water supply problem is more administrative than technical in nature. Too often the matter has been approached via a series of small projects requiring independent technical solutions and a large number of highly skilled and hard-to-find professional personnel. In fact, the more successful programmes have shown that each individual system should be treated as part of a larger framework using mass approach techniques to construct, operate and administer hundreds of systems. This means that *all* actions (technical, administrative and financial) must be coordinated at the central level—without forgetting that each project also needs strong local participation.

It must also be recognized that several years of groundwork will be needed to develop, coordinate, and refine techniques and to train technicians before the first system is built—and that as the programme grows the techniques must be redesigned and the technicians retrained.

Local participation

All the programmes of the region have actively sought the highest possible degree of local participation. In the initial promotion stages local water committees have been organized to promote the project, collect local contributions, etc. Once the project is completed the community generally elects a water board that is under the watchful eye of the national programme. The board is in charge of operating and maintaining the system, collecting the rates and undertaking minor expansions. Experience has shown that strong local participation is *essential* if the programme is to succeed. Therefore the full support of the community must be enlisted from the start.

This means that local leaders must be identified and engaged in the project. Too often it has been concluded that 'poorly educated' rural people lack the required skills to construct, operate, maintain and administer their own water system. But it has been shown time and again that with proper guidance community leaders can make meaningful choices, motivate others and provide the leadership required for success.

Emphasis on low-cost programmes

In developing the rurban programme the most common approach has been to first build those water systems which have the lowest costs. This has resulted in most of the systems having gravity supplies or wells, access by road, and a large (15% to 20%) community contribution toward the construction cost. The tendency has thus been to work in the 'richer' areas. The approach has been justified on the grounds that it permits the quickest flow of funds into the programme. This money can then be used for supplying water to areas with higher costs, thereby providing the greatest coverage in the shortest time. 'Problem cases' are resolved as funds and resources become available.

Public health v. public works

In most cases it was the sanitary engineers of the ministry of health who were the 'fathers' of the rural water supply programmes. Responding to their ministry's concern for rural health, they developed programmes making efficient use of limited resources and stressing the vital need for community participation. Then, in the course of assuring this participation, local health centre personnel (both promoters and sanitarians) became essential links in the effort to implement these plans.

Largely because financing was available through the Inter-American Development Bank, the rurban programmes have tended to grow much faster than the 'well' or 'rudimentary aqueduct' ones. As the rurban programmes have grown (thus requiring more capital and resources) they have tended to move out of the public health area and into the public works sector. This shift poses a new set of problems.

In sum, this is the critical juncture, where today's techniques must be scaled up to serve tomorrow's large-scale programmes. This implies two things: that multidisciplinary professionals are badly needed to develop programmes via which techniques, criteria and procedures can be applied by technicians on a mass scale; and that there must be thorough retraining of present staff in techniques and skills to be used in the future.

Use of urban concepts

Serious problems often result when programme designers try to 'scale down' urban concepts to fit rural situations. For example, because an urban water system is designed to make water instantly available in unlimited quantities, the rural designer may try to provide the same service in the rurban setting, this producing an overly large and expensive system.

Manpower considerations

The governments of the Americas have cited the following factors, in order of importance, as the major constraints on construction of water supply systems: (1) insufficient internal financing, (2) inappropriate administrative structures, (3) inappropriate financial frameworks, (4) lack of trained personnel, (5) inadequate or outmoded legal frameworks and (6) insufficient production of local materials.

Even though it is only fourth on the list, the personnel problem seems especially thorny. That is because this lack of trained manpower implies more than a need for extra training; it implies setting up conditions that can attract and hold the required personnel. At their 1972 meeting in Santiago the Ministers of Health said: 'All the health personnel in these [rural] areas merit relatively higher compensation for their efforts' (PAHO, 1973).

Another important consideration is that the worker in rurban programmes should be more of a generalist than a specialist. The reason for this is that the problems encountered involve many social and technical disciplines. Thus, each professional must be more closely aware of problems in related field and must be able to build 'bridges' to those problems that interface with his. Without this close and careful coordination, be it accomplished by 'systems analysis' or by using a small central staff, the rurban water programme quickly becomes chaotic.

Quite aside from the generalist–specialist problem, technical plans have often been implemented without thinking much about the technicians who will be required to make the programme work. For example, we need to train pump repairmen as we install pumps, or soon we will have an additional expense instead of a water-producing device.

The countries must seek to increase the number of professionals and technicians that enter this field. Moreover, these persons should be 'rural' experts trained in 'rural' techniques, for experience has shown that experts transferred from 'urban' areas tend to use inappropriate techniques that unnecessarily increase project costs.

Data gathering

In designing water systems, good population and consumption data is often critically important. When the programmes started in 1961, 'best guess' figures were used. In most cases populations were expected to at least double in 20 years and consumption was estimated at roughly 200–250 litres per capita per day. Over the years it has been found that these figures were too high and that they caused unnecessary investments. While prediction of future population size continues to pose problems, a growing body of knowledge has emerged on which to base more realistic consumption figures.

Another problem is that, in their rush to get started, programmes have frequently failed to obtain sorely needed data on potential water sources. Thus, many of them have initiated water surveys to locate potential sites, but limited funds usually condemn these investigations to be 'one step' in front of construction. The result has often been hasty decisions that were expensive to correct later on.

Rurban v. dispersed rural populations

In the past, priority was given to 'urban' areas, leaving a backlog of need in the 'rural' zones. But as the countries have realized the need for coordinated development the 'rural' problems have called forth increasing amounts of attention and resources.

The approach that has been used most frequently to date utilizes existing villages as 'poles of attraction', rather than concentrating attention on the more dispersed small farms. However, as solutions are found for the rurban areas, attention must be turned to the dispersed population. To meet this challenge, new approaches must be developed. For just as 'urban' techniques and approaches are of limited value in the rurban sector, it is to be expected that the rurban experience will only serve as a general guide for helping the dispersed populations. The few such 'dispersed' programmes now in existence are of such size that they can provide only limited data; but solutions must be found if effective 'balanced' water programmes are to be developed.

The vital need for safe rural water

Far too many in the rural areas are still without an adequate supply of water. To help remedy this the goals of the 1970s have been set, and now we need to find the ways and means to help the people involved as they strive to receive the benefits of safe water in their homes.

To achieve this ultimate goal—delivery of safe water as near as possible to its point of use—we must keep the consumer firmly in mind. His needs are the constant value in the equation. Our efforts must be directed at finding answers to his problems and *not*, as has too often been the case, at satisfying our preconceived notions of what we think the problems are.

Our immediate object is to supply safe water to all those in the rural areas who want it or need it—at a price they can afford and in a manner they will find useful. This must be done as quickly as is humanly, technically and financially possible; for too many in the rural areas have already been asked to wait for much too long.

11.4 REFERENCES

Davia, R. (1968). *Rural Water Supply Services: Community Financing* (Document REMSA/INF/12). Washington: Pan American Health Organization.

Donaldson, D. (1972). Rural water supplies in developing countries. *Water Resources Bulletin*, **8**, 391–398.

PAHO (1969). *Community Water Supply and Sewage Disposal Programs in Latin America and Carribean Countries.* Washington: Pan American Health Organization.

PAHO (1972). *Ten-Year Health Plan for the Americas* (Official Document 118). Washington: Pan American Health Organization.

PAHO (1973). *Annual Report of the Director for 1972* (Official Document 124). Washington: Pan American Health Organization.

WHO (1972). *Twenty Fifth World Health Assembly; Part 1: Resolutions and Decisions Annexes*, pp. 16–17. Geneva: World Health Organization.

IV

Sanitation

12

Sanitation and Low-Cost Housing

GERRIT VAN R. MARAIS

12.1 INTRODUCTION

Health is an essential component of the infrastructure of a country. Training and acquisition of skills take time; if life expectation is low, training takes a disproportionate part of the active life of the trainee and the country does not reap in full the investment in training. In the developing countries the State is interested in the most rapid development directly productive in wealth and desires to commit as much capital for this purpose as possible. Yet to what extent should the State assume responsibility in supplying those components regarded as conducive to good environmental health, i.e. housing, water supply, sanitation and other services?

The focal point of the problem hinges round the concept 'housing'. Housing can be defined as the environment to promote the physical, sociological and mental well-being of man within the family unit. Well-being, however, is a relative term and one man's well-being is not another's. In tropical developing countries having a high proportion of the population with low productivity and low income, with poor and non-existent health education, the relative concept of well-being as a measure of success of 'housing' does not provide a practical criterion for decision making. It is necessary rather to define the absolute basic requirements which 'housing' must satisfy. Three can be distinguished:

(1) Access to work.
(2) Water supply and sanitation.
(3) Shelter.

The order of these three is not immaterial and 'shelter' is consciously relegated to third position. It is the thesis of this paper that in 'housing' the 'house' is the least important.

This paper was originally published in *Progress in Water Technology*, **3**, 115–125 (1971). It is reproduced here in a shortened form by permission of Pergamon Press Ltd. © Pergamon Press Ltd., 1971.

Access to work

Without access to work there appears to be no justification for constructing a house. In a rural society habitation arises naturally near the place of work. In an urban society this is equally true but the location is more flexible depending on the speed, efficiency and cost of transportation. If access to work is difficult or expensive the journey to and from work is a constant drain on the energy, time, finances and efficiency of the low-income groups. Owing to the often dismal aspect of badly designed low-cost housing areas, there is pressure on the planner from the more affluent (and influential) urban dwellers to site low-cost housing away from their areas. This is a problem that presents itself sooner or later in all urban communities.

Water supply and sanitation

These two aspects of 'housing' go together for they are indivisible. The provision of a potable water supply is a priority which cannot be denied. What is not so obvious is that the provision of a satisfactory form of sanitation is equally vital.

Over the past ten years there has been a drive by the World Health Organization to provide potable water supplies to communities in the developing countries. Where implemented, it has significantly reduced the incidence of diseases such as typhoid, dysentery and cholera. This success has to a degree obscured the fact that increasing the water supply also increases the problem of its disposal. This point is well appreciated in the following quotation from the Indian Ministry of Health (1964):

In many towns where water supply was long since installed and a sewer system held up for want of adequate 'subsidy', the delay is costing the communities dear. Insanitation and mosquito nuisance have taken root and filariasis is becoming endemic over an ever widening urban area in the entire country. This is hardly a comforting thought. Ironically enough filariasis control is fast assuming an increasing importance as a health measure with prophylactics pressed into service. This is but fighting the shadow and not the substance.

Thus installation of water supply without wastewater disposal merely results in a shift from one dominant set of diseases to another. Such a shift develops only with time; in the interim it engenders a feeling of accomplishment in the unwary so that the true consequences may never be appreciated.

With limited financial resources, should water supply with sanitation be provided for a smaller, or water supply only be provided for a larger number of people? In this form the question is unreal for it is not a simple situation of have or have not but a graduation of needs. Rather one should commence by circumscribing the needs to identify the situations where the needs justify priority for assistance.

In a rural society the very dispersal of inhabitants is a powerful factor in reducing incidence of diseases due to insanitation. To achieve a tolerable standard of sanitation and water supply in this situation may require provision of the most elementary nature and is often attainable by individual or family effort. The cost may be only the labour of the individual. There is often a case for leaving things as they are. To insist on a more sophisticated system where a lesser one is adequate is to divert State capital from ventures which may eventually be of greater benefit to the whole country.

As the size and concentration of a community grows there comes a stage where individual effort no longer suffices. It becomes impossible for the individual to protect himself from the interaction of the insanitary practice of his neighbour on himself. Community effort is now imperative in both water supply and sanitation—the lack of either is equally fatal. In this situation it is no longer: 'Can the community afford sanitation?' but 'Has the community the best sanitation it can afford?'. Public money committed for this purpose should be allocated on the basis of water supply and sanitation adequate for the situation. The criteria for selecting the particular system are efficiency at lowest cost and the expectation of continuous function, not the sophistication of the system. If a community desires more sophisticated systems it must provide the capital out of its own resources and cannot look to the State for such aid. It is only by such harsh realism that the State can be equitable to all its citizens and yet leave as much capital as possible for development. As it is the bigger, denser communities which are the most vulnerable to insanitation, this is where the major effort at solution must be directed.

Acceptance of this philosophy will assist in getting health 'purists' to rethink their approach that only the latest and most sophisticated (often confused with high standard) installations should be allowed. It may also induce State purse strings to be loosened sufficiently to allow health measures, such as adequate sanitation, to safeguard the investments in training and the acquisition of skills. A budget which withholds adequate expenditure on sanitation is no worse than a 'health' policy which, by being inflexible in its demands for specific systems, places adequate sanitation for many communities beyond available funds.

Shelter

Examining causes of death in the tropics and subtropics from exposure and from lack of water supply and sanitation respectively, it is evident that exposure is a relatively minor cause whereas insanitation is a major one. Where there is a deficiency of public capital for 'housing' it seems logical that the available funds should be spent on providing those components of 'housing' which, from a community point of view, are most likely to bring about the maximum return in improved health and those which it is not possible for the individual to supply himself. On this basis the 'housing' needs that must be the prime responsibility of the community are access, water supply and sanitation, drainage and a plot for a house. Only secondary is the community's responsibility for providing a house.

A means of implementing this concept is the site and service scheme: the site plus services (roads, drainage, water supply and sanitation) are provided from public funds and the 'shelter' is provided by the occupier of the site. His contribution will depend on his financial resources and his interest. It may

234

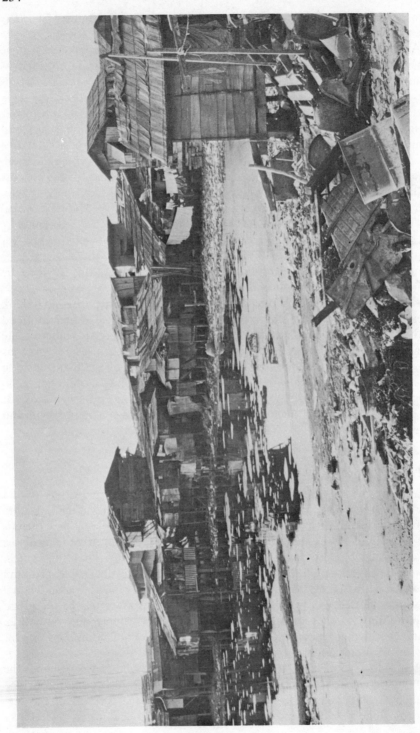

Urban housing in south-east Asia (photograph : courtesy P. Lacquian, IDRC)

be a crude shelter wherein he may live in physical discomfort but, from the communicable diseases' point of view, in a tolerably healthy environment. As the costs of services are usually much less than the costs of a house plus services more plots can be provided for the same capital expenditure so that overcrowding is less likely and easier to control. More people will also be able to rent or own their own plot. An important point about the site and service concept is that it devolves the contribution of the occupier on that aspect— the house—most likely to evoke his self-interest and endeavour. This is never possible with services in high density areas.

Site and service schemes usually present a very untidy appearance, due to the low standard of building by the occupiers. Untidiness does not make a slum; a slum is characterised by overcrowding from too high rentals making it imperative for individuals to band together in existing houses in order to afford the rental. It is ironical that the public-spirited by demanding that 'houses' must be provided may unknowingly be guilty of helping to create 'housing' shortages and slums.

When planning site and service schemes the end results must be clear in the mind of the planner from inception. Planning may often envisage ultimately the installation of individual water-borne sanitation and water supply, adequate roads, drainage and lighting. Initially it may be necessary to accept lower standards—for example pit latrines or unpaved roads—in order to deal with an interim situation or emergency. The planning must however be flexible so that improvements can be made as the financial situation allows without existing services being disrupted.

Planning on a lavish scale in terms of space or frontage may well result in substandard services which cost as much per plot as full services in a well designed, low-cost, high density area. Service costs are linearly related to the frontage width of plots, hence deep plots with narrow frontages are indicated. The services—light, water and sewerage—should also be located on the inner boundaries of the plots on the centre line of the blocks instead of in the street.

12.2 DETERMINATION OF 'HOUSING' NEEDS

Quantitative determination of 'housing' needs is extremely difficult. House-to-house surveys are normally completely misleading as house owners misinform on the number of residents for fear of penalization under regulations limiting the number of people per house. This also applies in illegal squatter settlements around a city. In the latter case useful information is obtained from aerial photographs which not only show the exact location of each shanty but also give a measure of the number of families involved.

An effective means of assessing the magnitude of the 'housing' problem is to attempt a knock-out blow in a typical town, not too large for the cost may be too high. The surveys show that 4000–6000 houses are required. A thousand are built and, say, four thousand site and service plots are prepared. Very likely a number of houses are not rented. This gives a sample by which the preference of the occupiers can be determined and of how much they are willing to pay in rental. By this procedure it is possible to discover the real needs of the people and their ability to pay instead of relying on postulations of the local authorities.

In attempts to satisfy each town's needs proportionally it often seems impossible to make an indent into the problem or to define it quantitatively; the situation looks insoluble. Because each town receives only a little help the real needs are obscured—whatever is built is snapped up in competition. Concentrating on one experimental scheme also makes it possible to bring to bear a greater variety of specialist skills, allows through investigation and experimentation with alternative layouts, sanitation systems and construction methods which can subsequently find application elsewhere. Piecemeal schemes tend to evade the issues and to perpetuate out-of-date layouts and substandard services.

12.3 EVALUATION OF SANITATION SYSTEMS

The standard of one latrine and one water tap per family has received international recognition, but the most suitable type of latrine or system to adopt in any particular situation remains for many developing nations a perplexing question. The water supply aspect is usually accepted with little resistance, but this is not so with the provision of the latrine. It is more expensive than the water supply, its need is not so immediately apparent (it is sometimes looked upon as a luxury), and money invested in it is not directly productive of material wealth. Experience with many sanitation systems in developing countries has often also been a dismal failure so that there is justification for opposition to their installation.

Before pushing for 'improved' sanitation one must be clear on expectation of success of a particular system. For this purpose it is necessary to enquire into the background, health education and level of technology of the people before evaluating a system in any particular situation.

Background

Most low-cost, high density housing areas in Africa are occupied by people who have moved from agricultural areas. Their behaviour pattern and habits are those of people living in a dispersed fashion where they are totally unaware of the dangers to health when living in close proximity. In a sanitary sense they have no health protective habits for urban living. Consequently they need in general very efficient systems which will work despite their lack of understanding.

Health education

In societies with a high general standard of health education, sanitation systems operate satisfactorily because of the safeguard of awareness in the users, that they know how to operate the system and to correct minor malfunctions. In societies where community health education is low this awareness is rudimentary so that there is often no effective attempt to correct even the most elementary malfunctions. In general, the lower the standard of health education the more necessary it becomes that the sanitation system will be self-operating and non-fouling.

Technology—social constraints

In technologically developed communities there is a tendency to equate efficiency with technological sophistication. Whereas this is normally true, sophisticated systems developed within these communities maintain their efficiency because of an 'infrastructure' of health education and the availability of operational 'know-how'. When such a system is transplanted to a different environment it does not necessarily follow that the same high standard of performance will be achieved on an enduring basis. One example will illustrate: with the flush system, toilet paper is in fact a major consideration, although because of its ready availability in richer communities it would not be considered to be a factor of any significance. However, in poor communities where corn cobs, stones, leaves, twigs, newspaper, cement bags, etc. are often the only cleaning materials readily available or within their means, the incidence of blockage increases sharply and additional supervision and expenditure are required to attain even spasmodic efficiency.

Communal facilities are rarely, if ever, satisfactory no matter what system is provided. There is no individual responsibility. In low-cost housing areas public latrines are usually provided because they are considered the most inexpensive. The price is paid in the consequences of the resulting low standard of sanitary conditions. Once a latrine is fouled, by misuse or accident, the next user may have no choice but to foul it further. Thus a chain reaction sets in and the latrine rapidly becomes unusable. Communal latrines may be up to 100 metres from some houses. Consequently at night the latrine is little used; this is particularly true if there is no street lighting. If the latrine itself is not well lit at night nobody uses it. To achieve even a minimum standard of cleanliness, strict control and constant attendance of cleaners are required; each time a cubicle is used it must be inspected and cleaned if necessary. Sanitary paper must be provided otherwise blockages due to stones, sticks, leaves and grass in flush systems are frequent.

With communal standpipes and communal ablution and washing facilities water waste can be appreciable. There is no individual responsibility to see that taps are closed and water consumption *per capita* may exceed that where each family has its own individual water supply. Invariably soakaways of communal ablution facilities fail.

12.4 CONCLUSIONS

What, then, are the *minimum* requirements for a satisfactory system of sanitation in low-cost, high density housing? One can put forward the following requirements: the system must be cheap, not communal, use little or none of the potable water supply for the operation, work despite misuse, require little supervision, not use soakaways, dispose of all the wastewater, treat the wastewater to a degree where it can be discharged with little subsequent danger to users, and require no mechanical equipment. One solution is the combined aqua-privy sewerage system developed in Zambia; a technological and economic appraisal of this and other systems is given by McGarry in Chapter 13.

A pertinent end to this paper is the following quotation from Vincent (1964): *'Considering the problems and real cost of attempting to maintain substandard sanitation, the question appears not to be can we afford to supply every house with its own water supply and water carriage system of sanitation, but rather do we want it? We are already paying for it'.*

12.5 REFERENCES

Indian Ministry of Health (1964). Recommendations. In: *Proceedings of a Seminar on Financing and Management of Water and Sewage Works*. New Delhi: Vigyan Bhawan.
Vincent, L. J. (1964). Improving the standard of existing housing. In: *Proceedings of a Conference on Urban Housing*. Lusaka: Ministry of Housing and Social Development.

13

Waste Collection in Hot Climates: A Technical and Economic Appraisal

Michael G. McGarry

13.1 INTRODUCTION: THE PROBLEM

In many ways, improvements in practices of disposing of excreta are crucial to raising levels of public health in developing countries. They have, however, lagged well behind recent advances made in water supply and, in contrast to what is needed, improvements in levels of sanitation accomplished to date are negligible and are likely to remain so at the current rate of effort and financing. Yet excreta disposal is an essential part of the environmental health services package. Water supply alone cannot provide full health benefits. In some cases, owing to the lack of adequate facilities for excreta disposal, an increased water supply may even cause the spread of disease. There are several reasons for this enigma, the more fundamental being: (a) The collection and disposal of human wastes is aesthetically displeasing and normally economically unproductive; (b) government commitment and motivation to improve levels of sanitation are lacking; and (c) social constraints on technology design have fostered the use of capital intensive, passive schemes which are both wasteful of natural resources and financially beyond the reach of over 90% of developing country people.

With regard to the first reason, consideration is given to reclamation and re-use of human wastes in Chapter 18; and with regard to the second reason, attitudes, approaches and incentives for improvements are discussed in Chapter 10. In this paper, I will try in summary fashion to review current knowledge of the impact of sanitation on public health and make comparisons between the various technologies which are available, their advantages and drawbacks.

13.2 WHY SANITATION?

For decades it has been assumed that the proper disposal of excreta will result in improvements in health, yet the incentive behind wastes removal from man's immediate environment has always been one based on the aesthetically unpleasant nature of faecal matter. Leaving aside aesthetics for the moment, let us examine more closely the effects of excreta disposal on health. Looking to the literature for hard facts, we find that there have been several empirical studies in which field data have been gathered in an effort to define what happens to public health, in particular to gastro-enteric morbidity levels, when a programme of latrine or sewerage installation is implemented. These were conducted in Guatemala, the USA, the Philippines, Colombia, India, Panama, England, Costa Rica, Egypt, Mauritius, Sudan and Venezuela.

It is understandable that before an investment is undertaken the outcome in terms of its costs and benefits should be predictable. Within this sector, however, there are very little comprehensive and reliable data by which a predictive capacity may be developed. Admittedly, there have been many investigations which have attempted to define the health–sanitation relationship but few have been able to separate out the impact of individual sanitation measures from the effects of economic status or cultural differences within the population being studied. It is also unfortunate that most of the comprehensive and reliable data were obtained, not in the developing countries themselves, but in low-income communities exhibiting high gastro-enteric disease rates in the USA. The conclusions drawn may not have cross-cultural application; besides, these studies focused on improvements in sanitation rather than the introduction of sanitation, the latter being more applicable to conditions in the developing country.

A study in Kentucky, USA (Schliessman, 1959) was able to demonstrate a significant reduction in stated morbidity rates with improved sanitation in low-income communities. Conflicting results were reported in Costa Rica (Moore *et al.*, 1965) where morbidity rates were found to actually increase when comparisons were made between populations having no latrines at all and those using pit privies. It was noted, however, that the no-latrine condition was geographically biased towards isolated rural areas; it is likely that population density influenced the results which suggests that, in practice, indiscriminate defecation in the fields is sometimes superior to confined defecation in latrines. Several studies have attempted to define the impact of sanitation on the incidence of shigellosis. Many concluded that shigellosis is inversely related to economic status although many other variables were confounded with economic levels of the populations under study (Moore *et al.*, 1965; Kourany and Vasquez, 1969).

The Kentucky studies included surveys of the human roundworm or ascarid, the incidence rate of which was found to be higher in children within the 5–9-year age group. Successive increases in ascariasis incidence and, by implication, severity were noted with reduced sanitation. Room crowding also appeared to encourage the spread of the worm regardless of the quality of sanitation facilities. The striking differences in ascariasis incidence rates between homes using inside privies and those employing inside flush toilets was observed in the Kentucky studies. This effect might well have been more to do with the availability of water in the toilet room and anal and hand cleansing practices than the actual mode of excreta removal from the toilet bowl. The Costa Rican studies illustrated a distinct drop in ascariasis rates with increases in economic status. The drop in incidence with use of privies was observed to be quite outstanding in that shigellosis rates actually increased, as described above, under identical conditions. Similarly, but far less evident, water availability had a notable beneficial effect on ascariasis incidence rates.

Few studies have included the effect of sanitation on incidence rates of hookworm and trichuriasis. However, those that do have illustrated in a general way that increased economic status and, by implication, improved sanitation does reduce the prevalence of these worms. In all, seventeen individual studies have attempted to observe the impact of sanitation; these are fully reviewed elsewhere (McGarry, 1975) and cannot be considered in detail here. Nearly all allude to health benefits through improvements in the level of general sanitation, including water supply. As noted above few were able to separate out effects of improved sanitation from those derived from raised socio-economic status. In three studies, negative or no sanitation impact on health was observed; however, reasons for these results were clearly identifiable. The Kentucky study demonstrated the benefits to be accrued through effective implementation of the 'sanitation package' including water supply. These conclusions are supported by historical evidence of the impact of urban water supply and sanitation on the incidence of typhoid in cities of the USA at the turn of the century (Kruse, 1966) and in England during the latter part of the industrial revolution (McKeown and Record, 1962). If little else, many of the more poorly designed studies have shown that stated morbidity rates and gastro-enteric bacterial and worm infestations are lower in the higher-income groups which have improved levels of sanitation.

It appears then that empirical evidence is basically not contradictory to our intuitive belief that sewers and pit privies do have a beneficial impact on health. However, there are major investments being made in such schemes throughout the world without adequate information on the benefits likely to result. Few cost-effectiveness studies are being made for technology comparisons and the engineer continues to insist on those requiring least maintenance, which are the most capital intensive systems.

13.3 APPROACH TO DESIGN

It hardly needs to be stated that defecation is a very personal act; habits associated with it are learned early in life; it is an important focal point of concern between mother and child. The rural peasant is loath to change personal habits and will resist such pressures as may be brought to bear from outside unless he is convinced of the superiority of the alternative method. To facilitate such changes as may be necessary the industrialized countries have adapted systems which do not involve manual transport or human contact with the excreta. Defecation takes place in as pristine and private an environment as is possible. The wastes are then flushed away with a minimum of odour and visibility. Such an approach is expensive, involving individual toilet rooms, intricate plumbing arrnagements and a complete subterranean network of

150 mm and larger diameter pipes and pumping stations. Transport of the solids through the pipe system requires large volumes of water which must then be treated before discharge into the environment downstream of the contributing population. The developed country national is willing to pay upwards of $ US 500/household in order to maintain such high standards of defecation practice and disposal. Funds are limited in the developing country; there, the householder is not only unwilling to pay for such facilities, he cannot afford to do so. And the municipality and central government can ill afford to subsidize such technologies indefinitely. It is essential therefore that alternatives are identified and utilized.

Any change in defecation practices which may be considered desirable by the health authorities must take full account of social attitudes and habits. This is amply illustrated by the reluctance of the Westerner, being used to the sitting position, to be faced with a necessity to squat during defecation; so too is it demonstrated by the urbanite who continues to practise indiscriminate defecation along the river banks despite alternative facilities being available in his home, an occurrence not uncommon in many parts of Asia. Such norms are not changed simply in response to the installation of alternative places to defecate; it takes a considerable length of time and an appreciation of reasons behind the need for change before old habits are altered. The low-income, peri-urban settlement populations adopt new practices more quickly than their counterparts in the rural areas. Traditional hierarchical authority patterns have been largely broken down in the urban centre and communications are relatively sophisticated and efficient. Urban acceptance of excreta collection systems is ameliorated by the fact that there are few alternatives.

The alienation of the sanitary engineer from the rural population with which he is trying to work aggravates the problems of introducing public health measures. Basically, the engineer and his medical counterpart are city oriented, having been educated at the university level; they are on a vastly different social and economic stratum to those whom they are attempting to assist. Another difficulty, and this is a very basic and important one, relates to technical university education curricula. Tunnel vision is amply assured by a purely technical education which prevents the engineer from relating to the social aspects of the problem, a condition which is quite as bad as the social scientist who, although seeing the social and technical needs, has no technical background with which to solve the problem.

Practically every aspect of rural excreta disposal projects seems to be preset to foster the technological 'quick fix' solution. The funds are most often centrally, and therefore urban, controlled. The programme must be large enough to adequately cover the numbers of villages to be 'helped'. The administrative personnel are more interested in numbers of facilities installed than in their effective use; seldom are post-project evaluations undertaken. There is little *rapport* between the urban oriented technician or administrator and the rural peasant. As a consequence standard technical 'packages' are likely to be imposed on the village without adequate concern for the peasant, his needs, desires, capabilities and norms.

It is necessary to have an adequate understanding of the social, cultural and organizational characteristics of the community with which one is working. Inducing change within the traditional society may well be a slow and arduous process, but it is possible. A rapid change can only be a superficial one and therefore short-lived. The introduction of a technology or concept without ensuring that the individual user understands and accepts the reasons why he is expected to alter his habits is bound to meet with failure in the long run, despite any initial burst of enthusiasm or respectful but ignorant concurrence with the idea. The media of change are normally the community leader and elders. These must be given the opportunity of participating if their support is to be acquired. The implicit imposition of concepts without their approval, such as may be imposed through preset government design criteria and standards, will be likely to run into opposition through not requiring community leader approval and thereby undermining the authority structure.

13.4 RURAL SANITATION

The pit-privy and bored-hole latrines

The pit-privy consists of a hand-dug pit over which is placed a squatting plate or slab, riser and seat. Around this is constructed a wall or shelter for privacy (Figure 13.1). The pit-privy is a minimum-cost solution providing for defecation with or without water use, excreta storage, digestion of waste solids and seepage of urine and moisture into the surrounding soil. Under normal circumstances one pit-privy is installed on the premises of each household. The pit-privy requires maintenance to ensure that it is kept clean, replacement of a lid over the defecation hole to prevent ingress of flies and earth filling with removal of the superstructure and slab to another dug pit when it becomes filled, which occurs after four to fifteen years of normal use.

Although technically sound, the pit-privy is not the panacea it is often assumed to be. For example, a latrine programme was undertaken in Brazil during the early 1950s which successfully installed nearly two thousand latrines in rural villages of the Rio Doce Valley—without cost to the local people. The programme was instituted through the 'guarda', a team of trained personnel having little previous educational background (Sanches and Wagner, 1954). After the project engineer had contacted the local health officer and other relevant authorities, the guarda would select households to receive privies and determine their location. 'During construction he would inspect frequently and make sure that every part was built according to the sanitation manual. When the privy was finished the guarda would turn it over to the house owners and instruct them on how to maintain it. After that, he would return to the house and while advising the people on other sanitary improvements he would make a new inspection and insist again on the privies being kept clean and in good condition'. Two years later it was discovered that few of the privies so installed were still in use *and some had never been used at all.*

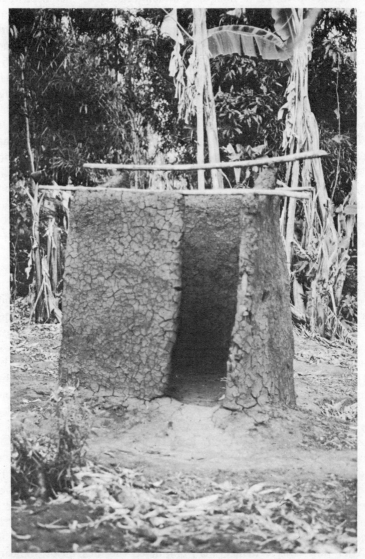

Figure 13.1 The pit-privy. This one, in the process of construction, has a dug hole 3 m deep and a mud and wattle superstructure; it is typical of pit-privies found in rural Malawi

However, shortage of funds for this programme soon necessitated the financial collaboration of the towns and cooperation of the house owners in providing labour and materials. Apart from financial benefits, this cooperative approach brought the local authorities closer to the problem and permitted the family to identify itself with its privy as something of value, having contributed to its construction.

Most other efforts to implement pit-privy programmes in rural areas without major sociological input have failed. Shelat and Mansuri have described many of the inherent difficulties of such programmes in Chapter 16; others have been described in the available literature by Wier *et al.* (1952) and Bruch *et al.* (1963). In most instances of failure the family makes initial attempts at using the privy as instructed by the visiting sanitarian or technician; with time, however, it becomes soiled by faeces and the user finds other places more attractive for defecation. When this happens the principle of concentrating excreta can have a decidedly adverse effect in that the latrine becomes a source of infection and so spreads the diseases it was originally intended to combat. The placement of boards over a deep hole with minimal provision for privacy, shelter and separation of sexes is used in Africa. Although in many ways superior to indiscriminate defecation, local practices include the deposit of anal cleansing material beside and not in the pit, which provides a feeding ground for flies. Also, the pit is allowed to fill to one foot below the slats before the village finds it necessary to dig a new latrine elsewhere; odours are ripe and fly breeding prolific under such conditions. Even this simple technology is subject to failure as illustrated in Figure 13.2.

The bored-hole latrine is in many ways similar to the pit-privy being based on the same principle and having identical outhouse superstructure. However, collection, containment and digestion is made in a much smaller diameter hole which is greater in depth. Being smaller in volume, the bored-hole's filling time or life length is shorter. However, the unit is easier to construct if auger boring equipment is available and appropriate soil conditions prevail. It is widely used in most tropical zones. Its use and maintenance are similar to the pit-privy as are the social constraints to its acceptance. The bored-hole's life is relatively short (1–2 years) so more frequent moves to new bored-hole sites are necessary. Where emergency conditions prevail as may occur in refugee camps the bored-hole has a distinct advantage in that numerous latrines can be easily and quickly installed close to residential shelters. The bored-hole is however confined to soils which are free of rocks and stones which cannot be removed by the auger. Care must be taken not to contaminate water supplies by means of penetration of the groundwater table used as a source of drinking water too close to the well. Under crowded conditions where housing density is high, as may be found in squatter settlements, both the pit and bored-hole latrines suffer the disadvantage of requiring open space: alternative sites for the pit's relocation and an acceptable distance from the home which minimizes odour nuisance.

The PRAI latrine

The PRAI latrine as developed in India is described in some detail by Shelat

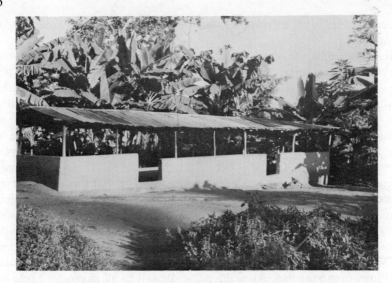

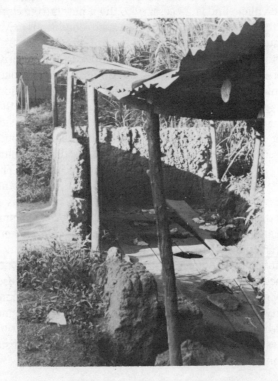

Figure 13.2 (Above) Communal pit-privies in West Africa. Conditions around the latrine are reasonably inoffensive. Traditional tribal authority is indispensible to the proper maintenance of such facilities. (Below) A failed communal privy, filled to the brim and alive with fly maggot but still in constant use by the male village population

and Mansuri in Chapter 16, as are the difficulties being encountered in its propagation.

The overhung latrine and the *feuillée*

The overhung latrine and the *feuillée* are sometimes necessary; most often they are undesirable methods of excreta disposal, both having greater potential for spreading disease than combating it. The overhung latrine is simply an outhouse superstructure with toilet seat or floor-hole located above the tidal flat, river, canal, lake or sea beach (Figure 13.3). Defecation takes place either directly into the water, for transport and eventual dilution, or on the mudflat or beach to await the tide. There are few, if any, alternatives for fishing villages of Asia which are supported by stilts embedded in mudflats. In such villages, many homes are as far as a kilometre from the nearest firm ground. Rubbish and household garbage are also deposited beneath the houses. This practice is satisfactory from the public health point of view if the water is saline enough to prevent its use as drinking water, if the faeces are always deposited in water and not on land, and if there is sufficient current for dilution. Unfortunately,

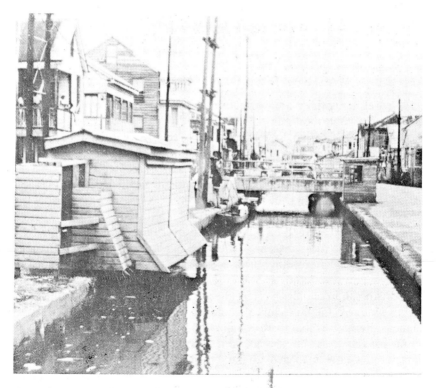

Figure 13.3 An overhung latrine in an urban area discharging directly into an open canal

freshwater rivers over which these latrines hang are commonly used as sources of drinking water, for personal cleansing, teeth brushing and bathing. Likewise the ideal waters under fishing villages are used for bathing recreation and cleaning fish.

The *feuillée* consists of a shallow hole dug into the ground into which faeces are deposited and lightly covered with soil after each use. A movable screen may be used to provide privacy. After filling, the hole is covered with earth and a galvanized iron sheet to prevent vermin having access. Unfortunately, the *feuillée* is rarely maintained in an hygienic condition; it quickly becomes unsanitary and offensive. Excreta, which often surrounds the hole, are breeding grounds for flies and also assist in the spread of disease, notably hookworm. The *feuillée* should only be used as an emergency and temporary method of excreta disposal.

Excreta composting and the biogas plant

Both composting and the production of methane through anaerobic digestion of excreta and farm wastes are means by which nutrients can be recovered and recycled as fertilizer back to the soil and plant. Additionally, the biogas plant produces natural gas usable in the home for lighting and cooking. Further consideration of both these approaches to excreta disposal are given in Chapters 17 and 18 respectively.

13.5 URBAN WASTEWATER COLLECTION

In the rural areas there are, in fact, as many modes of excreta disposal as there are acceptable locations to defecate. Not so in the town, where population density limits defecation to relatively few sites. In the country, privacy is afforded by the open field or nearby bush but, in town, defecation involves a search for privacy and an unsoiled aesthetically acceptable place for relief. Inadequate and poorly maintained communal facilities encourage open defecation turning river banks and woods into open latrines and every unlit alley and walled corner a place to defecate.

The pit-privy, the bored-hole, PRAI and overhung latrines which may be appropriate to the rural areas are, on occasion, also used in the city. Inappropriate subsoil, overcrowding, over-use, environmental contamination and offensive conditions within and around such latrines often negate their use. The individual householder has few alternatives; with little or no municipal or collective interest and no technical guidance he must fend for himself. The few technical alternatives that there are all require some level of municipal participation for effective implementation; these are discussed below. Many municipalities have managed to shirk their responsibility for urban excreta collection and disposal in the past; but there comes a point of environmental deterioration where the situation demands that the government must act to coordinate, implement and standardize a programme for wastes collection treatment and disposal. The methods used must be technically, socially and financially viable.

If costs are to be minimized technical efficiencies need to be compromised. Separate sanitary sewerage with sewage treatment may well be the best technical solution for sewage disposal, particularly as far as environmental benefits are concerned. In general, however, only the privileged class can afford such a high-cost solution. The government is then faced with subsidizing the remaining population—scarcity of funds and alternative uses of resources invariably dictate that sewerage be limited to the areas that can afford it and little is accomplished for the lower income groups, apart, that is, from the enactment of sanitary bye-laws which are seldom enforceable. All too often the wealthier suburbs are also subsidized at cost to the rest of the city. Politicians and consultants (particularly overseases engineers) are loath to propose alternatives to sewerage with which they are not familiar. As a consequence, master plans are drawn up to provide sanitary sewerage for the city centre with no improvement to the suburbs. As no alternatives appear to be forthcoming through the international consultancy system, it will be up to the nationals of the developing country to identify, adapt and test less costly approaches themselves. Government funds cannot be expected to subsidize all towns, yet conditions for most urban peoples in the less wealthy nations have become intolerable as population pressures mount each year.

In applying alternatives to sewerage and thereby reducing costs, certain cuts in technical efficiency must be accepted in order to make the system financially feasible to the population it serves. These may include the on-property and often unsanitary disposal of liquid effluent, from such units as the septic tank and aqua-privy, and also the inability to collect kitchen and bath waters, by the vacuum truck and vault system, and the compost toilet. In many cases such drawbacks are counteracted by other benefits such as the reduction of demand for water otherwise required for flushing and excreta transport through pipes. These and other aspects of the various alternatives applicable to the urban centre are considered below.

It must again be emphasized that social design plays an essential role in successful implementation of urban excreta disposal. The selected technology or mix of technologies must be socially acceptable. In selecting a less passive and reduced-cost method of excreta disposal there is always some trade-off which must be borne by the user. He should be given the opportunity of expressing his felt needs and opinions at each stage of design. Otherwise, if the system is planned in a vacuum in some government office (or worse still, in some consultant's office overseas) it is almost bound to run into difficulties related to social acceptance. Unfortunately, civil engineering design does not normally include social surveys and those responsible for planning the system are seldom familiar with the social sciences and have little knowledge of how to introduce such a component into design procedure. Likewise, the sociologist and anthropologist have seldom applied their skills to something so practical as excreta disposal design. Yet, if alternatives are to be identified and successfully adapted and

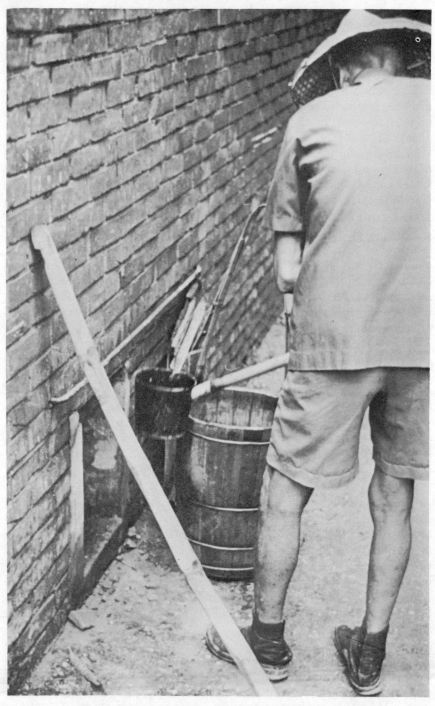

Household nightsoil collection (photograph: M. G. McGarry)

applied, the engineer and social scientist must be brought together in a team. In countries which are unfamiliar with alternatives to urban sewerage *in situ* trials will be required; if conclusions drawn from such trials are to be correct the investigations will need to be properly designed and conducted. The costs of conducting such pilot trials are minimal when compared to the savings to be made by installation of the reduced cost system thereby defined.

The septic tank

The septic tank is an on-site means of disposing of wastewaters from the household. Its construction, operation and maintenance is carried out solely within the confines of the private property, apart from infrequent desludging of the tank. As such it is often regarded as a panacea for sewage disposal by municipalities in that when operated properly the municipality need not be involved technically or financially; the system can be entirely supported by the individual house owner.

The septic tank consists of a large tank placed beneath the ground level in close proximity to the house from which it receives its influent of kitchen, cleansing and toilet wastewaters. Most of the solids in the waste settle in the tank as sludge and digest (ferment) on its bottom. The effluent leaves by overflow into a subterranean pipe or trench system which distributes it for percolation into the soil.

Unfortunately the septic tank has serious disadvantages. The first and most important one is that it is expensive, often costing more on a per household basis than separate sanitary sewers; its use is confined to the wealthier suburbs. The second is that it requires large areas of permeable subsoil through which it can distribute its effluent; where population densities are high the open spaces of land required for these purposes are too limited for its widespread use. Thirdly, in the majority of cases where cities have been built near rivers or in deltaic areas, the subsoil structure is too impermeable for the leaching of septic tank effluent; being unable to permeate the soil the effluent, still laden with pathogens, flows across the ground and, thereby hastening the spread of disease and not allaying it (Figure 13.4). Finally, and most insidious of all, the temptation of the municipality to rely upon privately owned systems during initial periods of urban growth may be too great and result in very costly reversions to other methods when population densities no longer allow septic tanks to function properly.

Other costs to be considered are those which affect the community as a whole. As often as not, vents on the septic tank are not effectively screened and the unit becomes an insect breeding ground. If a policy of endorsing septic tanks is followed in time by the installation of a municipal sewerage scheme there is a real danger of double costing, leading to public hostility if hook-up to the sewerage scheme is not offered entirely on a voluntary basis. Foresight is required to ensure that septic tanks are fully depreciated before sewerage schemes are imposed on the municipality.

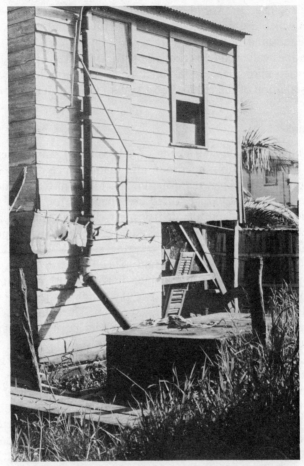

Figure 13.4 The septic tank in the foreground has been raised above ground level to accommodate flood conditions. The subsoil is clay and the tank leaky; board walkways are necessary to avoid contact with the ground which has become supersaturated with effluent

Conventional sanitary sewerage

Conventional sanitary sewers have only become widely used in the Western countries since the turn of this century. They have, however, gained such popularity that they are considered by most engineers to be the only 'acceptable' means of wastewater collection. There are many alternative methods of excreta collection which were used prior to the advent of sewerage and others that are successfully used in developing countries today. On the other hand, it is to be pointed out that there appears to be no better alternative to sewerage in the centres of the larger cities having high quantities of commercial and industrial wastewaters for disposal. Water-borne sewerage schemes are socially acceptable and technically efficient in removing wastes, but they are also often prohibitively expensive; on a household basis, they cost as much as or more than a television set.

The sewerage system begins upstream with the toilet, which is normally ceramic and requires 5–10 litres of water for flushing. The sewage (99·9 per cent water) enters the underground collection system outside the household via the house connection pipe leading to the street sewer. Moving down the 'collection tree' the sewage passes through manholes which provide access for inspection and cleaning into larger and larger lateral pipes, sub-branches and mains. As the accumulating flow builds up the downward slope of the sewer provides a velocity of flow sufficient to maintain solids in suspension. Using the river as a means of transportation and water supply, cities are built within a watershed. The river valley forms a natural drainage shed for the gravity sewer system, so that mains sewers are usually directed towards the river. Larger sewers known as interceptors are laid somewhat parallel to the river in order to intercept the mains' flow and transport it downstream of the city for treatment, discharge or re-use.

Sewerage systems are technically efficient and passive in that they require little maintenance and are relatively trouble-free. Any investment decision must take the relative cost of labour and capital into account. Sewerage systems are low in labour or maintenance costs but high in construction or capital costs. These cost characteristics are not compatible with the national economies of most developing countries, where there is a surplus of labour and a shortage of capital, particularly in the form of foreign exchange. Despite the unlikelihood of complete sewer systems being installed in developing urban centres, there is a continuing trend to provide aid to development funds for feasibility studies and sewerage master plans. Funds thereby spent are largely wasted but there are real reasons for this trend. Aid in the form of technical assistance is usually free, the money is spent on the donor country consultants and there is normally a high level of competence in designing sewers among developed country engineers. Likewise, the highly educated developing country planner tends to mimic Western preferences for capital intensive, advanced technologies. Although detailed plans may be drawn up for the whole urban population's sewerage, only 10% or perhaps 20% are eventually serviced. As a consequence, suburban, peri-urban and squatter settlements' improvements in sanitation are postponed for some distant time in the future.

From a water resource conservation point of view, sewerage systems are particularly inapplicable to arid areas. Conceptually, the process is one of depositing wastes in a ceramic bowl, diluting them with treated water for purposes of transportation down a complex system of underground piping for eventual collection at one point downstream of the city. This huge volume of wastewater must then be 'dewatered' for removal of sludge prior to its being treated. The liquid effluent being partially treated is wasted to the environment. In summary, our human waste is diluted, transported, concentrated again, treated and then wasted as is the water used for its initial dilution. The technology proposed is a capital intensive system within an economy which most often favours labour intensive solutions. From a system's point of view this does not make economic sense.

As has been mentioned above, despite its many drawbacks, the sanitary sewer scheme does find applicability in the dense urban centre as the only technology which can cope with the large volume of industrial wastewaters. Rapid industrialization has created a crucial demand for effective urban/industrial planning focusing on the use of industrial areas which facilitate the centralized collection and treatment of wastewaters. As far as is possible, industry, tourism and commerce should be directly responsible for the disposal of their own wastes: the point being made here is that scarce municipal funds allocated for wastewater collection should not be used up in subsidizing commerce and industry which should be capable of fending for themselves. Likewise such funds should not be put towards support of the wealthier suburbs at the expense of the low-income population. It is far better that they be allocated to the installation of lower-cost technologies and thereby reach a much larger population.

The bucket latrine

Collection of excreta in buckets, pans and baskets was common practice throughout the world long before sewerage was introduced. Whatever the mode of collection, the principle was the same: defecation was into a container which was removed for disposal (with or without treatment) at frequent intervals into local surface water bodies or on the land. Sydney, Australia, provides a modern-day example of perhaps the best operated system. There, tarred steel buckets are used. Collection of the bucket is made on a weekly basis during which a lid is fixed to the bucket before it is placed on a truck for disposal into the main gravity sewerage line for treatment and discharge to the sea. Each bucket is sterilized by retarring and returned to the household. The system is not offensive. This contrasts sharply with the method in which baskets are used to collect solid faecal matter only, the urine being allowed to drain away into open stormwater sewers or across the ground for eventual percolation.

Bucket collection is perhaps the cheapest method for excreta collection in terms of capital investment; it is highly flexible and does not require any major capital outlay by the householder. Municipalities on tight budgets are often tempted by low initial costs to establish a collection service with the aim of installing sewers later, but commonly find that the capital outlay required for sewerage is so excessive that they are forced to expand their bucket collection system. Operating costs are high, however, and the trade-off between capital and running costs sometimes (but in fact only rarely) favours sewerage.

The main reasons why the bucket system is undesirable as a method of excreta collection in developing countries are: (1) the collection procedure is nearly always aesthetically offensive; (2) the bucket is often washed in the immediate vicinity of the house with the result that excreta is splashed over the pavement and road; (3) the open bucket gives rise to odours and is accessible to vermin and insects; (4) the disposal site is almost always offensive and unhygienic, particularly where nightsoil is dumped and turned into the soil; and (5) there are less expensive methods of collection which are also labour intensive and more suited to developing country urban conditions— such as vacuum truck and vault system.

The aqua-privy

The aqua-privy comprises a watertight simple tank above which a toilet bowl is located. The household is protected from the contents of the tank by means of a water seal effected by a vertical drop-pipe extending from the toilet bowl down to and slightly submerged in the tank's contents. By these means, defecation is directly into the aqua-privy tank. Waste solids sink to the bottom where they digest as sludge over a period of time; the liquid used as flush water, low in volume as it is, passes out of the tank over a weir into an absorption trench or cesspit for percolation into the soil. The conventional design of the aqua-privy does not account for disposal of other household wastewaters. Also, it requires periodic desludging by vacuum truck.

The aqua-privy is widespread and successfully employed in Asia, where water is used for anal cleansing; daily washing of the toilet bowl is practised and the soil is adequately permeable for leaching the effluent away. It has not found such favour in parts of southern and eastern Africa where sticks, mudballs and stones are used for anal cleansing and maintenance of the privy is not carried out on a regular individual basis. Where water is not added to the tank, its liquid level soon falls below the vertical drop-pipe and flies are given access to, and odours emanate from, the tank; squat plates, soiled with excreta add to unpleasant conditions encouraging the user to defecate elsewhere. This situation has become so intolerable in one African country that the government has now officially banned the further installation of aqua-privies. The aqua-privy's varied popularity demonstrates the need to take social and cultural habits and constraints into account during design. Failure of an aqua-privy is illustrated in Figure 13.5.

The aqua-privy–sewerage system

This system has been developed and successfully applied in Zambia in order to overcome the inherent disadvantages of the aqua-privy such as its inability to cope with sullage waters, frequent failings of the water seal through in-

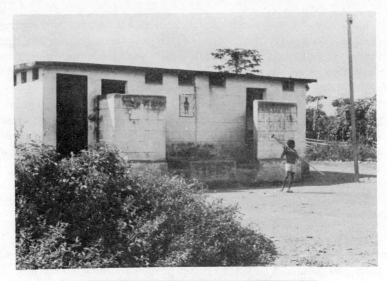

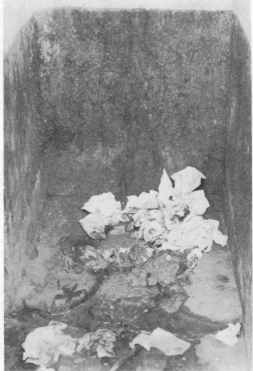

Figure 13.5 This aqua-privy was originally intended as a communal facility, but disposal of the liquid effluent into the soil has failed. The urban dwellers have little alternative but to continue using the facilities and rely on the greatly over-extended services of the municipality to pump out the tank contents. (Above) external view; (Below) internal view

sufficient water usage, the potential spread of disease caused by absorption trench failure and exclusion of its use from impermeable soils. All sullage waters from the household including wash and kitchen waters are allowed to pass through the aqua-privy vault and thereby maintain the integrity of the water seal. The much larger volume of water is passed out of the tank over a submerged weir into a sewer system—but one with a difference. As most of the waste solids have been settled out in the tank there is no need to provide velocities in the sewer collection system capable of maintaining them in suspension. The pipes are therefore smaller in diameter and at much reduced gradients thereby avoiding major trenching and pumping costs normally encountered in conventional sewerage systems. Where solid materials are used for anal cleansing, there is still the danger of clogging the down-pipe; this is much reduced in situations where a plentiful supply of piped water is immediately available for purposes of washing down the toilet.

In view of the health benefits to be accrued, piped water supply and washing facilities should be available in the immediate vicinity of the toilet. Where little water is used for toilet flushing or cleaning (10–20 lpcd) the danger of breaking the water seal can be overcome by tying several aqua-privies in series. Thus the effluent of one aqua-privy acts to maintain the water seal of several as it passes through the tanks. At the head of such a series, a communal washing facility or at least a public water supply standpipe should be installed to ensure adequate water is provided to the first tank.

The aqua-privy tanks can be designed so that they require desludging only once in about ten years. It is probable that much of the digested sludge passes out of the tank as light flocculated organic material with the effluent while some, being converted into gas by anaerobic digestion, escapes via the vent pipe.

Unfortunately, the aqua-privy–sewerage scheme is capital intensive; its initial capital requirements are sensitive to on-lot costs comprising the tank, toilet fixtures and, where used, the separate privy superstructure and washing facilities. In an effort to reduce these costs the tank itself can be made common between two to four families by constructing the privy over lot boundaries. Individual responsibility for maintaining the privy is assured by providing separate facilities and entrances above the common tank for each family. In comparison to conventional sewerage this system sets the costs of installing a tank on the property with its assoicated appurtenances and periodic tank desluding requirements against the benefits of shallow pipe trenching, low or nil pumping and essentially no additional water needed to maintain the water seal. This system holds considerable promise where a capital intensive passive technology is deemed necessary. However, care should be taken to assess relative costs on a case by case basis as both this and the conventional sewerage systems' costs are highly sensitive to local conditions.

The vacuum truck and vault

In China, human excreta has, for centuries, been looked upon as a valuable resource. Rather than growing cities being regarded as an undesirable cause of river pollution, they were viewed as a source of needed fertilizer where the farmer could purchase excreta from the housewife at relatively little cost and cart it to his fields. Whereas in Western thinking excreta are useless undesirable waste products to be got rid of as quickly and inoffensively as possible, the Chinese continue today to utilize excreta for agricultural development and by doing so provide a monetary incentive for pollution control. This has given rise to the use of a household vault both in China and Japan to store excreta with the small amounts of water used for anal cleaning and toilet bowl washing under or beside the house.

Preferably, water-seal low volume flush bowl is placed above the vault to provide protection to the household against the vault's contents. Simple water-seal squat plates are widely used in Asia which require only $\frac{1}{2}$–1 litre of water per flush. As is the practice in Japan, the vault's contents are collected by vacuum truck once every two to four weeks. Re-use of the excreta in agriculture is discussed in Chapter 18.

It is to be noted that the vacuum truck and vault system does not account for household wastewaters other than excreta. A trade-off needs to be evaluated in each application: does the reduction of installation and maintenance costs justify the environmental damage resulting from use of storm drains to transport kitchen and washing wastes? There are, however, several advantages in the use of this system. Apart from being less expensive than conventional sewerage and septic tanks, this approach is labour intensive and therefore likely to be more applicable to the developing country economy. The water-seal bowl and vault can be locally manufactured and sold as a market commodity. Collection by truck makes the system extremely flexible, a valuable asset in terms of urban planning; changes in land use patterns are as easily handled as redefining truck routes. Initial costs are low and benefits accrue immediately on initiating service to the household.

Again, care must be taken to ensure that the vault system is acceptable to the user; this implies field trials which are a worthwhile investment. Also, the municipality must be capable of maintaining a fleet of trucks for collection purposes. During the design phase it should be ensured that the transfer of technology which may be successful in one region is indeed applicable to another.

The compost toilet

Originally designed to suit country cottage use in Sweden, the 'Multrum' device is currently being appraised for possible use in tropical low-income conditions in Tanzania. This device comprises a vault with sloping floor into which is deposited excreta and compostable household refuse. Digestion takes place in the chamber under a mixture of aerobic and anaerobic conditions assisted by an air vent. Results of the East African trials are due to be published in 1977.

The chemical and other individual toilet units

The chemical toilet utilizes a tank in which strong basic chemicals are used to digest excreta deposited directly into the chamber. The liquefied effluent is either discharged with each use to an underground cesspit or removed by vacuum truck. Capital costs for the unit are high and chemical additives are required at regular intervals; as such it is only applicable to isolated cases of special needs where the required maintenance is assured and its relatively high costs can be met. There are several individual units which are becoming available on the commercial market. With few exceptions, all are under patent and complex in mechanical design, some requiring electrical energy and all needing regular maintenance. Invariably, initial costs are very high. The municipality considering such equipment for widespread application should evaluate each in the environment for which it is proposed. A healthy degree of scepticism during such appraisal is often rewarding.

13.6 THE TECHNOLOGY CHOICE: AN ECONOMIC COMPARISON

Choosing the technology for excreta collection is not a simple exercise. There are numerous variables which influence the initial cost of construction and running costs of each system. An example is given here which compares the conventional sanitary sewerage system, the aqua-privy–sewerage system, the vacuum truck and household vault system and the individual household septic tank. Of course, the comparison drawn below is only an example and the temptation to use it in absolute terms should be resisted. The unit costs employed have been drawn from a variety of sources in developing countries and therefore do not apply in any one given situation; however, the comparison between technologies and the methodology are of interest.

Density of housing and population will affect costs in that, on a unit basis, collection systems would be more intensively utilized in the concentrated city centre than in the fringe areas. Costs are sensitive to soil conditions. Installation of pipework in soft clay under high water table conditions can be very expensive. The cost of providing gravity sewerage would be less if the town were evenly sloped towards a sewage treatment plant than if it were located on flat or rolling topography. The cost of borrowing capital to construct the system (in terms and interest rates and period for repayment) will also have a bearing on annual charges levied against the householder.

Apart from these major influences there are variations in manpower costs reflected in construction and running expenses; design periods need to be carefully selected in order not to over-invest in excessive capacity; yet one's design must reflect urban growth lest the sewer's capacity be surpassed before the end of the design period is reached.

All this general information is of little use to the design engineer who, in searching for the most appropriate technology, is faced with a baffling array of inputs and interactions—none of them quantified. So, construction and running costs are calculated for the proposed system. For purposes of comparison annual costs may be calculated as costs per person per year; these are made up of the running costs (operation, maintenance and administration) and annual repayment made against the project initial capital loan for construction. This was done (McGarry, 1975) for the four technologies listed above. The separate sanitary sewerage system was based on conventional Western design criteria and incorporated pumping through a force main over a distance of two kilometres for treatment in waste stabilization ponds. House plumbing included a flush toilet and was assumed to discharge all domestic waste waters to the house connection. The aqua-privy and sewerage system employed sanitation units which were external to the house. These units included washing, shower and toilet facilities; all were located above a tank which received water-borne wastes acting to trap settleable solids and providing space for their digestion. The vacuum truck and vault system incorporated manually flushed toilets in every house. The excreta was collected on a manual basis by electrically driven carts using vacuum pumps; the excreta was transferred to larger tank trucks and delivered for treatment in ponds at a distance of two kilometres from the town limits. The septic tanks were designed on the basis of providing one day's retention and incorporated a flush toilet, a two-chamber septic tank and a tile field.

These technologies were applied to a model urban centre of one square kilometre in size. The topography was flat and the town's spatial organization was intended to simulate existing situations in the developing country. The variables of interest to this sensitivity analysis were population density (50, 100, 200 and 300 persons per hactare); interest rate (6%, 8%, 10%, 12%); repayment period (15, 20, 25 and 30 years); and subsoil conditions (soft and stiff soil). Costing out all combinations of these variables requires over 20000 calculations to be made, collated and evaluated—quite sufficient for our limited illustration. Under real conditions most of these variables would be set and so the calculations would be very much simpler.

In terms of capital costs, despite the fact that on-lot costs were higher in the case of the aqua-privy sewerage system, the greatly reduced trench excavation costs brought it to a price much below conventional sewerage at all population densities. The aqua-privy system has particular advantages in soft clays where network costs are half those of conventional sewerage. The vacuum truck and vault system, low in initial capital cost is clearly the least expensive, being some 29% of sewerage and 37% of aqua-privy and sewerage capital costs. Its advantage is increased where sewer systems need to be installed under the more difficult soft clay conditions. It should be noted that the vacuum truck and vault system does not account for sullage wastes but these can be transported using storm drains which are a necessary drainage infrastructure in any city under all technologies being considered.

By converting capital costs into repayment of loan costs on an annual basis, adding these to running costs and converting all into unit costs per person serviced, one can directly compare the technologies under study. Figure 13.6 illustrates the impact of loan conditions on annual unit costs. One might

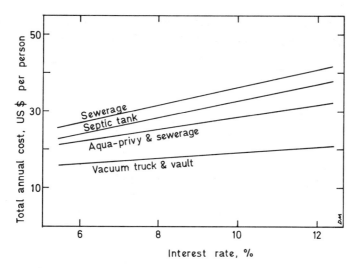

Figure 13.6 The effect of loan conditions and technology on total (capital and operating) costs of wastewater and excreta collection. Assumed conditions: population density of 50/ha 20-year repayment period and stiff soil conditions

expect that at reduced interest rates the capital intensive systems would gain preference over those with higher running costs. Although this is true in principle, it was not the case for the comparisons being made within the ranges considered here. The reduced running costs of the sewerage scheme did not make up for their higher capital costs. The aqua-privy sewerage systems' advantage stems largely from its lower capital costs relative to that of conventional sewerage where pumping is not a major factor.

It is noted again that, on a comparative basis, the vacuum truck and vault and aqua-privy–sewerage schemes are more attractive than conventional sewerage in soft clay than in stiff soil where the unit cost difference between these and conventional sewerage narrows slightly. This is simply a function of the greater cost of trenching in soft clay. The reduced pipe installation costs associated with the two cheaper schemes give them a greater advantage under adverse conditions. The consistently lower costs of the vault system are of interest to the planner in that under no population density covered does its unit cost rise above that of piped systems. There are, of course, several other variables which influence technology choice. Of interest are the selected project design life, population growth rate and their interactions with repayment periods and interest rates. It should be noted that, strictly for purposes of comparison, the interest rate should be the social discount rate, rather than at the rate which a concessionary loan might have been acquired for construction. The social discount rate reflects opportunity costs to other sectors of the national economy, whereas the concessionary rate often applied to aid-to-development loans may only reflect policies within international banks. Use of the concessionary loan rates in technology choice makes capital intensive solution look superficially more attractive as labour surpluses within the economy may call for labour intensive technologies.

13.7 CONCLUSIONS

This paper has attempted to cover the broad spectrum of technologies available to rural and urban areas of developing countries for hygienic excreta disposal, discuss advantages and drawbacks and compare four alternatives applicable to urban centres through a costing/sensitivity exercise. There are a few points which need to be emphasized even at the risk of repetition as they are not always self-evident to the planner, economist or engineer engaged in excreta disposal improvement programmes:

(1) Although empirical field data do not contradict our intuitive belief that sanitation does in fact have a beneficial effect on health, more field research is required to confirm such opinion: specifically, to separate out the individual effects of sanitation from other variables such as changes in social and economic status.

(2) Installation of a water supply system alone does not result in full benefits to health. Improvements should be effected through implementation of the whole sanitation package which also stresses the importance for changes in attitudes, hygiene and proper excreta disposal.

(3) Social design, that is the involvement of the proposed user and incorporation of his attitudes, beliefs, customs and habits in the design process, is as important to the acceptance and continued use of the installation, and therefore success of the programme, as its technical or engineering design. Most attempts to improve excreta disposal in rural areas have failed as a consequence of social rather than technical deficiencies in design.

(4) There are viable alternatives to the Western conventional water-borne sewerage scheme. These are in use in developing countries today. Because of its expense, conventional sewerage is applicable to only a small minority—the privileged class of the urban centre.

(5) Development aid in this sector, particularly those funds applied to the provision of master plans for urban sewerage, have often been of doubtful value in terms of opportunity costs. Overseas consultants have invariably been too limited in their range of experience in excreta collection devices which in general has been restricted to conventional sewerage.

(6) In opting for an alternative to sewerage, reductions in costs may be achieved —but most often at a cost to the user in terms of convenience, aesthetic qualities of the alternatives and technical efficiences. These trade-offs need to be considered and detailed cost effectiveness comparisons made before conclusions can be drawn. These may require pilot plant units to be set up to test such aspects as social acceptance, continued maintenance and financial viability.

(7) Redistribution of benefits from economic development can be effected

through the provision of excreta disposal facilities to lower-income groups. The practice of subsidizing sewers for city centres prevails, yet these are precisely the areas that can best afford to finance such facilities themselves. In fact such subsidies to the commercial sector and privileged classes from national budgets reverses the direction in which benefits should flow. In practice, the limitation of technology choice to water-borne sewerage invariably restricts provision of such facilities to the city centre, primarily as a consequence of the high cost and capital intensity of such schemes. As a result the funds available for such purposes are often depleted and no comparable improvements are made in the peri-urban areas or slums where they are needed most but where people are least able to afford them.

13.8 REFERENCES

Bruch, H. A., Ascoll, W., Scrimshaw, N. S. and Gordon, J. (1963). Studies of diarrheal disease in Central America, V: Environmental factors in the origin and transmission of acute diarrheal disease in four Guatemalan villages. *American Journal of Tropical Medicine and Hygiene*, **12**, 567–579.

Gotaas, H. B. (1956). *Composting*. Monograph Series No. 31. Geneva: World Health Organization.

Kourany, M. and Vasquez, M. (1969). Housing and certain environmental factors and prevalence rates of enteropathogenic bacteria among infants with diarrheal disease in Panama. *American Journal of Tropical Medicine and Hygiene*, **18**(6), 936–941.

Kruse, C. W. (1966). The minimum water service required for the promotion of health and well being (CWS/WP/66.2). Geneva: World Health Organization.

McGarry, M. G. (1975). *Developing Country Sanitation*. Report to the International Development Research Centre, Ottawa.

McKeown, T. and Record, R. G. (1962). Reasons for the decline of mortality in England and Wales during the nineteenth century. *Population Studies*, **16**, 94–122.

Moore, H. A., de la Cruz, E. and Vargas Mendes, O. (1965). Diarrheal disease studies in Costa Rica, IV. *American Journal of Epidemiology*, **82**(2), 162–184.

Sanches, W. R. and Wagner, E. G. (1954). Experience with excreta disposal programmes in rural areas of Brazil. *Bulletin of the World Health Organization*, **10**, 229–249.

Schliessmann, D. J. (1959). Diarrheal disease and the environment. *Bulletin of the World Health Organization*, **21**, 381–386.

Wier, J. M., Wasif, I. M., Hassan, F. R., Attia, S. M. and Kader, M. A. (1952). An evaluation of health and sanitation in Eygptian villages. *Journal of Egyptian Public Health Association*, **27**, 55–122.

14

Wastewater Treatment in Hot Climates

D. D. MARA

14.1 INTRODUCTION

The technology of wastewater treatment in hot climates is very different to that used in temperate climates. Advantage must be taken of the high ambient temperatures and due acknowledgement given to the need to minimize both costs and maintenance requirements. There are three realistic methods:

(1) Waste stabilization ponds
(2) Aerated lagoons
(3) Oxidation ditches

They are given in order of increasing complexity, and hence of decreasing preference (see Section 14.6). Aerated lagoons and oxidation ditches are thus usually reserved for use in large cities whereas ponds are suitable for all community sizes, from 'rurban' towns to the largest of cities. Ponds and aerated lagoons can be used for both waterborne and non-waterborne wastes, but oxidation ditches are suitable only for the treatment of sewage.

Wastewater characteristics

Domestic sewage is composed of (a) human excreta (faeces and urine, often termed 'nightsoil' when collected separately) and (b) sullage, which is the wastewater from sinks and baths etc. These wastes are principally organic; there are tens of thousands of different organic compounds present in sewage and it is impossible (and indeed meaningless if it were possible) to characterize them all. Since sewage and nightsoil are commonly treated by subjecting them to bacterial oxidation:

$$\text{Wastes} + \text{Oxygen} \xrightarrow{\text{bacteria}} \text{Oxidized waste} + \text{New bacteria}$$

it is customary to express the concentration of organic matter in terms of the oxygen required by the bacteria for their oxidation of the waste. This is the *biochemical oxygen demand* (BOD) of the waste, measured in milligrams of oxygen per litre of waste. Thus if we say that a waste has a BOD of x mg/l we mean that the concentration of biodegradable organic matter in one litre of it is such that the bacteria need x mg of oxygen in order to be able to oxidize it. (A slight complication is that BOD is usually measured as the 5-day, 20 °C value; this is some $\frac{2}{3}$ of the total oxygen required for complete bio-oxidation (the 'ultimate BOD'); in this book the term BOD refers to the 5-day, 20 °C value.)

The strength of sewage is usually judged on the basis of its BOD:

Strength	BOD (mg/l)
Weak	200 or less
Medium	350
Strong	500
Very strong	750 or more

The strength of a waste depends on two factors: the quantity of organic matter and the volume of water associated with it. The daily *per capita* output of organic wastes is some 30–50 g as BOD, about half of this being associated with faeces and urine and half with sullage. Thus for a *per capita* effluent flow of, say, 80 l/d and a BOD contribution of 40 g/hd. d, the BOD of the resulting sewage would be $(40/80) \times 1000, = 500$ mg/l. Nightsoil is considerably stronger as its volume is small, about 1–2 l/hd. d; if the nightsoil BOD contribution is 20 g/hd. d, its BOD is $(20/l) \times 1000, = 20\,000$ mg/l.

Why treat wastes?

Waste treatment has three vital aims:

(1) The destruction of the causative agents of those water-related diseases which are associated with domestic wastes (category 1 in Table 5.5). This is particularly important in areas where the major cause of morbidity and mortality is the improper disposal of human faeces.

(2) To convert the wastes into a readily re-usable resource and so conserve both water and nutrients (see Chapter 18).

(3) To prevent the pollution of any body of water (groundwater or surface water) to which the effluent escapes after re-use or into which it is discharged without re-use. The organic pollution of waters is especially undesirable as it interferes with (or may even prevent) the use of the water for drinking and other domestic, industrial or agricultural purposes; it interferes with aquatic life (notably fish); and it may drastically disrupt the ecology of the surrounding area (especially in arid zones).

Effluent standards

To achieve its aims wastewater treatment must produce an effluent of a certain quality. The required effluent quality should be established by a governmental agency; it then becomes the duty of the design engineer to ensure that his design can achieve the established standard. In the absence of a legal standard

Table 14.1 Recommended (minimum) effluent standards

	BOD (mg/l)	Faecal coliforms (per 100 ml)	Algae (per ml)
Effluent to be discharged into surface water[a]	< 25	< 5000	< 100 000
Effluent to be used for restricted irrigation[b]	—	< 5000	—
Effluent to be used for unrestricted irrigation[c]	—	< 100	—

[a]The available dilution is an important factor and this may be taken into account. The FC standard is not very strict but, since a conventional effluent contains some 5 000 000 FC/100 ml it represents a considerable degree of bacteriological purification. Pescod (1974) found that there was no adverse effect on a stream if the concentration of algae in it was below 100 000 cells/ml; a properly designed pond system should always produce an effluent with an algal count below this figure.

[b]Here only a FC standard is necessary, and this to safeguard the health of the labourers working in the irrigated area.

[c]The irrigation of vegetables intended for human consumption demands a very high FC standard (WHO, 1973).

the designer must still design the works to produce an effluent that (a) is suitable for its intended re-use (or will not pollute the receiving watercourse) and (b) will not constitute a risk to public health. Certain *minimum* standards can be identified (Table 14.1); in many cases a more stringent standard may of course be necessary.

Particular emphasis should be placed on bacteriological quality as judged by the faecal coliform count. Virus standards are not feasible in many areas simply owing to the difficulty of determining viral counts on a routine basis. Suspended solids standards are irrelevant in tropical developing countries, although they are often included (the reason for this is that they form part of the almost sacrosanct UK Royal Commission '20/30' standard, although there is no sound basis for the general application of this standard to hot climates; similarly, faecal coliform counts are omitted from many standards simply because they were not used by the UK Commissioners.)

14.2 PRINCIPLES OF WASTE TREATMENT

Waste treatment is a combination of physical, microbiological and (less usually) chemical processes. It is the job of consultant engineers to assemble a train of economic treatment processes that not only can produce an effluent of the desired quality but can also be easily maintained by the local available labour in a condition to be able to do this for its design life. This of course is obvious enough—or is it? A survey in Kenya showed that outside Nairobi, not one sewage treatment works functioned as designed and that this was primarily due to poor maintenance (Holland, 1973, personal communication).

The basic principles of the common waste treatment processes are briefly described below, principally for the benefit of non-engineering readers. Design procedures for the processes discussed in the remaining sections are given by Mara (1976).

Physical processes

Coarse solids such as rags, maize cobs and pieces of wood are usually first removed from the wastewaters by screening or comminution. A screen is a series of inclined bars placed across the sewage flow at intervals of 2–3 cm; the objects retained by the screen ('screenings') are removed once or twice a day by manual raking or, on large schemes, every 15–30 minutes by automatic raking gear; the screenings are disposed of by burial or incineration. Comminution is a method of solids disintegration (this is popular as it avoids the problems of screenings handling and disposal); comminutors are rotating horizontal screens (electrically powered) which have cutting teeth to chop up the screening until they are small enough to pass through the screen slots (about 1 cm).

Sedimentation is the most common physical treatment process. The removal of 'grit' (a term which refers to any heavy inorganic matter—sand, eggshells, glass etc.) is achieved by adjusting the velocity of flow of sewage to a value (0·3 m/s) low enough to permit the grit to settle out by gravity but not so low as to permit the lighter organic solids (which are highly putrescible) to settle out as well. Grit removal is desirable as it is highly abrasive and can damage (for example) comminutor cutting teeth and pumps as well as cause blockages in pipes. The effluents from aerated lagoons and oxidation ditches have very high concentrations of suspended solids (mostly bacterial flocs) and these have to be removed by sedimentation before discharge or re-use.

A flow measuring device such as a Parshall or Venturi flume should be provided after screening and grit removal.

Aerobic biological oxidation

Bacteria are the primary degraders of organic wastes. For the present purpose bacteria can be classified as to their ability to grow in air (strictly, in the presence of oxygen). Those that can are termed 'aerobes' and those that cannot are called 'anaerobes'. Aerobic biological oxidation and anaerobic digestion are the two microbiological treatment processes used, in one form or another, by sanitary engineers to break down organic wastes.

Bacteria break down wastes to provide themselves with the necessary energy to reproduce:

$$\text{Organic waste} + \text{Oxygen} \xrightarrow{\text{bacteria}} \text{Oxidized waste} + \text{Energy}$$

This energy is used to build new cells:

$$\text{Organic waste} + \text{Energy} \xrightarrow{\text{bacteria}} \text{New bacteria}$$

When their food is plentiful bacteria lay down within their cells food reserves; when food becomes scarce, these reserves are oxidized to provide the cells with sufficient energy to keep themselves alive:

$$\text{Bacteria} + \text{Oxygen} \xrightarrow{\text{bacteria}} \text{Oxidized waste} + \text{Energy}$$

This process is known as 'autoxidation'.

These processes of bacterial oxidation lead to the *mineralization* of organic wastes (their conversion to inorganic forms), for example:

$$\text{Organic-carbon} \quad + O_2 \xrightarrow{\text{bacteria}} CO_2$$

$$\text{Organic-nitrogen} \quad + O_2 \xrightarrow{\text{bacteria}} NO_3^-$$

$$\text{Organic-hydrogen} \quad + O_2 \xrightarrow{\text{bacteria}} H_2O$$

$$\text{Organic-sulphur} \quad + O_2 \xrightarrow{\text{bacteria}} SO_4^{2-}$$

$$\text{Organic-phosphorus} + O_2 \xrightarrow{\text{bacteria}} PO_4^{3-}$$

Bacteria are used by sanitary engineers to oxidize wastes because they are self-maintaining and self-adjusting chemical reactors that do the work at lower cost than can man with chemicals. Aerobic bacteria merely need an adequate supply of oxygen; this is provided by man in the form of mechanical aeration for aerated lagoons and oxidation ditches and by their fellow microbes, the algae, in the case of waste stabilization ponds.

Environmental factors

Bacteria need a neutral or slightly alkaline environment (pH 7–9). Toxic compounds (such as heavy metals) must be present in only minute quantities. Temperature is most important—most bacteria exhibit a maximum rate of growth somewhere in the range 20–38 °C and can double their growth rate for each 10 °C rise in temperature; growth slows down at temperatures above 45 °C and death often occurs above 55 °C (there are some bacteria which grow best below 10 °C or above 50 °C, some as high as 70 °C; but these are not normally found in tropical sewage).

Anaerobic digestion

Sewage solids are best treated in the absence of oxygen by two spontaneously appearing groups of anaerobic bacteria. The first group solubilizes the solids principally to organic acids, such as acetic acid, which are then converted by the second group to a mixture of carbon dioxide and methane. Methane is a useful fuel and is thus a potentially valuable byproduct of sewage treatment.

Anaerobic digestion is a slow process compared with aerobic oxidation, the time required being measured in weeks or months rather than hours or days. Temperatures above 15 °C are essential and the rate of digestion increases sevenfold for each 5 °C rise.

Chemical processes

Except in special circumstances (such as the reclamation of wastewater for drinking water; see Chapter 20) chemical process are only rarely used. Effluent chlorination (or ozonation) is common, for example, in USA and Israel; but elsewhere it is rare. A properly designed series of maturation ponds (Section 14.3) can achieve a high degree of bacteriological purification without the need for chemical disinfection.

Industrial and agricultural wastes

Many industrial and most agricultural (including food processing) wastes can be treated biologically. These wastes are often very strong indeed (for example, abattoir wastes are some ten times as strong as even strong sewage) and it is essential that they be allowed for in design, otherwise the works would quickly become overloaded. Toxic wastes, for example metal processing wastes and tannery effluents, usually require chemical treatment and a prudent local authority will insist on pretreatment before discharge into its sewers.

Waste stabilization ponds have been shown to function well when treating sewage containing 30 mg/l heavy metals (5 mg/l each of cadmium, chromium, copper, nickel and zinc), a concentration much higher than normally encountered in municipal sewage; their function was impaired, however, when the concentration was increased to 60 mg/l (Moshe *et al.*, 1972).

14.3 WASTE STABILIZATION PONDS

Waste stabilization ponds are shallow rectangular lakes in which raw (or screened) sewage is treated by natural processes based on the activities of

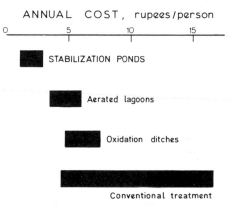

Figure 14.1 Annual costs of sewage treatment in India (from Arceivala *et al.*, 1972). These costs include amortization of the capital costs over 20 years at 6%

both algae and bacteria. They are without doubt the most important effective method of sewage treatment in hot climates—not only are they the least expensive (Figure 14.1) but they are considerably more efficient in destroying pathogenic bacteria and the ova of intestinal parasites. The importance of this latter advantage can hardly be stressed enough in tropical developing countries where water-related diseases, especially those associated with the improper disposal of human wastes, are responsible for a high level of both mortality and morbidity. This, combined with their low cost and their extremely simple maintenance requirements (see below), makes ponds the ideal form of sewage and nightsoil treatment in hot climates.

Stabilization ponds are widely used wherever there is land available for them. In USA, for example, one-third of all municipal sewage treatment works are ponds. Although ponds are widely used in hot climates, there is often consider-able local hostility to their introduction, a hostility largely based on ignorance and prejudice. Prejudice is often instilled by commercial salesmen peddling their wares of sophisticated package plants (imported often at great *per capita* cost); to achieve high sales they decry ponds as crude, odiferous and (most curiously of all) 'backward'. This ignorance and prejudice is now happily starting to disappear and much of the credit for this is due to the World Health Organization which has done a considerable amount to publicize their usage and inherent advantages (e.g. Gloyna, 1971).

There are four types of ponds—facultative and maturation ponds, anaerobic pretreatment ponds and high-rate ponds. These are discussed below.

Faculative ponds

The most common system in use is a faculative pond followed by two or more maturation ponds in series. The faculative pond is responsible for almost all the BOD removal. The term 'faculative' refers to a mixture of aerobic and anaerobic conditions and in a faculative pond aerobic conditions exist towards the water surface and anaerobic conditions in and just above the sludge layer. In the upper layers the pond bacteria oxidize the waste in their usual manner but the oxygen they use comes only partly from the atmosphere; it is mostly

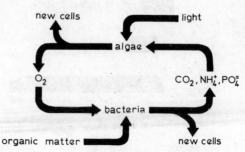

Figure 14.2 Symbiosis of algae and bacteria

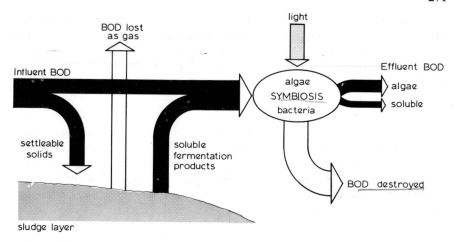

Figure 14.3 Pathways of BOD removal in facultative stabilization ponds (after Marais, 1970b)

supplied by the photosynthetic activities of the pond algae (these are so numerous that facultative ponds are bright green in colour). The algae in turn need carbon dioxide for photosynthesis and their demand for it exceeds its supply from the atmosphere; the balance is supplied by the pond bacteria. Thus there is an association of mutual benefit ('symbiosis') between the pond algae and bacteria (Figure 14.2); this is the main basis of waste stabilization in ponds. In the sludge layer which is formed over the entire pond bottom as the sewage solids settle under gravity, intense anaerobic digestion occurs. This is also an important part of BOD removal in the facultative pond as a considerable proportion (some 30%) of the influent BOD is released from the pond as methane gas; there is a feedback of soluble fermentation products from the sludge layer to the main liquid bulk of the pond. These pathways of BOD removal are summarized in Figure 14.3.

Photosynthesis is a light-dependent activity. This results in a diurnal variation of dissolved oxygen and pH and in the level in the pond where anaerobic conditions commence. The concentration of dissolved oxygen increases to a maximum (15–30 mg/l) in late afternoon and decreases to a minimum just before dawn (if the pond is overloaded the dissolved oxygen concentration may be zero for a considerable period at night). The pond pH follows a similar pattern reaching a maximum of perhaps 9·5–10 and falling to 7–7·5 at night; the increase in pH with photosynthesis is due to the release of hydroxyl ions from the dissociation of bicarbonate to release carbon dioxide for algal growth:

$$HCO_3^- \rightleftharpoons CO_2 + OH^-$$

Climate

In hot climates there is always sufficient light energy for algal growth. The principal effect of high solar energy is to increase the pond temperature and thus the algal and bacterial growth rates, hence the rates of oxygen production and waste stabilization. The effect of prolonged cloud cover is to decrease the pond temperature and hence the other factors mentioned. However, high temperatures increase the risk of stratification which reduces BOD removal.

Mixing and stratification

Vertical mixing ensures a relatively uniform distribution of waste, algae and dissolved oxygen. More importantly it is the only means by which non-motile algae can be transported into the top 15–30 cm of the pond which is penetrated by light (the 'photic zone'). Mixing is principally due to wind action—the depth to which wind-induced mixing is felt depends on the fetch, about 100 m being required for maximum effect in a pond 1·5 m deep. In the absence of wind-mixing, thermal stratification occurs: about 30–50 cm below the pond surface a thin static layer of steep temperature change (the 'thermocline') forms, above which there is some mixing but none below. Non-motile algae sink to the bottom of the pond where they exert an oxygen demand rather than supply it; above the thermocline the temperature rapidly rises (often above 30–35 °C) and the motile algae move away to a cooler depth. Thermal stratification leads to a vast reduction in the number of algae in the photic zone, hence a similar reduction in oxygen production and thus waste stabilization. Stratification can be overcome by wind action. Alternatively, in the absence of wind, temperature inversion has the same effect: in the evening the upper layers lose heat more rapidly than the layers below the thermocline and eventually they become cooler than the lower layers (which are insulated by the earth)—the upper waters then sink through the thermocline and the less dense lower waters rise through it. This daily cycle of mixing in ponds (Marais, 1966; Sless, 1974) is similar to the annual cycle in deep natural lakes in temperate climates; shallow natural lakes in the tropics, however, also exhibit a daily cycle (Viner and Smith, 1973). Stratification may also be overcome mechanically, by installing a circulating pump to take water from below the thermocline and eject it above it. The power requirements for mixing are not large: preliminary experiments in Cape Town showed that a 4 kW pump maintained a 10 ha pond in a well-mixed condition during the hot season (Marais, 1970a).

Depth

Pond depths are usually in the range of 1–1·5 m (Marais, 1963). Depths below 1 m do not prevent vegetation growing up from the pond bottom (this must be avoided to prevent the pond becoming a mosquito-breeding swamp), whereas if the depth is greater than 1·5 m the pond is predominantly anaerobic rather than aerobic; this is undesirable as it decreases the ability of the pond to withstand short organic overloads (slugs of high BOD). However, in cold areas (for example, at high altitude) and in arid areas, depths of up to 2 m are used to conserve thermal energy and reduce evaporation losses respectively.

Maturation ponds

Maturation ponds are used as second and third stages to facultative ponds. Their prime function is the destruction of faecal bacteria. They are also responsible for the quality of the final effluent. Whereas the size of the facultative pond governs the operating nuisance level of the series of ponds (principally odour), the size *and number* of maturation ponds control the effluent quality (both bacteriological and chemical) and hence the overall efficiency of the pond system (Meiring *et al.*, 1968); their function is thus fundamentally different from that of facultative ponds.

Maturation ponds are wholly aerobic and can remain so at depths up to 3 m (Marais and Shaw, 1961). Shallower depths are preferable as the destruction of enteroviruses is appreciably better at depths of 1–1·5 m (Malherbe and Coetzee, 1965). Two maturation ponds in series, each with a retention time of 7 days, are required to achieve an effluent BOD of less than 25 mg/l (Marais and Shaw, 1961). The exact number of maturation ponds required in any one situation depends on the desired reduction in faecal coliform numbers; each pond of 5–7 d retention is able to achieve a 90%–95% reduction in FC numbers (Marais, 1974).

In a facultative pond algal numbers are high because its environment is not suitable for the development of a large population of algal predators. In contrast algal numbers decrease markedly at each successive stage in a maturation pond system and an extended food chain is established with protozoa, rotifers, crustaceans and fish. This food chain is the basis for the aquacultural exploitation of waste stabilization ponds (see Chapter 18).

Anaerobic pretreatment ponds

The volumetric BOD loading on anaerobic ponds is so high (at least 100 g/m³ d, compared with 15–40 g/m³ d in facultative ponds) that the pond is devoid of dissolved oxygen. Few algae grow and the pond is often dark red or purple (rather than green) owing to the growth of the coloured anaerobic photosynthetic bacteria. Anaerobic ponds are essentially open septic tanks for solids settlement and digestion. They are used to treat large flows of strong wastes; septic tanks serve the same function for populations up to about 10 000 (Marais, 1970a).

Because of the high efficiency of BOD removal in anaerobic ponds (more than 50% after 24 hours' retention), their inclusion in pond schemes results in a considerable reduction in land requirements. The price paid for this economy of land is increased maintenance: anaerobic ponds must be desludged when half full of sludge, about once every 3–5 years (compared with every 10–20 years for facultative ponds and never for maturation ponds).

Odour release and prevention

Anaerobic ponds are often disfavoured because of fear of odour release. This fear arises from the illogical assumption that since overloaded facultative ponds smell then anaerobic ponds (incorrectly thought of as grossly overloaded facultative ponds) must also smell. However, a properly designed anaerobic pond does not smell, provided that its volumetric loading is less than 400 g/m³ d and that the concentration of sulphate ion in the raw waste is less than 500 mg/l. Under these conditions a stable alkaline fermentation with copious methane evolution is soon established and any sulphide present (formed as a result of bacterial sulphate reduction) is in the form of the odourless bisulphide ion rather than as the highly malodorous hydrogen sulphide gas.

High-rate ponds

High-rate ponds are designed to receive high loadings of settled sewage (for example, the effluent from anaerobic ponds). Their depth is very shallow, usually 20–40 cm so that the photic zone extends to (or almost to) the pond bottom. Under these conditions the conversion of sewage nutrients to algae is very fast—retention times of only 1–3 d are necessary to convert 1 kg of BOD to 1 kg of algae (McGarry, 1971). Since algae are 50% protein, the high-rate pond is a highly successful form of aquaculture (see Chapter 18). Removal of the algae from the effluent is essential, however, and it is the technology required for this (for example, flotation) which has so far limited high-rate ponds to experimental use. There is no doubt at all that in the future the high-rate pond will become increasingly more common; this must, however, await (despairingly, in all likelihood, for at least one, if not two, decades) until civil engineering consultants, regional planners, agricultural and fisheries officers decide to cooperate seriously in order to devise integrated schemes for waste treatment and the aquacultural and agricultural re-use of the treated effluent.

Pond layouts

A considerable number of single-pond installations have been built in developing countries over the last fifteen years. The provision of only facultative ponds is just plain bad engineering practice; *maturation ponds are essential.* As Gloyna (1971) states: 'The removal of BOD without regard to the destruction of disease-causing agents is inadequate'. The only acceptable pond layouts are thus:

> *either* 1 facultative + 2 (or more) maturation ponds
> *or* 1 anaerobic + 1 facultative + 2 (or more) maturation ponds

It has long been recognized (both in theory and in practice) that a series of ponds produces a better effluent than a single large pond of the same overall volume (see Marais, 1974). Marais (1974) showed that for maximum efficiency the retention time in each pond in a series of ponds should be the same. Mara (1975a) suggested that a series of 5–7 ponds each with a retention time of 5 days would be an extremely economical design if the effluent was to be used for unrestricted irrigation (i.e. should have a faecal coliform count less than

100/100 ml). The first pond would be anaerobic, the second facultative and the others maturation ponds; the design was based on a maximum influent BOD of 1000 mg/l and temperatures above 15 °C.

Pond facilities

The only facilities (additional to those already discussed in Section 14.2) required for ponds are for piping the flow from one pond to another. Several designs are given by Gloyna (1971) and Mara (1975b); an example is shown in Figure 14.4. The final effluent should pass through a flow-measuring chamber equipped with a vee-notch.

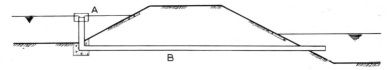

Figure 14.4 Simple interpond connection. A. scum guard; B. 150–250 mm dia. PVC pipe at 1 in 200 fall

Pond shape

Rectangular ponds are generally preferred; length to breadth ratios are commonly 2–3 to 1. Shindala and Murphy (1969) have shown that the performance of these ponds is superior to square and circular ponds and those of irregular geometry.

Pond base

Preferably ponds should be built on impermeable soil. Where seepage losses are expected to exceed more than about 10% the base should be sealed with polythene sheeting, puddled clay, bitumen or asphalt, whichever is cheapest. Seepage losses in unlined ponds decline with time if the soil is not too permeable as the sludge layer itself acts as a sealant.

Embankments

These are usually made with slopes of 1 in 2–3. They should be protected from wave erosion by precast concrete slabs or stone rip-rap laid at top water level; this also prevents vegetation growing down the embankment and so forming a suitable habitat for snails and mosquitoes.

Pond maintenance

Routine pond maintenance is extremely simple: cutting the grass on the embankments and removing scum from the pond surface. Arceivala *et al.*

(1972) have estimated the labour requirements for ponds in India as follows:

Population	Supervisors	Labourers
5 000	—	2
10 000	—	3
50 000	1	6
100 000	2	8

Sadly, however, pond maintenance, in spite of its simplicity, is often not done. Pond maintenance is of course *vital*. Often the reason for the neglect is that the labourers have little or no idea that they should attend to any maintenance jobs other than cutting the grass; nor can they recognize obvious malfunctions. A classic example of the latter is reported by Pickford (1973):

In Africa I recently visited a country's only substantial sewage treatment plant, a well-designed waste stabilization pond system. Virtually no flow was coming in. Following the sewer upstream led to a shattered pipe from which the whole flow, including that from a hospital, poured into a ditch. The accident had occurred sometime before, *but no one had bothered to do anything about it.*

Operator training is clearly essential.

14.4 AERATED LAGOONS

In temperate climates it was found that during winter the algae in waste stabilization ponds did not produce enough oxygen to satisfy the bacterial demand for it. Sanitary engineers therefore provided mechanical oxygenation (by means of floating surface aerators, Figure 14.5) to supplement the algal oxygen supply. They found, however, that within a few days of the aerators being switched on the algae in the pond disappeared and the bacterial flora became more flocculent and soon resembled activated sludge. It was thus that

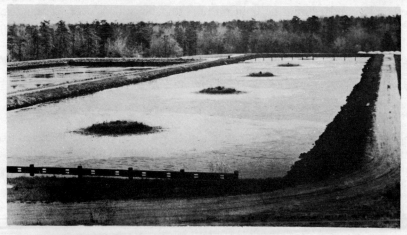

Figure 14.5 Aerated lagoon with five surface aerators (courtesy of Peabody Wells Inc.)

aerated lagoons, as mechanically aerated stabilization ponds are known, became recognized as a distinct treatment process in their own right.

In essence aerated lagoons convert sewage into bacterial cells:

$$\text{Wastes} + \text{Oxygen} \xrightarrow{\text{bacteria}} \text{Oxidized waste} + \text{New bacterial cells}$$

Depending on temperature this process takes some 2–6 days (4 days is the retention time most commonly provided). However, the cells ('sludge') so produced exert a high BOD and need to be removed before the effluent is discharged into a watercourse or used for irrigation. This is most simply achieved in a series of maturation ponds. The first pond in the series acts principally as a settling basin and a retention time of 5–10 days should be provided. The total number of ponds to be provided depends on the required reduction of faecal bacteria.

It is possible to use a conventional secondary sedimentation tank to remove the sludge from aerated lagoon effluent; in this case because the cells have been aerated for only 2–6 days they need further treatment before they can be placed on drying beds without creating an odour problem. This treatment is best done in an aerobic digester which is essentially a small aerated lagoon with a retention time of some 10 days. However, all these extra processes drastically increase the maintenance requirements. If, for reasons of land economy, a system like this has to be considered, the designer would be well advised to choose an oxidation ditch from which only small quantities of highly mineralized sludge are produced.

With 4 days' retention BOD removals of 85%–90% can be readily achieved in aerated lagoons (Dhalla, 1971). The removal of faecal coliforms is poor, only 85%–95%; further treatment in maturation ponds is usually necessary.

Preliminary treatment

Fine screening or comminution should be provided. This considerably helps lagoons performance as rags and similar materials do not foul the aerator propeller. Grit removal is usually advisable but primary sedimentation is not required.

Construction and maintenance

Aerated lagoons arc best built 3–4 m deep and with embankment slopes of 1 in 2. The aerators induce a very high degree of turbulence in the lagoon and it is thus essential to protect the embankments and lagoon bottom from erosion and scour. This may be achieved by providing a lining of butyl rubber (or similar material), masonry (set with cement or laid as rip-rap) or mass concrete.

The aerators require, of course, a reliable electricity supply; on large schemes standby diesel generators should be provided for using during failure of the mains supply. The aerators themselves are usually most reliable in operation and may only require periodic lubrication. Because of their high reliability

278

a skilled electrician is not required to be in constant attendance at the works (although there should be access to one in cases of failure).

14.5 OXIDATION DITCHES

An oxidation ditch is similar to an aerated lagoon in that the wastewater is oxidized by bacteria in flocculent suspension and that the oxygen required for bio-oxidation is supplied by mechanical aeration. It differs in three main respects:

(a) reactor geometry;
(b) type of aerator;
(c) sludge recycle.

Oxidation ditches are long continuous channels, some 1·5–2 m deep and usually oval in plan (Figure 14.6). Aeration is effected by horizontal cage rotors placed across the channel (Figure 14.7); these not only provide oxygen but also impart a flow velocity of 0·3–0·4 m/s to the ditch contents—this is sufficient

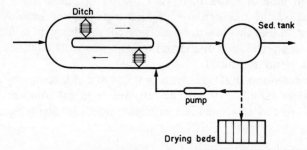

Figure 14.6 Typical oxidation ditch installation

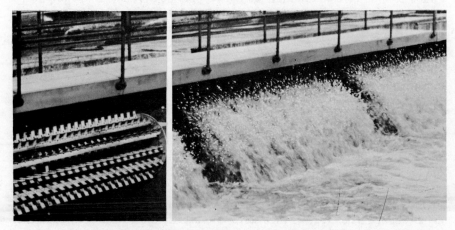

Figure 14.7 Cage rotors for oxidation ditch (courtesy of Whitehead and Poole Ltd)

to prevent the bacterial flocs from settling to the bottom of the ditch where they would rapidly decay.

The practice of sludge recycling is the major difference between aerated lagoons and oxidation ditches. To recycle the sludge some means of separating the sludge from ditch effluent must be available: a conventional secondary sedimentation tank is therefore provided. A sludge lifting wheel or screw pump must also be provided to return the sludge back to the ditch. The complete oxidation ditch installation is thus as shown in Figure 14.6. The advantages of sludge recycle are:

(1) The concentration of active cells in the ditch is much higher (some 3000 mg/l as compared with 300 mg/l in an aerated lagoon) so that the waste is oxidized more quickly, thus permitting much shorter hydraulic retention times (0·5–1·5 days rather than 2–6 days).

(2) The average length of time the sludge is under aeration in the ditch is much longer (20–30 days rather than 2–6 days) so that the amount of excess sludge that is produced is not only very small but also highly mineralized; it can thus be placed directly on sludge drying beds without fear of odour release.

In normal operation the BOD of the effluent from a properly designed (and properly maintained) ditch is consistently below 15 mg/l. The removal of faecal bacteria, as judged by the removal of faecal coliform bacteria, is poor—only about 90%–95%.

Preliminary treatment

To minimize maintenance on the ditch itself the wastewater should be screened or comminuted before it is admitted to the ditch. Grit removal is usually advisable but primary sedimentation is not required.

Construction and maintenance

The ditch is normally built in mass concrete or masonry with side slopes of 1 in 1½. Considerable maintenance is required: not only must all the electrical and mechanical plant be kept in perfect order but the plant operator has to maintain the concentration of suspended solids in the ditch in the range 3000–5000 mg/l; this is achieved by diverting the return sludge flow once or twice a day to the sludge drying beds, and although it is not unduly difficult to do this, the exact time period for which the sludge flow should be diverted has to be determined empirically for each ditch. The required level of maintenance and operator skill is thus considerably higher than that required for an aerated lagoon system.

Large populations

For populations above 15 000 the ditch is deepened to 2–4 m and is made with vertical walls of reinforced concrete. A more powerful rotor (the 'Mammoth' rotor), is used in place of the cage rotor shown in Figure 14.7. The largest ditch system presently in use is in Holland; it treats an industrial waste equivalent in strength and volume to a population of 250 000.

14.6 PROCESS SELECTION

If there is sufficient land available, waste stabilization ponds should always be regarded as the preferred method of sewage treatment in hot climates. The principal reasons for this may be briefly summarised as:

(1) Low cost.
(2) Extreme simplicity of operation and maintenance.
(3) Superior removal of faecal bacteria.
(4) Protein production in the form of algae, fish, ducks and crops (see Chapter 18).

Ponds do not require imported machinery and they therefore conserve foreign exchange. Although ponds require large areas of land, this is not completely disadvantageous as land is an extremely good investment for a municipality—ponds can often turn out to be a highly profitable real estate investment. As a town grows the municipality can sell the land used for ponds, the proceeds of the sale being used to extend the outfall sewer, to buy (cheaper) land further away from the town and to construct new ponds; with proper management there should be some moneys left over. This process can of course be repeated every 20 years or so.

For large flows anaerobic pretreatment ponds should always be considered as they significantly reduce the amount of land required (by about 50%); for smaller flows septic tanks may serve the same function. The level of maintenance required (although marginally above that for facultative and maturation ponds) is much less than that required for aerated lagoons and oxidation ditches as mechanical and electrical skills are not required.

Aerated lagoons are useful in certain situations where there is insufficient land for stabilization ponds. They should always be followed by a settling pond and, where necessary to reduce the population of faecal bacteria to the acceptable level, by maturation ponds. The most useful role for aerated lagoons is to extend the capacity of an existing waste stabilization pond system (Figure 14.8).

Oxidation ditches are used when there is insufficient land for an aerated lagoon system. Their major advantage is minimum sludge production but their disadvantages are high level maintenance requirements and, more seriously, poor removal of faecal bacteria. Maturation ponds are not used to improve the bacteriological quality of oxidation ditch effluent (if they could be, there would be sufficient land for the less expensive aerated lagoon system, so that a ditch would not be used in the first place). The only method available therefore

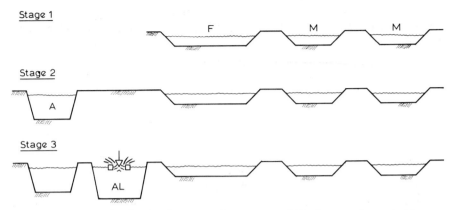

Figure 14.8 Stages in the development of a waste stabilization pond–aerated lagoon system. F. facultative pond; M. maturation pond; A. anaerobic pond; AL. aerated lagoon. At stage 3 additional maturation ponds will probably be necessary. In some cases septic tanks may replace anaerobic lagoons (usually for populations below 10.000)

for reducing the numbers of faecal bacteria in the effluent is chemical disinfection, usually either chlorination or ozonation. However, these are expensive processes which require considerable expertise in operation. This leads to the conclusion that oxidation ditches should only be installed when such expertise is available or when the effluent does not need disinfection (for example when it is to be discharged into the sea—sea water is itself a mild disinfectant—or used for the irrigation of industrial or fodder crops).

Disadvantages of conventional (temperate) sewage treatment in hot climates

Conventional sewage treatment works of the kind most commonly used in temperate climates consist of four separate stage:

(1) Preliminary treatment (screening, grit removal).
(2) Primary sedimentation.
(3) Secondary treatment (either activated sludge or trickling filtration followed by secondary sedimentation).
(4) Treatment of the large quantities of sludge produced in stages (2) and (3), usually by anaerobic digestion, followed by dewatering on drying beds.

A full description of these processes may be found in standard texts (e.g. Metcalf & Eddy, Inc., 1972) or introductory texts (e.g. Lumb, 1968).

Compared with waste stabilization ponds (and even oxidation ditches) conventional sewage treatment is a highly complex train of chemical engineering processes which are not only extremely expensive to both build and operate but also require a very high level of operator performance (which, at least in tropical developing countries, is better employed in manufacturing industries).

Odour is a problem almost always encountered in conventional sewage treatment in hot climates, especially those based on low-rate trickling filtration. Activated sludge plants are generally odour-free but these require an even higher degree of operator skill. Trickling filters are also ideal breeding places for *Psychoda* flies; under certain conditions dense clouds of these flies can emanate from the filters and make all human presence intolerable.

14.7 NIGHTSOIL TREATMENT

The best method of treating urban nightsoil is in facultative stabilization ponds. The pond depth should be maintained at 1·2 m by regular additions of river water (or groundwater) to counteract evaporation and seepage losses; nightsoil ponds need therefore to be sited near an adequate supply of fresh water (Shaw, 1963). At least two concrete inlet ramps (one at either end of the pond) should be provided to enable all the nightsoil to be discharged easily into (and well dispersed throughout) the pond; a pump should be also provided at each ramp to draw water from the pond to wash down the ramps and break up any scum mats which may form on the pond surface (Shaw, 1963). Maceration is advisable, particularly in large schemes, to ensure good dispersion and avoid the formation of sludge banks. Wherever possible the nightsoil pond should be sited so that it can be incorporated into any future installation of waterborne sewerage without the need for pumping.

In Lagos aerated lagoons have recently been installed for the treatment of nightsoil from some 14 000 households on Lagos Island (Hindhaugh, 1973). On arrival at the works the waste is screened, macerated, diluted with make-up water from Lagos lagoon and then treated in two aerated lagoons (each 3000 m² × 3 m with four 75 h.p. aerators); after treatment the effluent is discharged into Lagos lagoon. Aerated lagoons were chosen in this instance because there was insufficient land available on Lagos Island for ponds; to have built ponds on the mainland would have been to incur recurrently high transport costs. Indeed in order to minimize costs large municipalities will often need to establish two or more treatment works for nightsoil.

14.8 REFERENCES

Arceivala, S. J., Bhalerae, B. B. and Alagasamy, S. R. (1972). Cost estimates for various sewage treatment processes in India. In: *Low Cost Waste Treatment* (ed. C. A. Sastry). Nagpur: Central Public Health Engineering Research Institute.

Dhalla, M. S. (1971). Completely mixed aerated lagoons. *MS Thesis*, University of Illinois, Urbana-Champaign.

Gloyna, E. F. (1971). *Waste Stabilization Ponds*. Monograph Series No. 60. Geneva: World Health Organization.

Hindhaugh, G. M. A. (1973). Nightsoil treatment. *The Consulting Engineer*, **37**(9), 47–49.

Lumb, C. (1968). *An Introduction to Sewage Treatment* (2nd edition) London: Institute of Water Pollution Control.

McGarry, M. G. (1971). Water reclamation and protein production through sewage treatment. In: *Water Supply and Wastewater Disposal in Developing Countries* (eds. M. B. Pescod and D. A. Okun). Bangkok: Asian Institute of Technology.

Malherbe, H. H. and Coetzee, O. J. (1965). The survival of type '2' poliovirus in a model system of stabilization ponds. *CSIR Research Report 242.* Pretoria: Council for Scientific and Industrial Research.

Mara, D. D. (1975a). Proposed design for oxidation ponds in hot climates. *Journal of the Environmental Engineering Division, American Society of Civil Engineers,* **101** (EE2), 296–300.

Mara, D. D. (1975b). *Design Manual for Sewage Lagoons in the Tropics.* Nairobi: East African Literature Bureau.

Mara, D. D. (1976). *Sewage Treatment in Hot Climates.* London: Wiley.

Marais, G. v. R. (1963). A design chart for a series of oxidation ponds treating raw sewage and some remarks on the depth of the first pond. *Transactions of the South African Institution of Civil Engineers,* **5**, 241–245.

Marais, G. v. R. (1966). New factors in the design, operation and performance of waste stabilization ponds. *Bulletin of the World Health Organization,* **34**, 737–763.

Marais, G. v. R. (1970a). Overloading of oxidation ponds. *Paper presented at the annual conference of the Institution of Municipal Engineers of Southern Africa,* Salisbury.

Marais, G. v. R. (1970b). Dynamic behaviour of oxidation ponds. In: *Proceedings of the Second International Symposium for Waste Treatment Lagoons* (ed. R. E. McKinney). Lawrence: University of Kansas.

Marais, G. v. R. (1974). Faecal bacterial kinetics in stabilization ponds. *Journal of the Environmental Engineering Division, American Society of Civil Engineers,* **100** (EE1), 119–139.

Marais, G. v. R. and Shaw, V. A. (1961). A rational theory for the design of sewage stabilization ponds in central and South Africa. *Transactions of the South African Institution of Civil Engineers,* **3**, 205–227.

Meiring, P. C. J., Drews, R. J. L., van Eck, H. and Stander, G. J. (1968). A guide to the use of pond systems in South Africa for the purification of raw and partially treated sewage. *CSIR Special WAT 34.* Pretoria: Council for Scientific and Industrial Research.

Metcalf & Eddy, Inc. (1972). *Wastewater Engineering: Collection, Treatment, Disposal.* New York: McGraw-Hill.

Moshe, M., Betzer, N. and Kott, Y. (1972). Effect of industrial wastes on oxidation pond performance. *Water Research,* **6**, 1165–1171.

Pescod, M. B. (1974). Investigation of rational effluent and stream standards for tropical countries. *Research Report No. FE-476–2.* Bangkok: Asian Institute of Technology.

Pickford, J. (1973). Discussion. *Progress in Water Technology* **3**, 114.

Pradt, L. A. (1971). Some recent developments in nightsoil treatment *Water Research* **5**, 507–521.

Shaw, V. A. (1963). A system for the treatment of nightsoil and conserving tank effluent in stabilization ponds. *Public Health, Johannesburg,* **63**, 17–22.

Shindala, A. and Murphy, W. C. (1969). Influence of shape on mixing and load of sewage lagoons. *Water and Sewage Works,* **116**, 391–395.

Sless, J. B. (1974). Biological and chemical aspects of stabilization pond design. *Reviews on Environmental Health,* **1**, 327–354.

Viner, A. B. and Smith, I. R. (1973). Geographical, historical and physical aspects of Lake George. *Proceedings of the Royal Society of London, Series B,* **184**, 235–270.

WHO (1973). Reuse of effluents: methods of wastewater treatment and health safeguards. *WHO Technical Report Series No. 517.* Geneva: World Health Organization.

15

Entomological and Helminthological Aspects of Sewage Treatment in Hot Climates

Part A—Insect Breeding in Relation to Sanitation and Waste Disposal

B. R. LAURENCE

15.1 INTRODUCTION

Flies are found in immense variety throughout the world and they breed in materials as varied as the beach sand on the sea-shore and the pools of crude petroleum found in California. Patches of animal faeces are worlds unto themselves, with parasites, predators and dung-feeders living as a community together (Laurence, 1954) and different communities of insects are found in fresh water (Carpenter, 1928). Man-made environments with new innovations such as sanitation and waste disposal units are invaded and colonized by insects from the more natural breeding places. The insects are so numerous and variable that it is difficult to generalize about worldwide problems. Only a few species of insect are cosmopolitan in distribution and local problems depend largely on the specific insect fauna able to colonize the new man-made installations. Most problems are caused by flies, not only the housefly but mosquitoes and a great variety of other flies. Waste disposal provides two attractive materials for the development of insects—rich organic material and water. The kinds of insect found breeding in human waste disposal systems are, in consequence, those that breed in various forms of decaying organic material, including faeces, or those that breed in freshwater and show some degree of tolerance to organic pollution.

Relatively few kinds of insect are able to take advantage of the new opportunities for breeding provided by waste disposal but these few species often appear in very large numbers. The balance of a more varied fauna found in the natural breeding places may be lacking in the new man-made habitats (Crisp and Lloyd, 1954). Consequently the numbers of insects may build up to a level sufficient to cause a definite nuisance or even to endanger health. The presence of animal life in sludge and filter systems, where there is a mixed culture of organisms (including the insects), is also part of the process of purification and breakdown of the organic material (Lloyd, 1945). An abnormal increase in the numbers of an insect browsing at the expense of this biological community should be resisted or the balance in the community may be destroyed and the process break down (Pillai and Subrahmanyan, 1942).

15.2 THE IDENTIFICATION OF FLIES

The most common insects associated with sanitation and waste disposal are flies. These are two-winged insects (with the second pair of wings modified as knob-like balancing organs called halteres) and consequently all flies are placed in one group or order called the Diptera (*di* = two, *pteron* = wing). As in all insects, the adult fly has six legs and the body is divided into three parts, the head, the thorax (which carries the legs and the wings) and the abdomen. There are various kinds of fly and these are separated into families of related

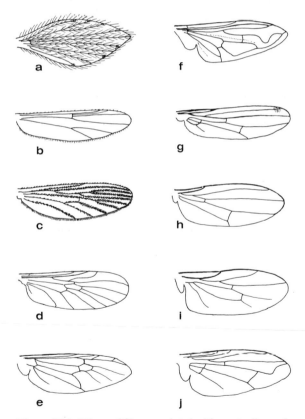

Figure 15.1 Wings of flies associated with waste disposal: a. Psychodidae; b. Chironomidae; c. Culicidae; d. Anisopodidae; e. Stratiomyidae; f. Syrphidae; g. Sepsidae; h. Ephydridae; i. Sphaeroceridae; j. Muscidae (not to scale; see text for size of flies)

kinds (given names ending with the suffix'-dae'). A particular kind of fly is given two names derived from Greek or Latin roots and this name is usually printed in italics. This is the specific name of the fly. For a formal treatment of the taxonomy of flies, both Oldroyd (1970) and Smith (1973) discuss the structure and give keys to the families. Only certain families and species of fly are associated with waste disposal systems and only these families are discussed here. The pattern of veins on the wings as well as the general appearance of the adult fly are the most useful ways of identifying the families (Figure 15.1).

15.3 THE LIFE HISTORY OF FLIES

The adult fly is the sexually reproducing phase (male and female) and the dispersal phase of the life cycle of the insect. Fly nuisance is caused by this dispersal of the adult fly from the breeding places. The eggs of flies are laid on

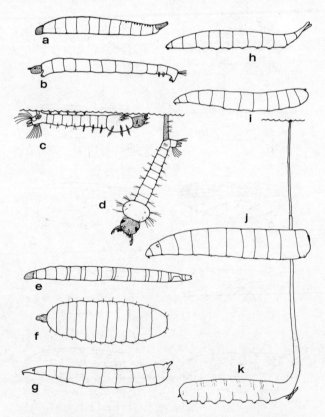

Figure 15.2 Larvae of flies associated with waste disposal:
a. Psychodidae; b. Chironomidae; c. Culicidae (Anopheline),
d. Culicidae (Culicine); e. Anisopodidae; f. Stratiomyidae;
g. Sepsidae; h. Ephydridae; i. Sphaeroceridae; j. Muscidae;
k. Syrphidae (not to scale; see text for size of larvae)

or in potential breeding material by the female and the young stages (known as larvae) emerge from the eggs and burrow or swim in the medium chosen as the larval habitat by the female fly. Sewage and other waste is attractive to certain flies as a breeding medium for the larval stages. The fly larvae feed and grow, with a number of moults (usually four), through a series of growth stages of increasing size called instars. Fly larvae are wingless and legless, with a segmented body, and they can be separated into two groups: (a) those with a distinct brown or black head capsule and (b) those without a head capsule prominent at the front end (Figure 15.2). At the fourth moult, the fully grown and fully fed fourth stage larva turns into the pupa. The pupal stage does not feed and resembles the structure of the adult more than that of the larva, bridging the difference in structure between the legless larva and the fully winged adult fly. In the higher flies, where the larva lacks the head capsule, the pupa is protected within the hardened, darkened last larval skin (known as a puparium). Fly larvae that are about to pupate tend to move out of the medium in which they have been feeding or to its surface and here the pupae may be found in numbers. Fly larvae are very adaptable with a simplified body form and some are associated with and adapted to life in the water (such as the mosquitoes and midges) while others (such as the housefly and its relatives) live on land, burrowing into their food, excrement or other organic material in decay. The families of flies tend to have the one or the other kind of larva, associated with either the water or the land. The individual species of fly within each family have specific preferences for certain types of breeding media as the larval habitat.

15.4 THE FAMILIES OF FLIES ASSOCIATED WITH WASTE DISPOSAL

The most common flies associated with waste disposal are found in 11 families. The wings of the adult flies are illustrated in Figure 15.1 and their larvae are illustrated in Figure 15.2. The most important families are the flies that transmit disease organisms from man to man, the mosquitoes, or family Culicidae, and the flies that breed in excremental material and also come into contact with man as adults by feeding on his food (the housefly and the blowfly, families Muscidae and Calliphoridae). Other flies cause a nuisance by the numbers of flies invading human habitation (families Psychodidae, Chironomidae and Anisopodidae), may land in food, and are known to cause contact and inhalation allergy in sensitized persons. In addition, other families of fly (Stratiomyidae, Syrphidae, Sepsidae, Ephydridae and Sphaeroceridae) are very common on sewage installations or in cesspits, but normally have little contact with man and are less of a problem except that they can cause confusion in problems involving the more important sewage breeding nuisances. All the flies play a part in the natural breakdown of waste materials but mosquito breeding in particular should be controlled in tropical countries, and so should any nuisance arising from the over-production of flies from the waste disposal system which invade human dwellings.

Flies causing disease

Family Culicidae

Adult: Medium-sized flies, 5–10 mm long, wing with margin and veins covered by flattened hairs (scales) and rounded at the tip (Figure 15.1c), bloodsucking flies with long forwardly pointing proboscis in front of head. Larva: Length 5–12 mm, with distinct head capsule, free swimming in the water either attached to surface film along length of body when undisturbed (Figure 15.2c—Anopheline larvae) or hanging from surface film by posterior siphon (Figure 15.2d—Culicine larvae).

These flies, better known as mosquitoes, are invaders of waste disposal systems from freshwater habitats. Adults of the Culicidae are often confused with the non-biting midges (family Chironomidae) but the presence of scales on the wings of the mosquito and its long forwardly pointing proboscis are good diagnostic features. The larvae are free-swimming and can usually be seen attached to the surface film where they respire, at the edges of ponds, streams and oxidation ponds. Few species of mosquito tolerate a high degree of organic pollution although any area of water that becomes progressively cleaner with an algal bloom or by mechanical aeration may then attract other species.

Mosquitoes transmit human diseases, the Anopheline group transmit malaria and in some parts of the world filariasis (elephantiasis) and the Culicine group transmit filariasis and a number of virus infections. The main mosquito vectors of epidemic yellow fever and dengue virus belong to the genus *Aedes*; these characteristically breed in small containers of water (tins, cisterns, motor-car tyres, coconuts etc.) and do not concern us here. The mosquitoes most able to breed in polluted waters are Culicine mosquitoes belonging to the genus *Culex*, notably the cosmopolitan *Culex fatigans* (sometimes referred to as *Culex quinquefasciatus* or *Culex pipiens fatigans* or *Culex pipiens quinquefasciatus*)which is the main vector of filariasis in towns in tropical countries, and *Culex tarsalis* which is a vector of encephalitis virus in America. This last species has been associated in particular with sewage stabilization ponds where the shoreline has shallow slope with emergent vegetation (Beadle and Harmston, 1958; Myklebust and Harmston, 1962; Rapp and Emil, 1965). Similar conditions would attract other species of mosquito in other parts of the world.

Culex fatigans, on the other hand, is a mosquito which has followed man's urbanization in the tropics and which thrives in polluted waters. Heavy breeding is found in pit latrines, septic tanks and sullage pits, drains, and in pools and rivers containing effluent from sewerage systems, in Asia (Singh, 1967), Africa (White, 1971) and the Americas (Burton, 1967). There is evidence that this mosquito is extending its range in West Africa and in the Pacific. The female of *Culex fatigans* is attracted by volatile compounds given off from the breeding places (Ikeshoji, 1966) where substances are also present which stimulate egg-laying once the female has arrived at the water surface (Ikeshoji

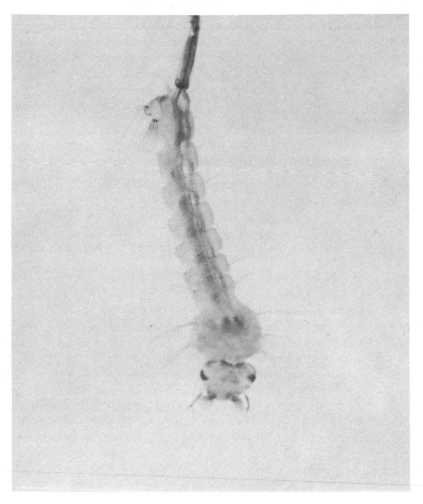

Larva of *Culex* attached to, and respiring at, the water surface. *Culex* mosquitoes are notable for their tendency to breed in polluted waters and are responsible for the transmission of filariasis and some viral infections. Actual length of the larva is 8 mm (photograph: S. A. Smith)

et al., 1967). Methane may also be an attractant (Gjullin *et al.*, 1965) and females are known to deposit eggs in waters too grossly polluted to support the larval stages (Subra, 1971). Breeding places are restricted to water in which substantial amounts of albuminoid nitrogen are dissolved (Ikeshoji *et al.*, 1967) and the optimum concentration for this species in laboratory experiments is 1000 p.p.m. of total solids (Parthasarthy and Kruse, 1954). Larval survival decreases in waters containing more solids. *Culex fatigans* is the main urban transmitter of the nematode worm *Wuchereria bancrofti*, where the disease in man is known as Bancroftian filariasis and where the most obvious clinical symptoms are elephantiasis of the legs and of the scrotum. Inadequate drainage and the impoundment of polluted waters near human habitation in towns in the tropics is resulting in increasing populations of the vector mosquito and increased incidence of the disease.

Family Muscidae and family Calliphoridae

Adult: Medium-to-large flies, 7–10 mm long, wing as in Figure 15.1j with bent vein behind wing tip, greyish body colour (Muscidae) or green (Calliphoridae). Larva: Length 10–12 mm, large maggot-like without distinct head capsule and no posterior siphon, each dark saucer-like plate (spiracle) on the posterior end with three snake-like slits (*Musca*) or with straight slits and an incomplete rim (*Chrysomyia*) (Figure 15.2j).

More commonly known as 'houseflies' (*Musca*) or 'blowflies' (*Chrysomyia*), the larval stages are found in excrement and in mixtures of excrement with decaying vegetable material. For the breeding of the housefly, *Musca domestica*, more solid, moist and fermenting materials are needed whereas other species of *Musca* breed in wetter materials. Competition with other larvae in nature, when the breeding medium is made more fluid, can reduce the number of houseflies (Kilpatrick and Schoof, 1959). Some species of the green tropical blowfly *Chrysomyia* also breed in excrement and latrines. Water disposal systems reduce the nuisance but exposure of faeces, manuring, unturned composts, and drying sludge, provide environments for these flies for breeding. All the flies that breed in human excrement are potential carriers of human faecal pathogens but the housefly *Musca domestica* and some species of *Chrysomyia* are especially important because of the adult behaviour. The adult fly will enter houses and shops readily and is attracted to human food as well as to excrement and garbage around the home. Human pathogens can be deposited whilst the fly is feeding, from the vomit drop produced to dissolve the food or in the fly faeces or from bodily contact with the fly. Other Muscid flies may be present out-of-doors but they do not show the domestic habits of the housefly *Musca domestica*. In the family Calliphoridae, some species of the green blowfly *Chrysomyia* have similar habits in tropical countries, attracted to both faeces and food. Smith (1973) surveys the flies in these two families.

Flies causing nuisance and allergy

Family Psychodidae

Adult: Small flies, 1–2 mm long, conspicuously hairy with hairy pointed wings (Figure 15.1a). Larva: Length about 5 mm with distinct head capsule and a distinct siphonal projection at the posterior end (Figure 15.2a).

The larvae of these flies are found in large numbers feeding on decomposing organic material, excrement, drains and filter beds. They are opportunist breeders and the larvae can develop quickly. Some species have a worldwide distribution. The most well-known pest of sewage treatment is *Psychoda alternata*, 'the trickling filter fly', a species with small dark spots on the wing margin at the end of the veins and also a highly adaptable species which has been found to breed in septic tanks, urinals, household drains, mudflats and decaying vegetation (Satchell, 1947). Other species of *Psychoda* have also been reared from larvae in bacteria beds, rivers polluted by sewage, drains and waste pipes. A related fly, *Telmatoscopus albipunctatus*, whose larva is markedly darker than those of *Psychoda*, is associated with latrines and sewage plants in the tropics (Forattini, 1973). Over-production of these psychodid flies from sewage purification units can cause trouble in the plant (Lloyd, 1945; Usinger and Kellen, 1955) and can also cause problems to the public as the flies disperse from the breeding area. Ordman (1946a, 1946b) and Phanichyakarn *et al.*, (1969) have recorded cases of bronchial asthma from south and west Africa resulting from inhalation of dust containing the remains of adult *Psychoda*. Skin tests of extracts of adult flies showed positive reactions in sensitized allergic patients. Steinhaus and Brinley (1957) have drawn attention to the presence of coliform bacteria in the larvae and adults of these and other 'nuisance' flies breeding in sewage, noting that the adult can deposit the bacteria in faeces after emergence and the flies can die in numbers in human food when the fly nuisance is extreme.

Family Chironomidae

Adult: Small-to-medium-sized flies, 2–8 mm long, wing bare transparent, rather thin, rounded at tip (Figure 15.1b), males have a pair of conspicuous plumed structures (antennae) projecting forwards from the head. Larva: Length about 5–14 mm with distinct head capsule, no siphon at posterior end but with short stumpy leg-like projection (pseudopod) immediately behind and below head (Figure 15.2b).

Unlike the more terrestrial Psychodidae, the larvae of this family of flies are typically inhabitants of freshwater lakes, rivers, ponds and streams, where they feed on organic detritus; some species spin silken tunnels and make use of a respiratory current, set up by characteristic undulations of the body, to draw in food. Some of the tube-dwelling larvae may cause a nuisance in sewage plant (Pillai and Subrahmanyan, 1942) where other species are inhabitants of the trickling filter fauna (Lloyd, 1945). One group of midges, the Chironominae, possess a blood haemoglobin which is efficient at low oxygen concentrations and some larvae can even respire anaerobically for a few hours. Consequently this group of flies are conspicuous in freshwater habitats with oxygen deficits, especially species of the large genus *Chironomus* (or *Tendipes*) which are numerous in oxidation ponds (Usinger and Kellen, 1955). The Chironomid midges pose problems similar to those produced by the Psychodidae. Over-production tends to interrupt biological processes in filter systems and, as well as the nuisance caused by the adult flies away from the breeding source, serious asthmatic and other allergic reactions in man have been found where skin tests with antigens prepared from Chironomid adults have been positive (Lewis, 1957).

Family Anisopodidae

Adult: Medium-sized flies, 5–7 mm long, wing rather broad with many veins (Figure 15.1d) and without scales. Larva: Length 10–15 mm with distinct head capsule, body segments divided into alternating long and short segments (Figure 15.2e).

Species of *Anisopus* are a nuisance entering human dwellings in large numbers (known as 'window flies'). The larvae of *Anisopus cinctus* are well known members of the filter bed fauna in temperate countries (Lloyd, 1945) where, in competition with other species, they may effect the efficiency of the percolating filter (Hawkes, 1955). The larvae of the Anisopodidae are found typically in animal faeces, decaying vegetation and other material with a high organic content.

Flies breeding in numbers in the sewage system

Family Stratiomyidae

Adult: Medium-to-large flies, 4–20 mm long, usually metallic or brightly coloured, wing with conspicuously thick and thin veins (figure 15.1e). Larva: Length 5–20 mm, very wide-bodied with small head capsule anteriorly (Figure 15.2f).

Species of *Hermetia* are well known to breed in privies and pit latrines (Furman *et al.*, 1959; Kilpatrick and Schoof, 1959) and other Stratiomyid flies breed in animal excrement. The presence of these large larvae breaks human excrement down into a more fluid condition which is less suitable for housefly breeding. As the adult flies do not enter houses in numbers to cause a nuisance, the presence of Stratiomyid larvae in sewage may be regarded as beneficial and contributing to the breakdown of the organic content.

Family Syrphidae

Adult: Medium-to-large flies, 6–15 mm long, brightly coloured or resembling hive bees, wing with a conspicuous loop in vein near wing tip (Figure 15.1f). Larva: Length 15 mm without distinct head capsule and with posterior end pulled out into very long, extensible siphon up to 30 mm or more in length (Figure 15.2k).

The larvae of the subfamily Eristalinae have the characteristic 'rat-tailed maggot' shape with a highly extensible siphon through which they respire at the surface of the water. They are scavengers in foetid waters containing much decaying vegetation, such as rot holes in trees or amongst the dense vegetation floating on tropical ponds, or animal material such as faeces and sewage sludge. The larvae are very prominent in pit latrines and in floating masses of sludge or at the edges of oxidation ponds (Usinger and Kellen, 1955). The adult flies hover motionless in the air ('hover flies') and rarely cause a nuisance.

Family Sepsidae

Adult: Small-to-medium-sized flies, 3–5 mm long, thin-bodied with rounded heads, body colour reddish or black, when alive commonly twisting their narrow wings (Figure 15.1g). Larva: Length about 5 mm without distinct head capsule, posterior end pulled out to form a short or long unpigmented siphon (Figure 15.2g).

Sepsid flies are produced in large numbers from animal faeces and from sewage and the adult flies can be found congregating on the surface of faeces and floating scum, or on vegetation surrounding the breeding area. These dense aggregation of flies outdoors may give rise to concern but they rarely enter human dwellings.

Family Ephydridae

Adult: Small-to-medium-sized flies, 2–4 mm long, found on the water surface, on floating sludge or on the shoreline in numbers, wing as in Figure 15.1h. Larva: Length 5–13 mm without distinct head capsule, usually with paired stumpy false legs on body and with long, often forked, siphon (Figure 15.2h).

These flies are known as 'shore flies' and are abundant at the edges of fresh-water lakes and ponds where the adults feed by scraping algae from the surface of the mud or on other insects trapped in the water film. They can be found by polluted waters including oxidation ponds (Usinger and Kellen, 1955) and in the filter system (Forattini, 1973). One species, *Teichomyza fusca*, is well known for its association with cesspits, urinals and excrement.

Family Sphaeroceridae

Adult: Small or medium-sized flies, 1–5 mm long, wing as in Figure 15.1i, hind legs with a very broad joint (metatarsus) before the last four joints (tarsi) of the leg. Larva: Length 4–8 mm, small maggot-like without a distinct head capsule and the posterior end rounded, without a siphon although there may be paired projections (Figure 15.2i).

As with the Sepsid flies, these small flies are found in very large numbers on faecal material, excrement or floating sewage scum. They are also found around the edges of freshwater and oxidation ponds (Usinger and Kellen, 1955) and species of *Limosina* have been found in sewage filters.

15.5 OTHER INSECTS

Although a description of 11 families of flies known to breed regularly in human sewage disposal systems may seem excessive, other insects in addition will be found attracted by the faecal material or by the water. Most will occur in smaller numbers below the nuisance level or in larger numbers under special conditions related to the habitat or to the local insect species. Discharge of sewage into rivers, for instance, may promote the breeding of certain species of blood-sucking blackfly downstream (*Simulium*) and overflow of faecal material into waterlogged soil provides a suitable breeding medium for some species of the biting midge *Culicoides*. However, relatively few other insects, other than some beetles and wingless springtails, are commonly associated with faeces, untreated sewage and sludge. Where the sewage effluent approaches more normal conditions, for instance in oxidation ponds with algal bloom and much floating or emergent vegetation, the insect fauna becomes much more diverse. Usinger and Kellen (1955) studied the fauna of oxidation ponds in America and found that these could approach more normal freshwater habitats, with surface-feeding predators (such as water beetles and pond skating bugs). Submerged beetles, corixids and dragonflies were also found. Many of these insects can be regarded as beneficial as they feed on other insects, including the disease-carrying Anopheline and Culicine mosquitoes (WHO, 1975) which may invade these more normal habitats.

15.6 CONTROL MEASURES

The less the human waste is diluted by water, the more the faeces fauna will predominate with the over-production of flies causing a nuisance, including the housefly *Musca* and the blowfly *Chrysomyia*, with the possible transfer of bacteria and other pathogenic organisms from faeces to human food. The wetter the medium, the more the freshwater fauna will predominate with the production of a variety of aquatic or semi-aquatic insects, predominantly flies as a nuisance and including the mosquitoes. It is advisable to consider potential problems associated with fly breeding during the construction of waste handling and treatment plant.

Fly nuisance and plant design

Preferably all large aggregations of sewage should be as far as possible from human habitation. Fly density decreases with distance from the breeding source, owing to dilution of the population and its mortality. Nuisance may be confined to workers on the plant itself or to its immediate neighbourhood; *Psychoda* are believed to travel ¾ to 1 mile (Lloyd, 1945). Landscaping, with the use of vegetation as a barrier, and taking into account prevailing wind movement which may assist fly dispersal, may prevent flies from dispersing too far. Lewis (1957) recommended barriers of trees between the Nile and areas of Khartoum where Chironomid midges from the river were causing nuisance and allergy in the Sudan. The more artificial the actual breeding place, the less attractive it becomes for the majority of the local insects. Theoretically, small plants can be made fly-proof but problems of maintenance and supervision, and the diversity of breeding species, present practical problems. Stabilization ponds in America attract a great variety of insects including the mosquitoes *Culex fatigans* and *C. tarsalis*. Heaviest production of *C. tarsalis*, which transmits encephalitis viruses from animals to man, was found in ponds containing aquatic or emergent vegetation (Myklebust and Harmston, 1962) and both Beadle and Harmston (1958) and Rapp and Emil (1965) recommended the removal of plant growth from stabilization ponds and also the maintenance of a steep bank profile (4:1 or 3:1) to prevent the growth of emergent vegetation and the shallow water favourable for mosquito breeding. A water depth of 4 feet with access for insecticide treatment is recommended. Clear, deep water is not so attractive to mosquitoes and other aquatic insect 'fringe-breeders' although floating scum may provide breeding material for the excrement fauna.

Insecticides

Insecticidal control methods require a balance between the elimination or reduction of disease-carrying and nuisance insects and the maintenance of micro-organisms (bacteria, protozoa) and the browsing macro-fauna (insects) essential to the breakdown of wastes in the sewage system. The insecticides chosen should eliminate the target insect but should not at the same time destroy the balance of the biological process. Even in latrines, Kilpatrick and Schoof (1959) found that insecticide treatment eliminated *Hermetia illucens* but not the more resistant housefly *Musca domestica*, resulting in an increase of housefly breeding in the more solid excrement found in the absence of the Stratiomyid fly. It is important that any insecticide used for control in the sewage plant should not effect micro-organisms adversely nor result in excessive insecticidal pollution in freshwaters at the outflow. The insecticide of choice depends upon its toxicity, persistence and availability (including costs). Chlorinated hydrocarbons such as DDT and benzene hexachloride (BHC) have been recommended in the past for sewage treatment, as well as chlorination (Lloyd, 1945; Hawkes, 1955; Busvine, 1966), but the insecticides are suspect for their persistence in the environment. The toxicity of organophosphorus insecticides to micro-organisms has been studied by Steelman *et al.* (1967) and Allegrini *et al.* (1973) and toxicity to fish by Chen *et al.*, (1972) and Darwazeh and Mulla (1974). Some insecticides are highly toxic under laboratory conditions and currently

296

the insecticides 'abate' and 'fenthion' show low toxicity to the other organisms and are effective against insects in polluted waters at dosages of 1 p.p.m. or less (Brown, 1967; Steelman *et al.*, 1967; Graham *et al.*, 1972). 'Abate' ('temephos') is less toxic to man. In small breeding areas, such as pit latrines, a granular formulation of organophosphorus insecticide may be the most convenient method of application (White, 1971).

Fish

At the lower, least polluted end of the sewage system, attractive to the greatest variety of insects (including the mosquitoes), it may be possible to introduce breeding populations of mosquito-eating fish (Sasa *et al.*, 1965). Local species of fish may be suitable which feed at the water surface, which survive and breed in the confined and polluted waters, which are small and not attractive as food to the local fishermen, and which can be transported from place to place. The most well known fish which prey on mosquito larvae are *Gambusia affinis* (known as the 'mosquito fish') and *Lebistes reticulatus* ('guppy'), but at least 13 other species of fish are known with the same desirable habits (WHO, 1975).

15.7 REFERENCES

Allegrini, J., Simeon, M. de B., Cousserans, J. and Sinegre, G. (1973). La lutte antilarvaire contre les culicides des fosses septiques, l'action du 'Dursban et du D.D.T.' sur la flore microbienne. *Cahiers O.R.S.T.O.M. série Entomologie Médicale et Parasitologie*, **11**, 101–106.

Beadle, L. D. and Harmston, F. C. (1958). Mosquitoes in sewage stabilization ponds in the Dakotas. *Mosquito News*, **18**, 203–296.

Brown, A. W. A. (1967). The present status of control of *Culex pipiens fatigans*. *Bulletin of the World Health Organization*, **37**, 297–299.

Burton, G. J. (1967). Observations on the habits and control of *Culex pipiens fatigans* in Guyana. *Bulletin of the World Health Organization*, **37**, 317–322.

Busvine, J. R. (1966). *Insects and Hygiene*. London: Methuen.

Carpenter, K. E. (1928). *Life in Inland Waters*. London: Sidgwick and Jackson.

Chen, P. S., Lin, Y. N. and Chung, C. L. (1972). Laboratory studies on the susceptibility of mosquito-eating fish, *Lebistes reticulatus*, and the larvae of *Culex pipiens fatigans* to insecticides. *Journal of the Formosan Medical Association*, **70**, 28–35.

Crisp, G. and Lloyd, L. (1954). The community of insects in a patch of woodland mud. *Transactions of the Royal Entomological Society of London*, **105**, 269–314.

Darwazeh, H. A. and Mulla, M. S. (1974). Toxicity of herbicides and mosquito larvicides to the mosquito fish *Gambusia affinis*. *Mosquito News*, **34**, 214–219.

Forattini, O. P. (1973). *Entomologia Medica Volume 4*. São Paulo: Universidade de São Paulo.

Furman, D. P., Young, R. D. and Catts, E. P. (1959). *Hermetia illucens* as a factor in the natural control of *Musca domestica* Linnaeus. *Journal of Economic Entomology*, **52**, 917–921.

Gjullin, C. M., Johnsen, J. O. and Plapp, F. W. (1965). The effect of odors released by various waters on the oviposition sites selected by two species of *Culex*. *Mosquito News*, **25**, 268–269.

Graham, J. E., Abdulcader, M. H. M., Mathis, H. L., Self, L. S. and Sebastian, A. (1972). Studies on the control of *Culex pipiens fatigans* Wiedemann. *Mosquito News*, **32**, 399–416.

Hawkes, H. A. (1955). The effects of insecticide treatment on the macrofauna populations, film accumulation and efficiency of sewage percolating filters. *Annals of Applied Biology*, **43**, 122–133.

Ikeshoji, T. (1966). Attractant and stimulant factors for oviposition of *Culex pipiens fatigans* in natural breeding-sites. *Bulletin of the World Health Organization*, **35**, 905–912.

Ikeshoji, T., Umino, T. and Hirakoso, S. (1967). Studies on mosquito attractants and stimulants. Part IV An agent producing stimulation effects for oviposition of *Culex pipiens fatigans* in field water and the stimulative effects of various chemicals. *Japanese Journal of Experimental Medicine*, **37**, 61–69.

Kilpatrick, J. W. and Schoof, H. F. (1959). Interrelationship of water and *Hermetia illucens* breeding to *Musca domestica* production in human excrement. *American Journal of Tropical Medicine and Hygiene*, **8**, 597–602.

Laurence, B. R. (1954). The larval inhabitants of cow pats. *Journal of Animal Ecology*, **23**, 234–260.

Lewis, D. J. (1957). Observations on Chironomidae at Khartoum. *Bulletin of Entomological Research*, **48**, 155–184.

Lloyd, L. (1943). Sewage treatment in a tropical city. *Nature London*, **151**, 646.

Lloyd, L. (1945). Animal life in sewage purification processes. *Journal of the Institute of Sewage Purification*, **1945**, 119–139.

Myklebust, R. J. and Harmston, F. C. (1962). Mosquito production in stabilization ponds. *Journal of the Water Pollution Control Federation*, **34**, 302–306.

Oldroyd, H. (1964). *The Natural History of Flies*. London: Weidenfeld and Nicolson.

Oldroyd, H. (1970). *Handbooks for the Identification of British Insects, Volume IX, Part 1, Diptera. Introduction and key to families*. London: Royal Entomological Society of London.

Ordman, D. (1946a). Bronchial asthma caused by the trickling sewage filter fly (*Psychoda*): inhalant insect allergy. *Nature London*, **157**, 441.

Ordman, D. (1946b). Sewage filter flies (*Psychoda*) as a cause of bronchial asthma. *South African Medical Journal*, **20**, 32–35.

Parthasarthy, T. and Kruse, C. W. (1954). Effect of organic matter in the control of *Culex fatigans* by D.D.T. larvicide. *Indian Journal of Malariology*, **8**, 33–43.

Phanichyakarn, P., Dockhorn, R. J. and Kirkpatrick, C. H. (1969). Asthma due to the inhalation of moth flies (*Psychoda*). *Journal of Allergy*, **44**, 51–58.

Pillai, S. C. and Subrahmanyan, V. (1942). Role of protozoa in the activated sludge process. *Nature London*, **150**, 525.

Rapp, W. F. and Emil, C. (1965). Mosquito production in a eutrophic sewage stabilization lagoon. *Journal of the Water Pollution Control Federation*, **37**, 867–870.

Sasa, M., Kurihara, T., Dhamvanij, O. and Harinasuta, C. (1965). Studies on mosquitoes and their natural enemies in Bangkok. Part 3 Observations on a mosquito-eating fish 'Guppy', *Lebistes reticulatus*, breeding in polluted waters. *Japanese Journal of Experimental Medicine*, **35**, 63–80.

Satchell, G. H. (1947). The larvae of the British species of *Psychoda* (Diptera: Psychodidae). *Parasitology*, **38**, 51–69.

Singh, D. (1967). The *Culex pipiens fatigans* problem in south-east Asia with special reference to urbanization. *Bulletin of the World Health Organization*, **37**, 239–243.

Smith, K. G. V. (1973). *Insects and Other Arthropods of Medical Importance*. London: British Museum (Natural History).

Steelman, C. D., Colmer, A. R., Cabes, L., Barr, H. T. and Tower, B. A. (1967). Relative toxicity of selected insecticides to bacterial populations in waste disposal lagoons. *Journal of Economic Entomology*, **60**, 467–468.

Steinhaus, E. A. and Brinley, F. J. (1957). Some relationships between bacteria and certain sewage-inhabiting insects. *Mosquito News*, **17**, 299–302.

298

Subra, R. (1971). Études ecologiques sur *Culex pipiens fatigans* Wiedemann. *Cahiers O.R.S.T.O.M. série Entomologique Médicale et Parasitologie*, **9**, 307–316.

Usinger, R. L. and Kellen, W. R. (1955). The role of insects in sewage disposal beds. *Hilgardia*, **23**, 263–321.

White, G. B. (1971). The present importance of domestic mosquitoes (*Culex pipiens fatigans* Wiedemann) in East Africa and recent steps towards their control. *East African Medical Journal*, **48**, 266–274.

WHO (1975). *Manual on Practical Entomology in Malaria Part 1*. Geneva: World Health Organization.

Part B—Helminthological Aspects of Sewage Treatment in Hot Climates

M. R. N. SHEPHARD

15.8 INTRODUCTION

At a conservative estimate, at least half the world's population is infected with one or more species of helminth parasite. In tropical countries, especially those with widespread poverty and low standards of hygiene, the rates of infection are considerably greater than this. Although the alimentary canal is the most frequent and familiar site of infection, certain helminth species also invade the blood, muscles, lungs, skin, liver and nervous system. While many people can carry fairly large parasite burdens without apparent ill-effect, certain helminths may cause disfigurement, blindness, anaemia, intestinal obstruction, impairment of the function of internal organs or death. Even the most harmless forms may deprive the human host of nourishment or weaken resistance to other infections.

15.9 GENERAL BIOLOGY OF HELMINTHS

Classification and morphology

The term 'helminth' is applied to parasites of the worm type, belonging principally to three biological groups—the nematodes (roundworms), trematodes (flukes) and cestodes (tapeworms). The phylum Nematoda includes both free-living and plant-parasitic species as well as parasites of man and animals. They have a typical elongated 'worm' shape, an alimentary canal with both mouth and anus and a body cavity; normally the sexes are separate. While free-living and plant-parasitic species are minute, nematode parasites of man are usually visible to the naked eye in their adult stage and some reach a considerable size. Trematoda and Cestoda are both classes of the phylum Platyhelminthes, which also includes Turbellaria (free-living flatworms). Trematoda are divided into the orders Digenea, which infect a wide range of vertebrate

Parts of this section are adapted from the author's review 'The Role of Sewage Treatment in the Control of Human Helminthiases', *Helminthological Abstracts, Series A*, **40** (1), 1–16 (1971) and are reproduced by permission of the Commonwealth Agricultural Bureaux.

hosts, and Monogenea, which almost exclusively parasitize fish. Trematode parasites of man are thus all Digenea, which typically have a flattened leaf-shaped appearance, two suckers for attachment, a gut which terminates in two blind-ended caeca and a life-cycle involving a snail, and possibly other animals, as intermediate hosts. Most trematode species are hermaphrodite (the schistosomes are an exception) and like all Platyhelminthes, they lack a coelomic cavity. Cestoda are characterized by a scolex with hooks or suckers for attachment, and a strobila, i.e. a ribbon of segments, each with a complete (hermaphrodite) set of reproductive organs. There is no alimentary canal. As with other helminths, the life-cycles of cestodes are complex and may involve one or two intermediate hosts, or none at all. Typically, there is a cyst-like larval stage which develops to the adult tapeworm when the intermediate host is consumed by the final host as food.

Adaptation to parasitism

All parasites show a remarkable range of adaptations to their unusual way of life and a close study of these is important in understanding their means of survival and transmission and thus developing possible methods of control. These adaptations may include: organs of attachment to enable the parasite to resist mechanical removal from the host; elaborate mechanisms for overcoming the host's immunological and digestive systems; digestive organs in the parasite reduced or absent owing to the freely available food supply; body shape related to the site of parasitism within the host; production of vast numbers of ova to increase the chances of transmission to other hosts; and often remarkable adaptations to the behavioural or ecological characteristics of the host or vector, in order to facilitate transmission. In addition, parasites of the intestinal tract have to survive in a largely oxygen-free environment, and their use of biochemical pathways not requiring oxygen has been closely studied, particularly in relation to the development of antiparasitic drugs.

Geographical distribution

Many helminth species parasitic in man, particularly the common intestinal nematodes, have a worldwide distribution. Others are limited by the inability of the ova or larvae to survive outside the host, owing to unfavourable environmental conditions. For helminths having one or more intermediate hosts, distribution will normally be governed by the limitations placed on the distribution of those intermediate hosts, or their contact with man, by climatic, geographical, ecological or sociological factors. Cultural variations will often play a significant part in helminth distribution, particularly in relation to associations between man and his domestic animals and local variations in diet. Thus, the Masai tribe of East Africa, well known for their close association with cattle, have particularly high prevalence of tapeworm infection, while the lung-fluke *Paragonimus westermanni*, acquired by eating raw crab, is commonest in countries such as Japan and Korea. In very general terms, both the prevalence and the variety of helminth infections of man appear to increase with proximity to the equator.

15.10 THE TRANSMISSION OF HELMINTHS

In order to understand the role of sewage in the transmission of helminth infections, one must first consider the variety of means which parasites employ to ensure their survival and spread. In many cases, the faecal route is of no significance. Certain nematodes, known as filariae, have a larval stage (the microfilaria) which is comparable in size to blood cells and circulates in the capillaries. These species are transmitted by blood-sucking insects in a similar manner to the malaria parasite. With other species, the parasite may release its ova or larvae to the environment by non-faecal routes; for example, the larvae of the guinea worm *Dracunculus medinensis* are released into water through skin ulcers. In many helminth infections, human beings accidentally 'break into' a cycle of transmission which is taking place in nature, but themselves play no further part in transmission; as far as the helminth is concerned, the human host is a 'dead end'. Thus, the cestode causing hydatid cyst, which can be fatal in man, is normally transmitted between dogs and domestic ruminants. Men become infected by the accidental ingestion of ova from dog faeces, but in order to continue the cycle, human viscera would have to be consumed by dogs, which is highly unlikely in most cultures.

We can assume that sewage treatment is only relevant as a possible means of control when helminth ova or larvae are passed in the faeces or urine of man and are then capable of infecting other human beings, either directly or after passage through one or more intermediate hosts. The principal helminth infections which come into this category can be listed thus:

Nematodes

> *Enterobius vermicularis* (pinworm)
> *Trichuris trichiura* (whipworm)
> *Ascaris lumbricoides* (roundworm)
> *Strongyloides stercoralis*
> *Ancylostoma duodenale* (hookworm)
> *Necator americanus* (hookworm)

Trematodes

> *Schistosoma* spp.

Cestodes

> *Hymenolepis nana* (dwarf tapeworm)
> *Taenia saginata* (beef tapeworm)
> *Taenia solium* (pork tapeworm)
> *Diphyllobothrium latum* (broad tapeworm)

It may be more convenient to classify these species not in terms of their taxonomic relationships but on the basis of their mode of transmission as in the following subsections.

Contaminative helminths *(Enterobius vermicularis* and *Hymenolepis nana)*

These are helminths requiring no intermediate host and whose ova or larvae are infective at the time they are passed in the faeces; they are normally acquired by mouth. Contaminative helminths are normally transmitted on soiled clothing, food, bedding etc., and an infected person can easily reinfect himself (autoinfection) or other people, particularly in conditions where individuals are crowded together and hygiene is poor.

Soil-transmitted helminths

These can be divided into those acquired by mouth *(Ascaris lumbricoides* and *Trichuris trichiura)* and those acquired by penetration of larvae through the skin *(Strongyloides stercoralis, Ancylostoma duodenale* and *Necator americanus)*. Ova of *Ascaris lumbricoides* require one to two weeks' development in the soil, and those of *T. trichiura* three to five weeks, before becoming infective. Infections are particularly common in rural areas where there is a lack of adequate means of sewage disposal, with consequent faecal contamination of soil around homes. *Ascaris* ova can survive in soil for months or even years, and are notoriously resistant to destruction. If nightsoil is used as a fertilizer, contamination of vegetables provides a further source of infection. Hookworm ova passed in faeces hatch within a few days releasing 'rhabditiform' larvae, which then moult to give infective ('filariform') larvae; these can survive for six to twelve weeks under favourable conditions but are quickly destroyed by desiccation, excessive moisture or direct exposure to sunlight.

Mollusc-transmitted helminths

All digenetic trematodes have a mollusc intermediate host. The schistosomes are by far the most important trematode parasites of man, infecting possibly 200 million people and causing damage, severe in chronic cases, to the liver, spleen and bladder; they differ from most other trematodes in that contamination of water by human excreta is a relevant factor in the epidemiology. In several other trematode infections, ova are passed in human faeces, but transmission is maintained in nature by other vertebrates (reservoir hosts) and even complete abolition of pollution by human excreta would not prevent infection. Examples of such trematodes and their reservoir hosts are *Clonorchis sinensis* (cats, dogs), *Fusciolopsis buski* (dogs, pigs), *Fasciola hepatica* (cattle, sheep) and *Metagonimus yokogawai* (cats, dogs, birds). In the typical digenean lifecycle, ova passed in the faeces hatch to release free-swimming miracidia, which penetrate the snail intermediate host. Within the snail, asexual reproduction takes place resulting in the release of tailed cercariae into the surrounding water. Infection of a new host by a cercaria can take place by active penetration of the skin of the host (e.g. schistosomes), by encystment on aquatic plants which are eaten by the host (e.g. *Fasciola hepatica*, *Fasciolopsis buski*), or by encystment on a second intermediate host, such as a fish or crab, which is then eaten by the final host (e.g. *Clonorchis sinensis*, *Paragonimus westermanni*).

Food-transmitted helminths

As indicated above, some trematode infections may be acquired by man in food (especially fish), but the principal food-transmitted helminths are the tapeworms *Taenia saginata*, *T. solium* and *Diphyllobothrium latum*. Man acts as the final host, harbouring the adult tapeworm, while a food animal (cattle, pig and fish, respectively, for the three species above) harbours the larval stage (known as the cysticercus in *Taenia*). For *T. saginata* and *T. solium*, there are no reservoir hosts and cattle or pigs must have been in contact with tapeworm ova from human faeces in order to become infected with cysticerci. In the case of *D. latum*, there are two intermediate hosts, *Cyclops* (an aquatic copepod) and fish. Besides man, fish-eating carnivores such as dogs and foxes also become infected and thus, as with most trematode infections, even totally effective sewage treatment would not necessarily prevent transmission.

15.11 THE EFFECT OF SEWAGE TREATMENT

All forms of sewage treatment consist of a sequence of physical, biological, and sometimes chemical, processes, aimed at removing dissolved and suspended organic matter. The choice of treatment system in a particular community, and the constructional and ecological organization of the plant, will be determined by geographical and climatic conditions, the nature of the sewage to be treated, and by economic considerations. The contribution of each stage of sewage treatment to the removal or destruction of helminth ova is discussed below.

Sedimentation

Provided sufficient time is allowed and turbulence is minimal, sedimentation gives a high rate of removal of helminth ova. Liebmann (1964) estimated that with a specific gravity of $1\cdot1$, helminth ova will settle at a rate of 2 to 3 feet per hour in static conditions, and thus for most tanks a sedimentation time of 2 hours should be sufficient. Liebmann also noted that *Taenia saginata* ova were the slowest to settle; in one experiment, 68% had settled after 2 hours and 89% after 3 hours. However, with the addition of a flocculating agent, 95% of all worm eggs had settled within 2 hours. Döschl (1972) found that flocculation with aluminium sulphate at 90 to 120 g/m^3 and sedimentation for at least

60 minutes was required for the removal of *Diphyllobothrium latum* ova.

Laboratory experiments by various workers, using columns of raw sewage, support the view that 2 to 3 hours sedimentation is sufficient for the removal of most helminth ova (Cram, 1943; Jones *et al.*, 1947; Newton *et al.*, 1949). With regard to settlement rates in operational sewage works, Schmidt and Wieland (1950) found that 80% of helminth ova were removed in the settlement tanks as Stuttgart, while Bhaskaran *et al.* (1956) reported that at a sewage works in India with a retention period of 2 hours, 75% of *Ascaris* ova, 60% of *Trichuris* ova and 70% of hookworm ova were removed.

Biological filter

Since the principle of this process is to encourage biological activity, one would not expect the environment to be particularly hostile to helminth ova; this is borne out by the relatively low removal rates observed. For example, Vishnevskaya (1938) reported that at Kharkov, USSR, *Ascaris lumbricoides* ova, present at 60 per litre in raw sewage, were reduced to 20 per litre by sedimentation, but from there only to 13 per litre after bacteria bed treatment.

Experiments by the three groups of workers mentioned above showed that addition of helminth ova of various species to the influent of laboratory-scale bacteria beds resulted in the recovery of about 25% to 40% in the effluent within a few hours, suggesting that this form of treatment did not give satisfactory removal rates. Bhaskaran *et al.* (1956) reported that a pilot-plant bacteria bed in India gave 98% to 100% removal of *Ascaris* and hookworm ova, but it appeared that observations were made after secondary sedimentation and it is probable that most removal took place here rather than in the bacteria bed itself.

Being a relatively stable environment, the bacteria bed can provide an ecological niche for larger organisms, both vertebrate and invertebrate, which may be significant in the transmission of helminth infections. Flies which breed in the beds, and birds which scavenge on them, have been suggested as possible carriers. It has been demonstrated (Silverman and Griffiths, 1955) that helminth ova can pass through the alimentary canal of seagulls and still retain their viability; this may be one means by which cattle pasture becomes contaminated with *Taenia saginata* ova. Free-living nematodes also occur in bacteria beds and although harmless in themselves, it has been shown (Wolf, 1971) that they can carry pathogenic bacteria and must be considered a potential hazard in the re-use of water from treated effluents.

Activated sludge

In studies on the effect of activated sludge treatment on helminth ova, effluents have usually been sampled after both aeration and sludge separation. Quite high removal rates have been observed, probably due to physical removal during settlement rather than any adverse effect of aeration. Bhaskaran *et al.*

(1956) found that at two sewage works in India, activated sludge treatment removed 93% and 98% of *Ascaris* ova, 91·8% and 100% of *Trichuris* ova and 81·5% and 96% of hookworm ova. Rowan (1964) reported that activated sludge treatment in Puerto Rico, including primary and secondary sedimentation, reduced the concentration of *Ascaris* ova by 97% to 100% and *Schistosoma mansoni* ova by 99·7%. Jones *et al.* (1947) noted that an experimental tank proved a very favourable hatching medium for *Schistosoma japonicum* ova. Since a hatched miracidium must find a snail intermediate host within a relatively short time, this may prove helpful in preventing transmission, provided there are no snails in the outflows or nearby watercourses.

Waste stabilization pond

In laboratory trials, Lakshminarayana and Abdulappa (1972) found that hookworm larvae were completely eliminated in less than 2 days in a facultative pond, and sludge samples did not show any viable ova; in a maturation pond, however, filariform larvae were recovered for up to 16 days. The authors considered that lack of oxygen was the principal lethal factor, although Cram (1943) found viable hookworm ova in anaerobically digesting sludge for considerable periods. In an operational works at Nagpur, India, consisting of a three-pond series, ova of *Ancylostoma duodenale*, *Hymenolepis nana* and *Ascaris lumbricoides* were regularly present, and those of *Trichuris trichiura* and *Enterobius vermicularis* occasionally present, in the raw sewage. In the final effluent the only helminths present were occasional filariform larvae of *Ancylostoma duodenale*. A corresponding accumulation of helminth ova in the settled sludge of the first pond was found, suggesting that removal was due to simple sedimentation. Studies in Rhodesia and South Africa have confirmed that helminth ova are normally absent from the final effluent of waste stabilization ponds (Hodgson, 1964; Meiring *et al.*, 1968).

Kawata and Krusé (1966) studied the effect of laboratory-simulated waste stabilization ponds on ova and miracidia of *Schistosoma mansoni*. Completely anaerobic ponds were found to inhibit the hatching of ova by a mean value of 77·3%, while there was no inhibition of hatching in facultative or aerobic ponds. Ova recovered from the sludge of the anaerobic pond after 4 hours showed only 9% hatchability, and after 8 hours hatchability was zero. Miracidia survived for a maximum of 6 hours in anaerobic pond water and 10 hours in aerobic pond water, compared with 18 hours in tap water. Under anaerobic conditions, the schistosome snail vector *Australorbis glabratus* did not lay eggs and the mean survival period was 20 days, with none surviving beyond 42 days. In the facultative pond, the snails survived and reproduced as if under normal conditions. From their results, Kawata and Krusé recommended the inclusion of a preliminary anaerobic chamber in stabilization pond design to suppress hatching of schistosome ova. However, since the maximum survival time of hatched miracidia is much less than the normal retention period of stabilization ponds, this alone should be sufficient to prevent transmission, provided that vector snails are absent from the maturation ponds and outflows.

Sludge digestion and drying

Helminth ova removed from sewage by the processes so far discussed have not necessarily been destroyed. They can still cause human infection depending on what form of sludge treatment is employed and for what purpose the treated sludge is used. Most treatment plants include anaerobic sludge digestion with the production of methane gas either as a separate stage or as an integral part of other processes.

The degree of destruction of helminth ova during digestion appears to be closely related to the temperature achieved, since other apparently hostile factors, such as lack of oxygen, have little effect on helminth ova. For most helminth ova and larvae, the critical lethal temperature is between 50 °C and 55 °C (Nolf, 1932; Keller, 1951). In digestion plants where these temperatures are not achieved, helminth ova frequently survive for long periods. Cram (1943) found that in experimental sludge digesters at 20 °C and 30 °C, the viability of *Ascaris lumbricoides* ova was little affected during the first 3 months and 10% were still viable after 6 months. In the same experiment it was shown that hookworm ova could still hatch after 64 days digestion at 20 °C and 41 days at 30 °C. Jones *et al.* (1947) and Newton *et al.* (1948) found that at normal summer temperatures (24–29·5 °C), a 3-week retention period in digesting sludge ensured the absence of *Schistosoma japonicum* ova, while at winter temperatures (6·5–18·5 °C), 10 weeks' sludge digestion was required. Newton *et al.* (1949) reported that at 24–29·5 °C, 50% of *Taenia saginata* ova added to digesting sludge were still apparently normal after 60 days and 10 to 15% after 200 days. Reyes *et al.* (1963) studied the effect of both aerobic and anaerobic digestion on *Ascaris suum* ova and worked out a time–temperature curve for the loss of viability. It was found that the sludge was free of ova after 20 days at 45 °C in the aerobic system and after 30 days at 38 °C under anaerobic conditions.

Digested sludge is usually dried by exposure to the air in shallow beds. Ova of different helminth species show considerable variations in their resistance to desiccation. *Ascaris* ova are exceptionally resistant and have been shown to survive for at least 7 years in drying sludge (Kozlova, 1965). It has been estimated that the moisture content of sludge must be reduced to 5% or less to bring about any significant destruction of *Ascaris* ova, a level that is impracticable under most conditions (Cram, 1943; Hogg, 1950). *Trichuris* ova are somewhat more sensitive than those of *Ascaris*, but still show considerable resistance. Hookworm larvae are known to be fairly susceptible to desiccation under normal transmission conditions. In sludge, hatching of hookworm ova is inhibited by the anaerobic environment, but during drying hatching takes place as aerobic conditions are re-established. Cram (1943) found that in drying sludge, hookworm larvae developed to the infective stage and remained alive for up to 62 days or until the moisture content dropped below 10%. *Schistosoma japonicum* ova appear to survive in sludge-drying beds for not more than 3 weeks irrespective of moisture content.

Tertiary treatment

In some sewage works, purified effluents are subjected to final cleansing measures such as filtering through sand or disinfection by chlorination. However, these measures are by no means universal even in the more sophisticated treatment plants, and are probably inappropriate to the simpler economies of most tropical countries. It is worth noting, nevertheless, that sand filtration is generally considered to be one of the most effective means of removing helminth ova. Removal rates approaching 100% have been found for ova of *Ascaris* and hookworm (Cram, 1943), *Schistosoma japonicum* (Jones *et al.*, 1947) and *Taenia saginata* (Newton *et al.*, 1949; Silverman and Griffiths, 1955).

By contrast, chlorination, although effective against some water-borne pathogens, cannot be relied upon to destroy helminth ova. Those of *Ascaris lumbricoides* are particularly resistant (Iwańczuk and Dożańska, 1957). Jones and Hummel (1947) found that miracidia of *Schistosoma japonicum* were considerably more susceptible to chlorination than their ova.

15.12 THE AGRICULTURAL UTILIZATION OF SEWAGE

The use of purified sewage effluents for irrigation and digested sludge as a fertilizer are both of considerable agricultural importance, especially in the poorer areas of the world. However, as has been seen, most sewage treatment processes cannot guarantee the complete absence of helminth ova. It is difficult to strike a balance between the relative importance of different criteria in the well-being of a community. Some may feel that the possibility of occasional nematode infections is a small price to pay for the undoubted benefits of increased soil fertility. However, a complete neglect of the dangers is likely to have serious repercussions. It is well known that the agricultural use of insufficiently treated sewage can cause helminth infections, either by the contamination of vegetables, especially those eaten raw, with helminth ova, or by the direct infection of agricultural workers. A severe outbreak of ascariasis at Darmstadt, West Germany, attributable to vegetable contamination and aggravated by a general post-war lack of hygiene, was described by Baumhögger (1949) and Krey (1949).

Purified effluents treated by conventional methods should be largely free of helminth ova; untreated sludge or nightsoil are the most likely sources of infection. Various methods of disinfecting the sludge have been suggested, of which composting or digestion is the most familiar. In general, the greater the temperature and the longer the digestion period, the greater the destruction of ova. If temperatures around 55 °C can be achieved, helminth ova are rapidly eliminated. As an alternative to digestion, chemical treatment of sludge against helminth ova using sodium nitrite (Kozai, 1960, 1962) or thiabendazole (Kutsumi and Komiya, 1965) have been found to be effective.

Romanenko (1967, 1971) investigated various methods of introducing sewage into soil by means of subsurface irrigation, deep ploughing or special injection drills, thus obtaining the agricultural benefits without the danger of contaminating vegetables. Although successful, the capital cost of most of these methods would appear to be prohibitive.

15.13 THE POSSIBILITIES OF CONTROL

Faecal transmission does not automatically mean sewage transmission. As has been seen, ova of contaminative helminths are acquired from soiled hands or clothing, or even inhaled in the air, and it is personal hygiene rather than sewage treatment that will reduce the rate of transmission. With soil-transmitted helminths, the main problem is the prevention of faecal contamination of soil in areas of human activity. While the provision of sewage treatment facilities is an important contribution, the solution must be seen in broader social terms. Hookworm *(Necator americanus)* infection is particularly characteristic of tropical countries with large plantations of sugar, coffee, bananas etc. For workers on these estates, the incentive to use proper sanitary facilities, even if these are available, is slight since there is plenty of cover for defecation closer at hand. The sites used tend to be moist and shady, precisely the kind of environment favouring development of the larvae. Furthermore, latrines which are poorly constructed or improperly used are more likely to aggravate the spread of hookworm than control it; contamination around the base of such a latrine would give a more concentrated focus of infection. Encouraging people to wear shoes might be a more effective and cheaper solution.

With pork and beef tapeworm, there is a fairly straightforward life-cycle and relatively few complicating factors in the epidemiology, with the result that sewage treatment provides a good opportunity to break the cycle of transmission. Other means of prevention include meat inspection, adequate cooking of pork and beef, and keeping cattle and pigs away from sewage outflows. By enforcing these measures, many countries have now virtually eliminated tapeworm infection and there is no reason why others should not do so, except where there are particular cultural situations which invalidate normal control measures.

Increasingly, it is being realised that campaigns against helminth infections based on a single control method are remarkable only for their lack of success. Instead, a wide range of weapons—drugs, vector control, education, sanitation—must be mobilized and employed in accordance with the epidemiological characteristics of the particular infection. This applies especially to schistosomiasis. While sewage treatment may enhance the effectiveness of other measures, by itself it is both impracticable and ineffective as a means of control.

Schistosome-infected persons usually live in such close association with water that the complete prevention of pollution is virtually impossible. Furthermore, Macdonald (1965) showed statistically that, because of the ability of the parasite to reproduce asexually within the snail, even reducing the amount of excreta reaching water by a factor of 15000—representing a very high standard of sanitation—would have no effect on the prevalence of schistosomiasis in a community. By comparison, the provision of a piped water supply, by greatly reducing the frequency of contact between human skin and contaminated water, would make a much greater contribution to control.

Control measures against schistosomiasis must be aimed at altering environmental conditions to the permanent disadvantage of the parasite. Besides those measures already mentioned, treatment of infected persons with anthelmintics, destruction of snails with molluscicides, designing watercourses to prevent the likelihood of human contact, educating vulnerable communities about the dangers of infection—all will no doubt contribute to the eventual conquest of this disease. But where these measures are applied in a haphazard and uncoordinated way, their success is only transitory. To be permanently effective, they must be harmonized in a programme of integrated control.

15.14 REFERENCES

Baumhögger, W. (1949). Die Spulwurmerkrankungen in Darmstadt und Hessen vom Abwasseringenieur gesehen. *Zeitschrift für Hygiene und Infektionskrankheiten*, **129**, 488–506.

Bhaskaran, T. R., Sampathkumaran, M. A., Sur, T. C. and Radhakrishnan, I. (1956). Studies on the effect of sewage treatment processes on the survival of intestinal parasites. *Indian Journal of Medical Research*, **44**, 163–180.

Cram, E. B. (1943). The effect of various treatment processes on the survival of helminth ova and protozoan cysts in sewage. *Sewage Works Journal*, **15**, 1119–1138.

Döschl, R. (1972). Versuche zur Sedimentation der Eier des Fischbandwurmes *Diphyllobothrium latum* durch das Flockungsmittel Aluminiumsulfat. *Inaugural Dissertation, Ludwig-Maximilians-Univ., Munich*, 70 pp.

Hodgson, H. T., (1964). Stabilization ponds for a small African urban area. *Journal of the Water Pollution Control Federation*, **36**, 51.

Hogg, E. S. (1950). A preliminary study of ova and cysts in Cydna digested sludge. *Journal and Proceedings of the Institute of Sewage Purification*, Part 1, 57–58.

Iwańczuk, I. and Dożańska, W. (1957). Wpływ chlorowania na przeżywalność jaj *Ascaris suis* w ściekach miejskich. *Acta Parasitologica Polonica*, **5**, 429–448.

Jones, M. F. and Hummel, M. S. (1947). Studies on schistosomiasis. The effect of chlorine and chloramine on schistosome ova and miracidia. *National Institute of Health Bulletin, US Public Health Service*, No. 189, 173–179.

Jones, M. F. et. al. (1947). Studies on schistosomiasis. The effects of sewage treatment processes on the ova and miracidia of *Schistosoma japonicum*. *National Institute of Health Bulletin, US Public Health Service*, No. 189, 137–172.

Kawata, K. and Krusé, C. W. (1966). The effect of sewage stabilization ponds on the eggs and miracidia of *Schistosoma mansoni*. *American Journal of Tropical Medicine and Hygiene*, **15**, 896–901.

Keller, P. (1951). Sterilization of sewage sludges. II. The influence of heat treatment on the ova of *Ascaris lumbricoides* in sewage. *Journal and Proceedings of the Institute of Sewage Purification*, Part, 1, 100–109.

Kozai, I. (1960). [Re-evaluation of sodium nitrite as an ovicide used in nightsoil. 1, 2, 3.] *Japanese Journal of Parasitology*, **9**, 202–210; 519–528; 529–540. (In Japanese.)

Kozai, I. (1962). [Re-evaluation of sodium nitrite as an ovicide. 4.] *Japanese Journal of Parasitology*, **11**, 400–410. (In Japanese.)

Kozlova, M. V. (1965). [Treating sewage deposits at filter stations against helminths.] *Materialy Nauchnoi Konferentsii Vsesoyuznogo Obshchestva Gel'mintologii*, Part I, 117–120. (In Russian.)

Krey, W. (1949). Der Darmstädter Spulwurmbefall und seine Bekämpfung. *Zeitschrift für Hygiene und Infektionskrankheiten*, **129**, 507–518.

Kutsumi, H. and Komiya, Y. (1965). Effect of thiabendazole as an ovicide on helminth eggs in nightsoil. *Japanese Journal of Medical Science and Biology*, **18**, 203–224.

Lakshminarayana, J. S. S. and Abdulappa, M. K. (1972). The effect of sewage stabilization ponds on helminths. *Proceedings of Symposium on Low Cost Waste Treatment, 27–29 October, 1969*, Nagpur, India: CPHERI. 290–299.

Liebmann, H. (1964). Parasites in sewage and the possibilities of their extinction. *Proceedings of 2nd International Conference on Water Pollution Research, Tokyo*, Vol. II, 269–276.

Macdonald, G. (1965). The dynamics of helminth infections with special reference to schistosomes. *Transactions of the Royal Society of Tropical Medicine and Hygiene*, **59**, 489–506.

Meiring, P. G. J., Drews, R. J. L., Van Eck, H. and Stander, G. J. (1968). A guide to the use of pond systems in South Africa for the purification of raw and partially treated sewage. *CSIR Special Report WAT 34*, Pretoria: National Institute for Water Research.

Newton, W. L., Figgat, W. B. and Weibel, S. R. (1948). The effect of sewage treatment processes upon ova and miracidia of *Schistosoma japonicum*. II. *Sewage Works Journal*, **20**, 657–664.

Newton, W. L., Bennett, H. J. and Figgat, W. B. (1949). Observations on the effects of various sewage treatment processes upon eggs of *Taenia saginata*. *American Journal of Hygiene*, **49**, 166–175.

Nolf, L. O. (1932). Experimental studies on certain factors influencing the development and viability of the ova of the human *Trichuris* as compared with those of the human *Ascaris*. *American Journal of Hygiene*, **16**, 288–322.

Reyes, W. L., Krusé, C. W. and Batson, M. S. (1963). The effect of aerobic and anaerobic digestion on eggs of *Ascaris lumbricoides* var. *suum* in nightsoil. *American Journal of Tropical Medicine and Hygiene*, **12**, 46–55.

Romanenko, N. A. (1967). [Sanitary and helminthological evaluation of some new methods for treating sewage sediment used in agriculture.] *Meditsinskaya Parazitologiya i Parzitarnye Bolezni*, **36**, 184–189. (In Russian.)

Romanenko, N. A. (1971). [Sanitary and helminthological evaluation of new methods of irrigation with sewage.] *Meditsinskaya Parazitologiya i Parazitarnye Bolezni*, **40**, 361–362. (In Russian.)

Rowan, W. B. (1964). Sewage treatment and schistosome eggs. *American Journal of Tropical Medicine and Hygiene*, **13**, 572–576.

Schmidt, B. and Wieland, F. (1950). Bietrag zur Frage des Wurmeiergehaltes von Abwässern und Klärschlamm. (Experimentelle Untersuchungen in der Kläranlage der Stadt Stuttgart.) *Zeitschrift für Hygiene und Infektionskrankheiten*, **130**, 603–612.

Silverman, P. H. and Griffiths, R. B. (1955). A review of methods of sewage disposal in Great Britain, with special reference to the epizootiology of *Cysticercus bovis*. *Annals of Tropical Medicine and Parasitology*, **49**, 436–450.

Vishnevskaya, S. M. (1938). The degree of dehelminthization of sewage at the Kharkov biostation. *Meditsinskaya Parazitologiyu i Parazitarnye Bolezni*, **7**, 450–454.

Wolf, H. W. (1971). Biological problems with reused water. *Journal of the American Water Works Association*, **63**, 181–185.

Rural Sanitation: Editorial Introduction

In response to the World Health Organization's 1970 questionnaire, 61 developing countries provided the following information about the provision of excreta disposal facilities in rural areas. In 1970, only 8% of the rural population had adequate disposal facilities and it was hoped to increase the number served by 327% by 1980. To achieve this enormous improvement an investment of US$ 1033 million over ten years is required (assuming a cost per user of only US$ 4) which represents an investment of US$ 103 million per year. Current investment in rural sanitation is running at only US$ 12 million per year and so clearly current progress holds out little hope that targets will be reached.

Poor excreta disposal practices promote a large number of important infectious diseases. Following the classification of disease given in Chapters 1 and 5, they will promote all faecal–oral diseases (Category 1, Table 5.5), all water-based diseases (Category 3, Table 5.5) and hookworm. Certain infections, most notably some forms of schistosomiasis, are prevented with reasonable economy only by the correct disposal and treatment of human wastes.

The problems of village sanitation are not primarily technical in nature since the methods of disposing of human wastes in small communities engaged in agriculture are well known. The problems are social, institutional and, more than anything else, motivational. To have a pit latrine is not enough—one must use it. To use it one must perceive some tangible advantage from using it—an advantage to hygiene, or to health, or to modesty or, in cases where human wastes will ultimately by applied to the land, an advantage to agricultural productivity. To build 1000 pit latrines is relatively simple and inexpensive. To ensure that 5000 or more people actually use the pit latrines and keep them in a hygienic condition may pose enormous problems. The answer, in most cases, must lie in the adoption of waste re-use systems with obvious benefits to the villager. The sanitary worker in the village is then in a position of saying not 'always use the latrine because it's good for you' but rather 'always use the latrine because it will enable your excreta to be put to some productive purpose' such as fish pond enrichment or agricultural fertilization.

16

Problems of Village Sanitation in India

R. N. SHELAT *and* M. G. MANSURI

16.1 INTRODUCTION

The real prosperity of India depends on the development of over 566 000 village communities. In Gujarat State, for example, out of a total population of 20 633 350, over 15 316 736 persons live in 18 584 villages. The bulk of this village population lives in villages of less than 5000 population (Table 16.1).

It is a very sad reflection on our development plans that most village people continue to live in insanitary conditions without even the elementary necessity of life—wholesome water. This paper briefly reviews the existing conditions of village sanitation and suggests possible methods of improvement. The purpose of the paper is to provoke discussion on some of the questions of village sanitation which require *immediate* attention.

Table 16.1 Village Population in Gujarat State[a]

Population	Number of villages	Total population
Below 200	3202	362 915
200 – 499	5302	1 819 031
500 – 999	5299	3 799 585
1000 – 1999	3301	4 511 498
2000 – 4999	1332	3 848 552
5000 – 9999	141	889 394
Above 10 000	7	85 761
	18 584	15 316 726

[a]1961 National Census.

This paper was originally published in the Journal of the Institution of Engineers of India. It is reproduced here in a slightly modified form by permission of the Institution of Engineers of India. For this paper the authors were awarded a Certificate of Merit by the Institution. © The Institution of Engineers of India, 1971. Reprinted from the Journal of the Institution of Engineers (India), volume 52, No. 2, pt PH1, October 1971, pages 21–24.

16.2 SURVEY OF EXISTING CONDITIONS

Rural water supply

Water is essential for life, health and sanitation. Man can live for over two months without food but can rarely live for more than three days without water. The first step in village sanitation is, therefore, obviously the supply of wholesome water. Rural sanitation methods too will depend largely on the method and quantity of water supplied to the community.

Prior to 1951, only three villages covering 10 000 people had a piped water supply in Gujarat State. At the start of the Third Five Year Plan in 1961 provision was made to supply water to 80 000 people in 32 villages. By 1966 however only $2\frac{1}{2}\%$ of the village population had in fact been supplied with piped water. A preliminary survey by Bhatt (1968) indicated that Rs 430 million will be required to provide for the bare minimum supply of water to all villages in Gujarat. If the population increase is taken at 550 000 persons per year, out of which say 350 000 are in villages, an additional amount of about Rs 35 million will be needed for this yearly increase in population alone. At present the woefully low figure of about Rs 17·5 million is spent each year on water supply and sanitation. How can the target of wholesome supply of water to all villages ever be achieved at this rate?

Village sanitation

Although it may be surprising, very little systematic data are available on existing methods of village sanitation. To get some idea of existing conditions, the appropriate authorities such as the public health divisional officers of the State Public Works Department, district health officers, sanitary inspectors of Primary Health Centres and other officials were contacted; and on-the-spot inquiries were made in the villages near Surat. The results of these inquiries and information obtained therefrom are given in the following paragraphs.

In Gujarat, very few towns have any worthwhile sewerage scheme. Even district towns like Broach and Bulsar do not yet have a sewerage scheme. Important towns like Dakora, Kapadvanj, Sojitra and almost all other towns of Gujarat have no scientific water-carriage system for the collection and disposal of sewage.

On enquiry from the Sanitary Inspector of Surat area (which comprises 52 villages) and the District Health Officer of Surat it was revealed that the bulk of small village communities uses the open field as a latrine, although some have community latrines. In fact, even where latrines are available, the villagers prefer to use the open field. This is perhaps partly due to very poor maintenance of the latrines and their surroundings and partly because the villagers are not used to latrines. The Government of Gujarat has worked out a scheme which can provide a standard Bavla type bowl and a concrete slab over the pit on payment of only Rs20 by the owner. However, the response

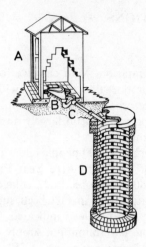

Figure 16.1 Planning Research Action Institute (PRAI)-type latrine: A, latrine building (1 × 1.2 × 2 m); B, latrine pan with steep slope, 0·6 m long; C, soil pipe with water seal; D, brick-lined pit (3 m × 1 m dia.) with concrete cover and openings to permit seepage of liquid wastes

to this scheme is poor. Even a lot of persuasion has failed. A latrine constructed by compulsion is quite often not used.

Some villages have basket-type latrines. Efforts are being made to convert these to PRAI-type latrines (Figure 16.1). According to the State-aided scheme, this can be done at a cost of only Rs150 out of which the owner will be required to pay Rs75 and the rest will have to be contributed equally by the village, taluka and district panchayats. Response to this scheme however does not appear to be very encouraging (Table 16.2).

Inquiries in Umra and Piplod villages were very revealing. Both these villages are directly adjacent to Surat City and are in fact very much urbanized. In Piplod, which has about 200 houses, there are hardly 15 latrines. In Umra, which has a population of over 1500, conditions are very similar. The bulk of the population uses open fields to answer nature's call. As these villages are on the bank of the Tapi River the bank has become badly polluted. Even a socially privileged and educated villager who has a latrine in his house told the investigator that he preferred to go to the field rather than use his latrine. Such conditions persist in spite of the fact that these villages are almost urban areas and the villagers fairly affluent.

16.3 PROBLEMS OF VILLAGE SANITATION

It is evident from the above discussion that the sanitary conditions in our villages and even in many small towns present a dreadful picture and it is a wonder how people live in such places. But quite often people are forced to live in this manner because the local authorities do nothing positive to change the situation. Stagnant pools of water, garbage carelessly strewn about, refuse freely littering the streets, ill-conceived and traditional insanitary habits of living and many other examples of insanitation are a common picture of our rural life. In these contexts the major needs of village communities are:

Table 16.2 Progress of latrine construction in Surat District

Taluka	Number of villages in taluka	Total population as per 1961 Census	1965				1966				1967				1968				1969				Total			
			Balvas type	Flush type	PRAI type	Septic type	Balvas type	Flush type	PRAI type	Septic type	Balvas type	Flush type	PRAI type	Septic type	Balvas type	Flush type	PRAI type	Septic type	Balvas type	Flush type	PRAI type	Septic type	Balvas type	Flush type	PRAI type	Septic type
Choryasi	11	140 133	—	—	—	—	—	—	—	—	6	—	—	—	—	—	—	—	—	23	—	8	6	23	—	8
Kamrej	15	62 822	26	—	—	—	32	—	—	—	30	—	—	—	26	—	—	—	6	—	—	—	120	—	—	—
Olpad	4	79 444	—	—	—	—	—	—	—	—	—	—	—	—	—	—	—	—	2	7	—	—	2	7	—	—
Mangrol	5	95 367	3	—	—	—	7	—	—	—	—	—	—	—	3	—	—	—	2	—	—	—	15	—	—	—
Mandvi	12[a]	93 805	—	—	—	—	—	—	—	—	—	—	—	—	—	—	—	—	—	—	—	1	—	—	—	1
Bardeli	8	90 608	1	—	—	—	62	—	—	—	102	—	—	—	9	—	—	—	11	—	—	—	185	—	—	—
Pulsana	23	41 807	—	—	—	—	2	—	—	—	110	—	—	—	171	—	—	—	21	—	—	—	294	—	—	—
Mahuwa	14	65 533	—	—	—	—	55	—	—	—	3	—	—	—	—	—	—	—	6	—	—	—	64	—	—	—
Walod	7	42 828	—	—	—	—	16	—	—	—	11	—	—	—	8	—	—	—	4	—	—	—	39	—	—	—
Vyara	19	119 100	—	—	—	—	1	—	—	—	58	—	—	—	53	—	—	—	32	—	—	—	144	—	—	—
Songadh	[b]	76 870	—	—	—	—	—	—	—	—	—	—	—	—	—	—	—	—	—	—	—	—	—	—	—	—
Uchchal	[b]	31 535	—	—	—	—	—	—	—	—	—	—	—	—	—	—	—	—	—	—	—	—	—	—	—	—
Nizar	[b]	58 801	—	—	—	—	—	—	—	—	—	—	—	—	—	—	—	—	—	—	—	—	—	—	—	—

[a] Figures do not give total number of villages, but only those with some form of sanitation.
[b] Details are not available.

316

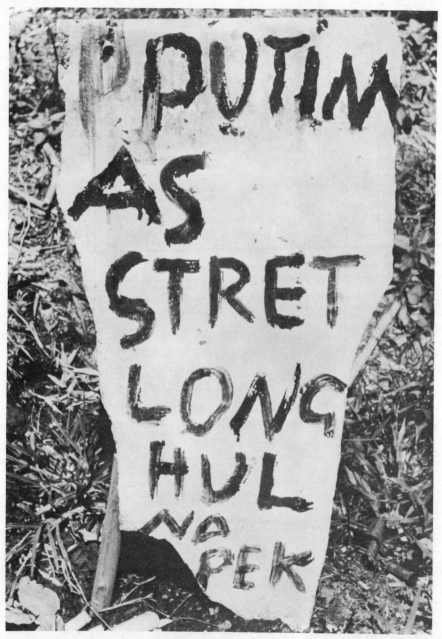

A sign placed outside a pit latrine in a village in Papua New Guinea. If this advice was generally followed the problems of rural sanitation would be largely overcome. The language is New Guinea Pidgin, also called Neo-melanesian, and may be translated as follows: *as* = posterior; *hul* = hole; *long* = at; *na* = and; *pek* = defecate; *putim* = place (verb); *stret* = precisely (photograph: courtesy W. H. Ewers, University of Papua New Guinea)

(1) Supply of wholesome piped water to each house or at least by a few stand-posts at suitable points.

(2) Arrangements for the collection and disposal of dry refuse and the provision of suitable surface drains.

(3) Construction of latrines and systems for collection of nightsoil, its treatment and disposal.

(4) Education of the villagers to make them conscious of the advantages of a healthy sanitary environment.

16.4 EXCRETA COLLECTION, TREATMENT AND DISPOSAL

The method of excreta collection, treatment and disposal of for a village community of, say, less than 5000 persons would obviously depend on the method of water supply, the quantity supplied and its location and above all its financial resources. The methods followed in places where piped water supply is provided would be obviously unsuitable where such facilities are not available.

Communities without piped water supplies

The problem in small villages can be tackled by any one of the following methods dependent upon local circumstances—type of soil, position of the water table and locally available resources.

Construction of sanitary latrines

Construction of standard sanitary latrines, preferably of the PRAI type (Figure 16.1), has been found to be quite suitable for small village communities. Among its other advantages, the following may be mentioned: it is easy to convert the basket-type latrine to PRAI-type, thus eliminating nuisances of daily collection of nightsoil; it gives reasonably satisfactory service with an absorption pit about 3 m deep and 1 m diameter, and with limited use of water in a porous soil; and its construction cost is below Rs 200. Basket-type latrines are likely to contaminate local water supplies and adequate precaution must be taken where such possibilities exist.

Construction of septic tanks

Latrines with septic tanks may also be suitable where resources are available. Particularly for village communities where community latrines are provided outside the villages, septic tanks of an improved design and with suitable provision for effluent disposal may be constructed for groups of latrines.

Conservancy systems

In spite of the known disadvantages of the conservancy system where latrines

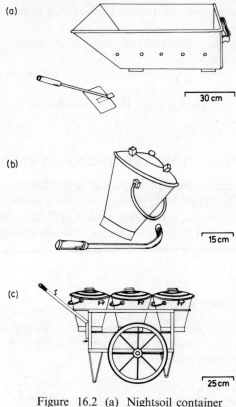

Figure 16.2 (a) Nightsoil container (made from 24 gauge galvanized iron sheet) and scraper. (b) Nightsoil bucket and scraper (c) Wheelbarrow for three or six buckets. (Designs by Department of Social Welfare, Ahmedabad)

of the above type are not suitable owing to a high water table, unsuitable soil conditions, proximity to housing or the possibility of contaminating water sources, it will be desirable to improve the conservancy system to make it at least comparatively more hygienic. In this connection the following steps should be taken: the excreta container must be of an improved standard design and should be supplied by the local authority; employees should be provided with standard scrapers, boots and handgloves; and wheelbarrows or preferably rickshaws should be used for carrying the waste. Figure 16.2 gives details of these implements. Disposal of the waste can be conveniently done by composting (Chapter 17); alternatively ponds may be used (Chapter 14).

Communities with piped water supplies

Although it is desired that more and more villages should come under this category, for the present only very few villages which are located near urban areas, pilgrim places, health resorts, educational centres, market centres, mining centres, etc. will fall into this category.

In such villages, sewage should ideally be collected by a regular network of sewers and treated and disposed of by any of the methods described in Chapters 14 and 18 (see also Chapter 13).

16.5 CONCLUSIONS

It is clear from the above discussion that when there are many urban communities without a hygienic water-carriage system and when 90% of village communities do not have a safe water supply, the provision of a scientific water-carriage system for the collection of sewage and its treatment will have to wait for some considerable time. It would, however, be criminal to neglect village sanitation any further. In the circumstances the minimum that should be done is to provide at least an adequate number of sanitary latrines in each village and make necessary provisions for their maintenance. Much can be achieved by making the villager sanitation-minded. The village can be kept clean if community effort is directed toward that end by proper education.

16.6 REFERENCE

Bhatt, D. B. (1968). Review of public health engineering achievements in Gujarat State. *Paper presented at the 48th Annual Convention of the Institution of Engineers of India, Ahmedabad.*

Note: A 'taluka' is an administrative unit within a district and a 'panchayat' is the principal representative local body at district level.

Solid Waste in Hot Climates

JOHN PICKFORD

17.1 INTRODUCTION

In 1973 I spent two days with Shri S. Mitra, the City Engineer of Calcutta. He told me that of all the troubles with which he had to deal in that infamous concentration of squalor and disease, the problem which seemed most intractable was solid waste. What he showed me convinced me of the validity of his claim. Around the streets there were piles of rotting vegetable waste left because of 'labour-trouble'. Half his fleet of vehicles were in workshops undergoing repairs or waiting for spares. Many of those still in working order were so dilapidated that they frequently broke down and were so unsuitable for their purpose that they left a trail of rubbish along the streets. The tips, some ten metres or more high, seethed with pickers. Hundreds of men, women and children spent their days scavenging amongst the rotting wastes of the city. Their work was shared by goats, dogs and over-size rats. Their number was only exceeded by the number of flies, who swarmed in their thousands around everyone and everything.

Since then there have doubtless been improvements; there have been many studies and reports and proposals, and there was certainly a determination to deal with refuse in a better way. And of course Calcutta is not typical of all hot cities; for two hundred years it has been renowned for its beggars, its crowding, its odour and its disease. However, it is an excellent caricature of all hot cities; just as a cartoonist draws a politician with exaggerated nose and teeth so Calcutta portrays the difficulties of solid waste everywhere.

17.2 SOLID WASTE DATA

Of all material with which an engineer has to deal perhaps least is known about solid waste. By its very nature it is removed from its source as quickly as possible without bothering too much about what it measures, weighs or looks like. Even in Britain, where on the whole waste is dealt with in an efficient and unobtrusive way, half a dozen 'average national analyses' of refuse show half a dozen proportions of, say, paper, and future trends are even more uncertain.

In Britain and some other industrial countries by far the greater part of domestic waste is collected, treated and disposed of by local authorities, and a reasonable proportion is now weighed. In hot countries the dangers of insanitary disposal of waste are greater, but a variable proportion reaches municipal hands, where its quantity can only be guessed. For example in India the towns of Mysore and Sarat both have a population of about 300 000, but Mysore reports more than four times as much town refuse as Sarat; Ahmedabad and Jamnapur both have a population of about 100 000, but Ahmedabad claims a hundred times the weight of refuse that comes from Jamnapur.

Solid wastes are 'useless, unwanted or discarded materials that arise from man's activities and are not free-flowing' (WHO Expert Committee, 1971). The extraction and processing of industrial raw materials produces far greater quantities of solid waste than come from people's homes. For example in Britain the china clay industry alone dumps nearly three-quarters as much solid waste as all the houses in the land. When gold, diamonds and other precious materials are extracted, as in Sierra Leone, Ghana and South Africa, only a tiny proportion is useful and the remainder is waste. However, with the exception of some special wastes which we will consider later, this type of industrial waste has little effect on health and is sometimes at places far removed from centres of population.

On the other hand, the wastes associated with manufacturing industry are often dealt with in similar ways to domestic waste. The workers in factories form the population of towns and produce waste at home. Domestic and factory waste may be tipped together, or they may compete for limited disposal space.

Domestic wastes

Everyone has waste from food preparation and sweeping, although the quantity and type of waste varies. In rural areas and in many towns in hot countries there are always hungry goats to help with disposal, and their efforts are aided by dogs and birds. In wet climates there is often a great mass of leaves used for wrapping food. Except in the most prosperous places where gas or electricity are used, food is cooked by fuel—usually wood or charcoal—and ashes have to be disposed of.

Other types of domestic waste increase with prosperity. There is little waste in the shantytowns, the bustees, the squatter settlements, the 'spontaneous settlements' that are so prominent a feature of third world cities (see, for example, Dwyer (1975)). Waste paper is hardly seen here, but in the United States it amounts to more than half the domestic refuse. Such tins and bottles as are used by the poor are kept and re-used; in industrial countries metal and glass each amount to nearly a tenth of the refuse.

Waste from offices and shops is strictly 'commercial', but it is usually collected with domestic refuse. The waste from the market in an agricultural area in hot countries is largely vegetable, including the leaves often used for wrapping purchases. Where there is more money there is more paper and cardboard— from packing, from offices, from computers.

Table 17.1 Composition of town refuse

Place	World range	Bangkok, Thailand	Bangkok, Thailand	Calcutta, India	Calcutta, India	Deshapara, India	Delhi, India	Dubai	Enugu, Nigeria	Ibadan, Nigeria	Ibadan, Nigeria	Madras, India	Nagpur, India	Nagpur, India	Poona, India	UK	USA
Date	1971	1957	1970	1970	1964	1970	1974	1973	1973	1972	1972	1970?	1970?	1970?	1970?	1968	1972
Note (see below)	1	2	3	4	5	6	7	8	9	10	11	12	13	14	15	16	17
Fruit and vegetable	5-90	47·5	2·6-5·1	16·0	14	20	20·3	40				57	3·8	4-6	68	1706	
Leaves, grass, straw wood, coconut shells									83	80·7	9·6		12·9	4-6			9
Food wastes	0·25-55	0·7	6-75	18·0		21			9·1	9·1	70·3						14
Paper and cardboard		4	7-13	3·2	2	1	5·9	25·5		3·4	10·0	4·8	2·0	3-6	8·7	36·9	55
Rags		5·4	0·3-0·6	3·6	4		3·6	8·0	4·1	4·1	1·6	3·8	0·6	3-7	1·6	2·4	3
Glass, crockery, bones		1·9	1·6-6·9	7·4	4	1	0·6	5·0		0·5	2·5	0·5	0·2	0·3-0·8	0·6	9·1	9
Metal, tins		2·3	0·8-1·3	0·7			0·6	12·5	2·3	2·3	5·9					8·9	9
Plastics	0·1-7			0·6			0·5	4·5				0·6			0·7	1·1	1
Dust, ash, cinder		24·1		41·6	69	57	6·0						0·3	0-2		21·9	
Miscellaneous		14·1			7			4·5	1·0							2·1	
Moisture content				41			14·7			43-65			42	10-32			
Weight per person kg/d	0·2-3			0·51	0·39	0·32	0·31			0·4-0·6		0·56			0·3	0·80	2·6
Density kg/l	0·1-0·5		0·163-0·335	0·52-0·57	0·46	0·38	0·47			0·28		0·435			0·298	0·157	
Volume per person l/d				1·08	0·8	0·85	0·66			1·4		1·29			1·0	5·1	
Calorific value kJ/kg				6300		1400	6600					6700	5300	4600	7100	8000–10 500	

(The composition rows above are given as % by weight (generally wet weight).)

1. WHO Expert Committee (1971).
2. Surveyor (1958).
3. Information from Professor M. B. Pescod.
4. Central Public Health Engineering Research Institute (1970).
5. Ghosh et al. (1964).
6. Rao et al. (1970).
7. Bijlani et al. (1974).
8. Information from J. D. and D. M. Watson.
9. Information from Enugu Municipal Council.
10. Ibadan Old Town. Oluyemi (1972) and Oluwande (1974).
11. Ibadan reservation. Oluyemi (1972).
12. Information from CHERI.
13. Bhide and Muley.
14. Bide, Mottghave, Patel and Gautam.
15. Information from CPHERI.
16. Department of the Environment (1971).
17. Davoll (1972).

Most of the waste from hotels, restaurants, barracks, boarding schools and hospitals is domestic in nature. Factories also provide domestic-type refuse from canteens and offices.

All this material together constitutes town refuse. Its variability in nature and quantity can be seen from Table 17.1. Unfortunately, for reasons already outlined, these data are unreliable and only cover a few places. Little information is collected; less is published.

Disposal of wastes

We will consider various aspects of the collection, treatment and disposal of solid wastes in later sections, but it is useful to notice now that all waste ends in one of two ways: it may be put to some useful purpose or it may be dumped. Re-use may occur at the place where the waste comes from, as when goats eat banana skins or an empty tin can is used as a drinking cup. Even when treatment is intensive, as in a modern refuse incinerator, there is a residue which has to be put somewhere. Fortunately, as we will see, dumping when controlled can achieve a useful purpose by reclaiming low-lying or derelict land.

Industrial solid waste

The waste from factories varies as much as their raw material and products. There are often packaging, offcuts and spoiled material and unwanted by-products. Oil refineries produce a great deal of solid bituminous waste; in many factories there are residues from fuel used for power or the incineration of chemicals.

In industrial countries such as Britain the quantity of industrial waste exceeds domestic waste (Butcher, 1973). 90% of British industrial waste is similar in composition to domestic waste but frequently individual components are large and difficult to consolidate in a controlled tip. In detail the composition of industrial waste in Britain is as follows (Ministry of Housing and Local Government, 1970):

General factory rubbish uncontaminated by factory process wastes	10%
Relatively inert process wastes	83%
Flammable process wastes	1%
Acid or caustic wastes	4%
Indisputably toxic wastes	2%

So only a small proportion, 7%, needs special consideration. In hot countries the scope of industry is usually much more limited, but the proportion of troublesome waste is probably even lower than in Britain, except when one particular industry dominates. This occurs in Kano with its vast hide tanneries and in many cities with oil refineries.

Flammable wastes, if mixed with other refuse, can set fire to the whole, and some process wastes can become explosive if mixed with other material. Some wastes have an effect on the skin and must obviously be confined to places where scavengers cannot reach them. The poisonous or toxic wastes need very special consideration; if they reach underground water it can become unsafe for generations.

Agricultural solid waste

Normally crop residues and animal manure are returned to the land, but in recent times concentrations of activity have resulted in a concentration of waste that cannot be absorbed by the land. A fruit or vegetable cannery, for example, has a large discharge of unwanted material. This creates difficulties if the factory is in an urban area. Similarly, intensive threshing of grain in towns may generate waste straw for which there is insufficient local use. In some cities poultry and pigs are kept in factory-like conditions where there is no local site to spread manure.

In hot countries slaughtering of animals and dressing of carcases is usually done near the market for the meat—in the towns and cities. Unless there is a local processing plant, the unusable parts must be removed and covered quickly if nuisance is to be avoided. Quite a large quantity is involved. For example, in Dubai it is estimated that the unusable waste from a sheep is 4·7 kg, from cattle 32 kg and from each camel 90 kg.

Other urban wastes

Construction wastes can be dealt with on-site in most rural areas but as buildings increase in size and complexity the waste gets more. A multi-storey building often has two or three stories underground producing a vast quantity of excavated material. Fortunately this is useful for covering a controlled tip and in any case the majority of building waste is inert. An exception is gypsum plaster which can give off a foul smell when dumped in water.

Hospitals, clinics and dressing stations have wastes which are obviously dangerous unless treated carefully. Special incinerators have been developed (British Standards Institution, 1959, 1970), or contaminated material may be placed in the core of controlled tips. This contaminated material consists of surgical dressings of all kinds (especially those from suppurating sores), afterbirths, and surplus drugs. Disposable syringes are now commonly used and are a dangerous attraction to children if freely discarded.

Storm drains are used as receptacles for rubbish in all but the tidiest of tropical cities. Because of the high intensity of rainfall they are usually roadside channels rather than underground sewers and have to be constantly cleared of accumulated sand which is often highly contaminated with domestic waste and excreta. In Calcutta over three hundred tons of material is removed from storm drains each day; this is more than 20% of the weight of town refuse collected daily.

Street cleaning, especially in central market areas, is important to make towns attractive. Litter-strewn streets are an affront to civic pride: the use of litter bins should be encouraged by a vigorous public education programme. Whether litter is deposited in bins or dropped by the roadside it still has to be collected regularly. With litter there is bound to be quantities of stones, dust, debris fallen from passing vehicles and usually animal excreta.

Abandoned vehicles are a considerable problem and many municipalities make arrangements for their removal to scrap yards. Scrap tyres are a particular danger in the tropics as they can contain water which is a breeding ground for mosquitoes.

Nightsoil in rural areas is often deliberately mixed with vegetable waste to form compost. Similarly a municipal compost plant may mix nightsoil and refuse, although they are collected separately (see Section 17.7 below). Wherever there is no water-borne sewerage system nightsoil is likely to be dumped with other solid waste.

17.3 THE EFFECTS OF SOLID WASTE MISMANAGEMENT

'Solid wastes management is an important facet of environmental hygiene and needs to be integrated with total environmental planning' (WHO Expert Committee, 1971). Its storage, collection, treatment and disposal can lead to short-term risks; in the long term there may be dangers arising particularly from to the chemical pollution of water supplies.

Wilson (1974) said that the problems connected with refuse storage in buildings were insects, rats, fire and odour. These problems are also associated with the progress of refuse to its final resting place and we will consider them first.

Insects

A common transmission route of bacillary dysentery, amoebic dysentery and diarrhoeal disease is from man's faeces by flies to food or water and thence to man (Rajagopalan, 1974). Flies thrive on food wastes and in the United States 90% of the housefly population in cities breed in open garbage cans (Wilson, 1974). If nightsoil or unprotected latrines are close to refuse the disease route is wide open, but distance is no trouble—flies can travel up to ten kilometres.

Refuse dumped on the ground results in infestation with fly eggs and larvae which have been found up to 50 mm below the surface.

The breeding of mosquitoes in discarded tyres has already been mentioned; they can find as good a place in empty tin cans or jam jars.

Rats

The main source of food for rats and other small rodents is refuse, and in rubbish dumps they quickly proliferate and spread to neighbouring houses. The diseases for which rats may be a reservoir make a horrifying list: 'plague, murine typhus, leptospirosis, histoplasmosis, rat-bite fever, salmonellosis, tularaemia, trichinosis, and many other diseases' (WHO Expert Committee, 1971).

Fire

Hot ashes added to combustible refuse are the greatest danger at source, and fires in uncontrolled tips have been known to burn for months or even years. Usually the fire starts with the objectionable practice of open burning of refuse, but it can spread accidentally from cooking fires used by scavengers. Occasionally fires have begun spontaneously from the heat given off by decomposition or by glass on an open tip acting as a lens for sunlight. Flammable industrial waste increases the danger of fire, and fire can convert inert waste such as old tyres to toxic material.

An additional danger with fire is that if large quantities of water are used to put it out, there can be leaching of toxic material to underground water.

Odour

Passing through the crowded parts of a humid tropical city a traveller is immediately aware of the pervading odour, which is as characteristic as the myriads of children uninhibited by the restraints of industrial society. Some passers-by do not find this odour unattractive; others consider it a revolting stink. It is due to the combination of rotting vegetation and faecal matter—solid wastes indiscriminately discarded.

When this stink persists all day and night it constitutes a major environmental nuisance, which can be avoided by removing all waste before it becomes putrid and by covering dumps as in a controlled tip.

A more difficult and even more unpleasant stink can arise from the release of hydrogen sulphide where refuse is deposited in water and this will be considered again in Section 14.7.

Other effects on health

Apart from diseases for which insects and rats are carriers the handling of refuse can cause illness to workers, especially if nightsoil contaminates the waste. A survey in India (Central Public Health Engineering Institute, 1973) showed that at Bhopal up to half the samples of refuse in the slum and poor quarters and at the disposal site contained roundworm ova. A smaller but still substantial proportion of samples from slum, poor and middle-class areas had whip-worm ova. In another Indian survey worm infections in stool specimens from refuse workers were three times those of the control group (WHO Expert Committee, 1971).

The accident rate amongst refuse workers is also high as a result of lifting heavy loads and dealing with mechanical equipment.

Atmospheric pollution

When refuse is burned in the open, a pall of dense black smoke often covers the site and neighbouring land so that its position can be located from miles around. Old-fashioned incinerators without air-cleaning equipment are little better except that the chimney ensures that the smoke is carried further afield— and can be seen from greater distances.

Apart from the particulate matter that constitutes 'smoke', the gaseous discharge from incomplete combustion may include sulphur dioxide, nitrous oxide and various noxious gases. If PVC is a constituent of the refuse the gases may include hydrogen chloride.

Environmental degradation

Uncollected refuse and insanitary tips in full public view are eyesores. If tourism is important such aesthetic nuisance may reduce the number of visitors, with resultant economic loss. There can be depreciation of the value of property near to a badly-kept tip or incinerator, or even along routes frequented by inadequately-covered refuse vehicles. Spillage from vehicles, bad smell, increase of flies and rats, and windblown dust, paper and plastic are all harmful to the locality.

On the other hand, refuse can be used in a well-planned controlled tip to improve low-lying and derelict areas, and property values may then increase to the vicinity.

Water pollution

When rain passes from an open refuse dump to surface water there is inevitably pollution. Floating solids are unsightly, organic matter exerts an oxygen demand, and pathogens can create a health danger downstream. Unless the water table is high or underlying rock is fissured, groundwater will hardly be affected. However, dumps should not be too close to shallow wells; twelve metres is suggested as a minimum distance in permeable sand or gravel.

On the other hand, avoidance of groundwater pollution is of paramount importance in the siting of refuse tips, and is dealt with in Section 17.6.

Waste of resources

During the last few years there has been increasing awareness in industrial countries that the vast and growing quantities of refuse are an indication of wasteful use of resources. Separation of valuable material in refuse is supported by conservationists. In developing countries everything of value is already separated for recycling.

17.4 ON-SITE STORAGE AND COLLECTION

Individual households

The ideal arrangement is for each household to have its own container with a tight-fitting lid. Refuse should be removed regularly and frequently. In the humid tropics waste food can become putrid very quickly and consequently there should be daily collection, and it is rarely wise in hot countries to have less than two collections a week. The cost of frequent house-to-house collection is high and must inevitably be beyond the means of many municipalities even if it were possible.

Since the early 1950s there has been considerable discussion about the merits of using paper or plastic sacks for household storage of refuse. The advantages of the sack system are improved hygiene and the elimination of double journeys for the collectors (Ministry of Housing and Local Government, 1967). The disadvantages are increased cost, increased volume, unless the refuse is compressed in collection vehicles, and damage to sacks by hot ashes and sharp-edged objects. Sacks also provide attractive fodder for goats. They are rarely used in hot countries except for high-income low-density residential areas.

Refuse dumps

For high-density housing it is usual to provide refuse dumps. Often these are merely convenient pieces of spare ground on the roadside. Refuse is scattered by wind, goats and children. After collection of the main mass of refuse some still remains as a breeding place for flies whose eggs and larvae penetrate the ground. Such dumps cry out for improvement.

A good type of communal refuse container is made in Lagos. It is a covered metal box which can hold about ten cubic metres of refuse. Sliding panels enable the container to be completely closed after refuse has been dumped. The container is removed by a special vehicle which brings an empty, cleaned replacement container. Smaller covered containers are locally made in Nairobi and are emptied into refuse collection vehicles using a purpose-made lifting device on the side.

Trailers made of sheet metal with reinforced edges are suggested by Rajagopalan (1964). The width is about 2 metres, the depth varies from 750 mm to one metre and the length is variable. This trailer has an open top and one end is hinged with a rubber sealing gasket. It can be towed to a tip by a tractor and the contents discharged by shovelling or by lifting the towing eye. In other places large open-topped cylindrical containers are used.

When refuse is wet it is debatable whether drainage holes should be provided. If they are, the ground beneath becomes saturated with foul-smelling and polluting liquor. If they are not the metal is quickly corroded, even if a good protective coating is provided.

Concrete refuse bins have been criticized because they are difficult to clean. However, metal containers also retain a layer of refuse unless they are removed from site and their cleaning is carefully supervised. A concrete, masonry or block 'bin', if provided with a roof and impermeable walls and floor, and if properly cleaned when refuse is removed before it overflows, is a considerable improvement on an open dump. What is probably the best type has low walls so that children can deposit refuse inside; the roof can be supported by columns at the corners. Attempts to make masonry refuse containers fly-proof have not usually been successful. Unless it is easy to put refuse inside the building it is deposited outside; any cover which requires effort to close is left open; fly-proof netting is easily damaged and more often left torn than repaired.

Multi-storey buildings

A number of dustbins or sacks can be provided either on each floor or at ground level; communal containers of the type provided for high-density housing are suitable. The burden of carrying waste from upper floors can be avoided by using chutes. A building constructed in the Girgaum area of Bombay about 1890 had a 900 mm × 900 mm chute with window-size openings at each floor to receive refuse (Central Public Health Engineering Research Institute, 1971). Modern chutes are often made of 380 mm diameter pipes, with a 100–150 mm ventilating pipe extending from the highest hopper to about two metres about the roof. Inlet hoppers can be purpose-made to prevent tenants pushing large objects down the chute. The chute should discharge into a metal bin in a fly-proofed chambers constructed with impermeable surfaces for easy cleaning. The bin may be mounted on wheels.

Industrial premises

Replaceable containers are convenient for storage and removal of factory waste. A standard charge can be made for removing a full container and providing an empty one.

Medical waste

Unless medical waste can be incinerated on site, contaminated material, including the afterbirth from home confinements, should if possible be kept and collected separately from other refuse. Some authorities issue coloured plastic bags to enable this material to be distinguished at the tip (Department of the Environment, 1974).

Methods of collecting domestic refuse

Where there is collection from individual premises and good road access the bins can be emptied directly into collection vehicles. Refuse dumps are sited near road access whenever possible. Difficulties arise where vehicles cannot get near to collection points; houses may be too close together or pathways too steep, too uneven, or too much crossed by open drains. In Amman some three hundred thousand refugees—about half the total population—occupy land on seven hills which are mostly inaccessible to motor transport and refuse has to be carried up to four kilometres. Here easily-cleaned rubber sheets two metres square are used by refuse collectors. In other cities collection of refuse from squatter settlements and other crowded areas is in baskets or sacks or wheelbarrows.

The inclusion of liquid wastes in refuse add to the difficulties of collection. Some local authorities in Britain have made bye-laws prohibiting any liquid, including waste oil, to be mixed with refuse (Department of the Environment, 1974). Legal sanctions are unlikely to be much use in congested areas, but something can be done by public health education.

Refuse collection vehicles

In industrial countries the tendency in recent years is to use larger vehicles with some form of mechanical compression to increase the density and hence the payload. These may be appropriate for some well-planned city centres in developing countries, but generally smaller and simpler vehicles are better. Despite protests by the City Engineer of a large tropical capital, the Council insisted on purchasing two heavy compression-type vehicles. At the start of the next rainy season both vehicles were immediately bogged down on the tip and could not be used again while the rains lasted. The capital of a nearby country purchased eleven compression vehicles. A couple of years later only two were in service; the remainder were in the depot waiting for spare parts. Nairobi has a number of compression-type vehicles which are kept in service although they are expensive to maintain.

Rajagopalan (1974) points out that the collection method should avoid spillage and trucks should be of adequate capacity with suitable covers and facilities for tipping or unloading with ease. Manoeuvrability for narrow and winding roads is important.

Standardization of vehicles in a fleet makes for easier maintenance. The cost of maintaining old vehicles may well exceed the annual cost of replacement and a programme for regular replacement, after say eight years or 150000 kilometres, may well prove economical. Daily washing of vehicles and regular repainting with bituminous paint reduce corrosion and also improve the 'public image' of the refuse service. There is advnatage in keeping vehicles and collection under single control rather than making use of a separate motor department (Central Public Health Engineering Research Institute, 1970).

Optimum use of the collection crews' time can be achieved by a relay system, which is especially worthwhile if haulage distances are long. For example, collection can be in trailers with a lesser number of tractors.

Although double-handling of refuse should generally be avoided, the system of transfer loading and bulk transport is justified if the journey to a tip is greater than about twenty kilometres (Department of the Environment, 1971). Where collection vehicles are small because of narrow streets, transfer loading may save money for shorter journeys.

At a transfer station refuse is placed in large vehicles or railway trucks which take it to the distant tip. Occasionally water transport is an acceptable alternative to road or rail. If the refuse is compressed, an economically heavy load can be carried. The best construction for a transfer station is a ramp leading to a concrete paltform where the smaller vehicles discharge. Refuse falls, or is pushed, through holes into the transfer vehicles which wait on a roadway or railway track about five metres below. The whole station should be enclosed to prevent the spread of light rubbish by wind (Department of the Environment, 1971). The vehicles or wagons should be covered with tarpaulin sheets extending half a metre down the sides and tied securely. By using transfer loading it is possible to use tips a long way from city centres; it has been reported that one American city proposed to take its refuse 550 km by train (Countryside in 1970, 1970).

Planning storage and collection

About 80% of the total cost of dealing with refuse goes to collection and storage (WHO Expert Committee, 1971). Proper planning and supervision are therefore essential to get as efficient a service as possible from the money available. Good public relation can lead to community participation. For example, in Jeddah there has been a successful 'keep waste off the ground' campaign.

17.5 TREATMENT AND DISPOSAL OF REFUSE

Evaluation of alternatives

The following points should be considered:

(1) The quantity and character of the refuse, and likely changes.
(2) Land available for final deposit.
(3) Constraints on the temporary and ultimate use of possible tipping sites.
(4) The health of the public and refuse workers.
(5) The need to restrict the use of mechanical equipment in developing countries.
(6) The need for compost due to the soil structure and the type of agricultural activity.
(7) Potential use of power or heat obtained by incineration.
(8) The cost of possible methods.

Survey of reclamation sites

Refuse is a valuable material for the reclamation of land. Initially all potential tips within 15 km of the town should be examined and listed. If necessary the survey may be extended to 75 km or even further, bearing in mind the possibility of transfer loading. Sites especially suitable for reclamation are worked-out surface mineral excavations—quarries, gravel pits and the like—and low-lying swamps and marshes. The hydrogeology of sites should be examined to check the likelihood of pollution of water supplies. Other factors to be noted are the proximity of residential areas, the direction of the prevailing wind and access by road, rail or water. Large numbers of birds are always attracted to refuse tips, so areas near airports are to be avoided because of the danger of bird-strike.

One of the best-known examples of land reclamation is the Otterspool scheme at Liverpool in England. Since 1926 fifty hectares of attractively land-scaped public park have been provided on what was formerly marshland. Reclamation schemes have provided additional land for towns and cities all over the world. In Sekondi in Ghana a large area has been reclaimed from low-lying, mosquito-ridden swamps. Several substantial buildings (including an abattoir, brick kilns and the City Engineer's depot) have been erected on the land. There is no evidence of subsidence.

Composted refuse

Composting converts the fermentable organic content of refuse to a soil conditioner. It is a recycling process, returning organic matter to the earth and there are no specific land requirements except for rejects—material which cannot be converted.

The value of compost has often been over-estimated. There is evidence against the use of compost as a fertilizer. Some agricultural experts consider it to have little value as a soil conditioner as it requires about 75 tonnes per hectare. It is bulky and the cost of transport and spreading is high. If the refuse includes factory wastes there is a danger of excess metals such as zinc (Department of the Environment, 1971).

When the Bangkok composting plant was built it was claimed that 'sales will more than cover the cost of the plant and its operation, and profits will be set against the cost of refuse collection' (Surveyor, 1958). In fact, not all the installed capacity has been used; there is little sale of compost because there is plenty of fluvial silt in the area.

The highest selling price for compost is in Israel and even here the cost of production in mechanized plant is four times the sale value.

In the United States, Terman and Mays (1973) found that large quantities of compost—up to 360 tonnes per hectare—can be applied to grassland and cropland, and result in positive yield responses. However, the value of the increased crops was only about 7% of the cost of composting, and it was concluded that the process is of little value apart from getting rid of refuse.

On the other hand, high intensity rainfall and rapid run-off result in the erosion of humus from a great deal of tropical land. This may be replaced by compost, which has good moisture-retaining capacity and is not so easily washed away as chemical fertilizer (Central Public Health Engineering Research Institute, 1971). It helps to improve the soil structure and to control soil erosion (Department of the Environment, 1971).

The manurial value of compost can be increased by adding nightsoil or sewage sludge. Two solid-waste problems are dealt with at once. After applying a refuse/nightsoil compost at 20 tonnes per hectare, Archarya (1939) obtained up to 2·7 times more sorghum than on unmanured soil.

Non-mechanized methods of composting can be used in developing countries where labour is abundant. There is a great saving in capital and operating costs. Refuse in developing countries is more suitable for manual composting and the resulting material is of higher quality than that obtained in a fully-mechanized plant.

Use and cost of alternatives

Table 17.2 shows that tipping is the most popular method of dealing with refuse in industrial countries.
Some comparative net costs are given in Table 17.3

Table 17.2 Methods of treatment and disposal

	% of authorities		% tonnage
Method	United States[a]	Great Britain[b]	UK[c]
Crude tipping	84	7	0·8
Controlled tipping	6	80	⎰25·5[d]
(sanitary landfill)			⎱63·2[e]
Incineration	8	6	9·1
Pulverization ⎱	2	⎰6	1·1
Composting ⎰		⎱1	0·3

[a]Davoll, 1972.
[b]Association of Public Health Inspectors, 1972.
[c]Department of the Environment, 1971.
[d]'Semi-controlled' tipping.
[e]Properly controlled tipping.

Table 17.3 Approximate net costs of treatment and disposal of refuse

Method	Great Britain	India[a]
Crude tipping		1
Cheapest controlled tip	1	
Controlled tip	1–2	3·3
Pulverization	2·5–4	
Manual composting		(no profit, no loss)
Mechanized composting	5–7	2·9
Incineration	5–10	9·2–12.0

[a]The Indian figures assume that compost can be sold to farmers or gardeners.

17.6 LAND RECLAMATION BY CONTROLLED TIPPING

The principle of controlled tipping is that layers of refuse are compacted and covered by a layer of inert material. Americans call it 'sanitary landfill'. To allow for proper compaction the layers should not exceed 2·4 metres in depth. To provide an adequate seal the 'cover' should normally be at least 200 mm thick. If the refuse includes large irregular objects it may be necessary to increase the thickness of the cover. On the other hand, a cover thickness of less than 150 mm may be satisfactory if the refuse has been pulverized (see Section 17.8).

The compaction and the cover control the tip in the following ways:

(1) Limit the odour emission.
(2) Prevent light refuse being blown away by wind.
(3) Prevent the emergence of fly larvae.
(4) Prevent the breeding of flies.
(5) Allow rat control to be easily applied.
(6) Reduce the risk of fire.
(7) Make the tip less attractive to birds.
(8) Provide good conditions for the biological degradation of organic matter in the tip.

Biological degradation of organic matter is carried out by micro-organisms which are already present in refuse. During the first few days the temperature may rise to 65 °C or higher, and then gradually drop. The high temperature destorys pathogens in the refuse. The waste products of the micro-organisms include gases such as carbon dioxide and methane. These are diffused slowly and harmlessly through the surface.

Operation of tips

All exposed surfaces of the tip—top, sides and ends—should be quickly covered by inert material. The usual practice is to cover the top and sides of freshly-tipped refuse as soon as possible, and certainly not later than at the end of the working day. The working face (the advancing end of the tip) should ideally be covered at the end of the working day. However, in most controlled tips the working face is only covered at weekends or holidays, or when the tip is completed.

Small bulldozers such as a D4 are often used on large tips to spread refuse and covering material. One D4 bulldozer can deal with about 500 tonnes of refuse in an 8-hour shift. The working life of a bulldozer is about 10 000 hours, equivalent to four or five years' operation (Central Public Health Engineering Research Institute, 1971). Their weight, moving about on the completed parts of the tip, help compaction. If a bulldozer is not available, a tractor loader-shovel can be used. This can do other work on the site such as carrying cover material. Refuse should be tipped from the collection or transfer vehicles on top of the tip. The bulldozer or tractor then pushes the refuse over the edge.

Sides of the tipped refuse should be sloped at one vertical to three horizontal so that the bulldozer can operate on the slopes.

Large articles, such as furniture or kitchen equipment are usually broken up by scavengers in developing countries. If big pieces remain they should be crushed and dumped in the core of the tip—not less than one metre from the top or two metres from the side. Fish, animal waste, abattoir waste, dead animals, waste from hospitals and other noxious material should be tipped in front of the tip face and immediately covered with other refuse.

Generally a large tip can be better controlled than a small one. By using a central tip for a number of neighbouring communities it may be possible to purchase a bulldozer or tractor while this would not be economical for small individual tips. Where a single large site is not available a wheeled tractor is sometimes used on a number of local sites, travelling by road from one to another. Controlled tipping is possible without any mechanical plant at all. Movement of vehicles compacts the refuse to some extent but it is more difficult to keep the tip tidy. Levelling by hand obviously creates health dangers for the workers.

Compared with industrial countries, refuse in developing countries is usually dense and there is less danger of light material being blown away. Where there is substantial content of loose paper and light plastic in refuse it is important to erect fences around the tipping area to catch this material during windy weather. Bamboo and grass matting are suitable materials for the fence. Watering of roads and the surface of the tip during dry weather reduces the dust nuisance.

The use of the tip should be planned to reduce the exposed sides and ends as much as possible. One method is to divide the area into strips each say 20 metres wide. Tipping is first carried out on alternate strips, providing cover on both sides. When the intermediate strips are used no cover is required at the sides.

Surface water

No surface water should pass through a tip. Dig a ditch along the upper side of a tip area about ten metres from the edge of the proposed tip, and so divert any water flowing across the surface following rainfall. If it is impossible to divert existing streams around the tip, construct a culvert with manholes reaching above the ultimate level of the tip surface. Sulphate leachate from refuse corrodes concrete pipes, so surround the culvert with clay or other impermeable material. Make the culvert strong enough to carry the weight of superimposed refuse.

Leachate from tips

The importance of avoiding pollution of groundwater has already been mentioned. Fortunately, in normal permeable soil, bacteria do not penetrate more than twelve metres (WHO Expert Committee, 1971). Fissured rock may give a comparatively free passage for leachate to reach groundwater. A hydrogeological survey is therefore essential if there is the slightest danger of pollution of water used for public supply. This is especially important if toxic industrial waste is deposited on a tip. Some chemicals are resistant to natural purification processes and may contaminate a water source for many years once they have entered the aquifer. Such pollution is comparatively rare, even in an industrial country like Britain where there is a large amount of factory waste. A recent survey in England and Wales showed that only 51 out of 2494 landfill sites presented serious pollution risks to aquifers (Gray *et al.*, 1974).

Tipped material can be divided into three groups according to their effect on groundwater:

(1) Inert solid wastes with no risk to groundwater. These include wastes from construction and demolition of buildings, and inert process wastes from industry.
(2) Wastes with potential to cause pollution by increased concentration of organics and inorganics to levels where water becomes unfit for drinking. These include domestic refuse, cesspit contents, nightsoil, sewage sludge and most industrial wastes.
(3) Toxic material including oil.

The leachates from group (2) may have a high biochemical oxygen demand (BOD) and high concentrations of ammoniacal nitrogen, chlorides and sulphates. Water supplies will usually be safe if the leachate from a dry tip passes through about 15 metres of granular material and is then diluted by mixing with other groundwater. A distance of 800 metres between a tip and abstraction is usually enough for this dilution.

Leachate is caused by rainwater passing through the tipped material. The first rain is absorbed in the tip and experiments in England showed that there was no percolate until about 200 mm of rain had fallen—a delay of three or four months (Ministry of Housing and Local Government, 1961). During this time the refuse is partly stabilized so that the leachate is less offensive than it would be if the refuse were all fresh. With tropical rain the delay is much less during wet seasons. After the initial delay less than half the rain passed out of the tip; the remainder was absorbed or evaporated. The first percolate contained 10^8 coliforms per 100 ml, the BOD_5 was 6000 mg/l, ammoniacal nitrogen concentration was 700 mg/l, sulphides 29 mg/l and chlorides 1700 mg/l. After one year coliforms were only $10^3/100$ ml. After two years there were no coliforms; ammoniacal nitrogen and sulphide concentrations were both 2 mg/l, but the chloride concentration was still quite high—573 mg/l. Throughout the two years there was an irregular variation of sulphate: the lowest concentration was 2 mg/l and the highest 1800 mg/l. Several authors have noted the increase of hardness, sulphate and chloride in aquifers receiving leachate from tips.

In laboratory tests at Nagpur, India, leachate from refuse showed rapid improvement. In two weeks chlorides dropped from an initial concentration of 1500 mg/l to 200 mg/l and hardness from an initial 2700 mg/l to less than 500 mg/l. After a month the chlorides and hardness were both around an acceptable 100 mg/l. Organic removal was slower, the BOD_5 falling from an initial 5900 mg/l to 1000 mg/l in $2\frac{1}{2}$ weeks and to less than 10 mg/l after three months.

Stander (1960) reported on the seepage from a refuse dump on the Witwatersrand in South Africa during a three-month period of heavy rainfall. The concentration of total alkalinity as $CaCO_3$ was 1010 mg/l, total dissolved solids was 3470 mg/l, ammoniacal nitrogen as N was 21·9 and sulphates as SO_4 was 880 mg/l.

A tip may be built up of successive layers one on top of another. An interval of three months between the placing of layers allows the lower layers to consolidate and their organic content to stabilize with the gases dispersing through the surface. The leachate from the newly tipped top layer has to pass through previously deposited material before reaching the original ground. The lower layers then act as a kind of reservoir/filter so that the leachate through the whole tip is reduced in quantity and in concentration of polluting substances other than chlorides and sulphates.

There are three ways of preventing undesirable leachate from reaching the groundwater.

(1) Where the underlying strata are fissured a layer of sand or gravel may be put at the bottom of the tip. This acts as a filter. Biological degradation of organic matter and natural reduction of bacteria occur.

(2) An impermeable barrier may be put at the bottom of the tip. Clay or plastic sheeting covered by a protective layer of sand are suitable. The leachate should be collected and discharged to sewer or special treatment facilities. Alternatively it can be pumped and sprayed on the surface of the tip to control dust.

(3) The cover may be imprevious to prevent rain reaching the tipped waste. Clay can be used. The surface must be given a slight fall and vegetation should be encouraged to reduce run-off and desiccation. Drying cracks and settlement of tip material often destroy the impermeability of the cover. If the seal is maintained gases given off during stabilization of refuse will be trapped. The cover may be lifted as a dome and then fractured.

Cover

Any inert material may be used.

(1) On natural low-lying or desert sites a shallow trench can be dug for the first section of the tip and material stockpiled. Cover is then obtained by excavating ahead of tipping until the whole site has been filled. The stockpile from the first trench is used to cover the last section of tip.

(2) Near large towns and cities builders are often very willing to dispose of solid construction waste on refuse tips.

(3) Inert industrial wastes may be available. If coal is used at local electricity power stations large quantities of ash may be available. At Sekondi and Kumasi in Ghana, sawdust from local mills provides an excellent cover. A smooth even surface has been obtained.

(4) Stabilized material from old tips makes a satisfactory cover.

Nairobi has no difficulty in finding sites or cover. Generally, abandoned quarries are taken over. More than enough cover is delivered by contractors who are given a free tip for excavated material obtained during construction work. This is mainly black cotton soil and is stockpiled near the quarry. At large tips refuse is received throughout the 24 hours. Cover is moved from the stockpiles by day-shift workers using a tractor-shovel.

Tipping in water

Dry pits are preferable but may not be available. Anyway the purpose of a land reclamation scheme may be to raise the level above marshy swamps. Pollution is bound to occur if refuse is tipped into water. Decomposition below the water level is anaerobic. Sulphate-reducing bacteria may release foul-smelling hydrogen sulphide. If the water is shallow, as on marshland, the gas is absorbed by the upper part of the waste material. Care should be taken to keep the working face of the tip as near vertical as possible. If tipping is into deep water, as in a water-filled gravel pit, control of odour is more difficult. Chromate waste from local industries has been successfully used. Aeration is not effective when the temperature is above 12 °C. Chlorination requires large quantities of bleaching powder—about four tonnes per hectare for water three metres deep.

Siting of tips

We have already seen that a survey can enable solid waste to be useful by reclaiming old quarries or low-lying land. Where operation of tips is properly controlled nuisance can be greatly reduced. A study of the hydrogeology can fix suitable sites in relation to possible pollution of drinking water supplies.

There remains the question of public opinion regarding the distance of the tip from houses. Rajagopalan (1974) rules that disposal sites should be at least a kilometre downwind of municipal limits. In Britain a distance of 200 metres is acceptable in certain circumstances (Department of the Environment, 1971). With careful management a site can be quite close to built-up areas.

Wind-blown refuse should be controlled by fences or by raising an embankment around the site. In windy weather refuse should be tipped at the end of the tip away from houses or in bays formed in windless weather.

The entrance should be attractive. Vehicles, and especially their wheels, should be cleaned before leaving the tip.

Plant trees or shrubs, or raise embankments, as a visual screen.

Start tipping near to roads and work away so that the tip face cannot be seen by the public.

Keep the completed tip tidy, putting it into temporary use as soon as possible. Plant grass, shrubs or flowers.

Inspect frequently for infestation by insects and vermin and take corrective action.

17.7 COMPOSTING

In rural areas vegetable waste has been composted since ancient times. Micro-organisms, already present in the waste, stabilize organic matter to produce a land conditioner. We looked at the value of composted refuse in section 17.5 above.

The heat generated by the activity of the micro-organisms causes the temperature to rise, and many organisms thrive in the thermophilic range 45 °C to 65 °C. When the temperature is above 50 °C pathogens are quickly destroyed. For example *Salmonella typhi* does not grow above 46 °C. At 55 °C it dies in 30 minutes, at 60 °C in 20 minutes (Gotaas, 1956).

In India two methods of composting nightsoil/refuse mixtures have been developed. In the *Bangalore method* alternate 150 m deep layers of vegetable waste and thinner layers of nightsoil are spread in a trench about a metre deep. At first aerobic organisms use the air trapped around the waste but the mass soon becomes anaerobic. Decomposition is then slower and it takes six months or more to produce a good compost. In the *Indore process* layers of nightsoil and vegetable waste are alternated in the same way either in a trench or to form a mound above ground called a windrow. This is kept aerobic by turning regularly for two or three months. Then the compost is left for another month or so without turning, the whole process thus taking about four months.

Mechanized plants

Mechanical composting plants have been developed but it is now appreciated that stabilization in windrows is still essential. The best 'mechanical' process is to pulverize the refuse in a rotary drum (see Section 17.8) and then place the pulverized 'fines' in windrows which are turned once a month; after 3 months, the now stabilized compost is screened to separate glass and other inert material. This process gives a high-quality product, but it may not be economic in developing countries owing to the relatively high capital cost of the rotary drum pulverizer.

Factors affecting composting

Moisture content should be 40% to 60%. If the material is too dry or too wet the process is slowed down. When there is more than 60% water the anaerobic bacteria are stimulated and unpleasant smells are given off.

Temperature should not rise above 70 °C. If it does, degradation is slowed down. A lower temperature is required for a high paper content (Jeris and Regan, 1973). Temperature may be reduced by turning the material over. *Carbon/nitrogen ratio* is reduced during composting. Decomposition of vegetable matter with high C/N (e.g. potato) is quicker than vegetable with low C/N (e.g. cabbage) under both aerobic and anaerobic conditions (Saxena and Patwardhan, 1965). An initial C/N ratio of 30 is best for the micro-organisms and gives a ratio of about 20 in the product. In experiments on Calcutta refuse with an initial C/N ratio of 35·4 the material was stabilized to a C/N of about 23 after three weeks. The moisture content was maintained at 60% and the material was turned every three days (Central Public Health Engineering Research Institute, 1970). Ghate *et al.* (1966) reported experiments at Roorkee, India. Mixtures of refuse with nightsoil and animal manure took about three weeks to stabilize.

Wind lowers the temperature and reduces the moisture on the windward side of composting heaps. It may be necessary to add water to maintain a satisfactory moisture content.

Flies can be controlled by turning the outside of windrows to the middle. If flies are creating a nuisance it may be necessary to turn the refuse daily.

Composting in windrows

Fully mechanized plants involve shredding, grinding and mechanical separation of high-density solids. The refuse from industrialized cities may require this treatment because of the high content of paper, glass and tins and because labour is not available.

For cities in developing countries the windrows system with crude refuse is usually much more appropriate. Refuse is discharged to form windrows, long piles of refuse about two metres high. Every few days the windrows is turned by hand or tractor-shovel. Working from the end of the windrow where tipping started the material is moved to form another windrow a few metres away. After about three weeks the compost is stabilized. It is turned at least three times—perhaps as many as ten times. Moisture content can be reduced by turning; if it drops too low, add water or sewage sludge.

Windrows can be formed on open land and the whole operation carried out by hand. However, for large cities some mechanization may be desirable. The windrows can be formed on a concrete floor, controlling the pollution of groundwater and reducing health dangers. A semi-mechanized plant has been proposed for Delhi (Bijlani *et al.* 1975). A tractor-shovel will be used for turning the windrows. When composting is complete the compost will pass to a plate conveyor from which contraries such as tin cans may be picked by hand. Dense particles can be removed in a ballistic separator, or by passing the refuse along an inclined belt conveyor.

17.8 OTHER TREATMENT PROCESSES

Separation

We have already noted that in developing countries much less re-usable material is discarded. At all stages, from the individual premises to the final tip, refuse is examined by scavengers. This is an unhealthy practice, but is only ended by prosperity, as in cities like Singapore.

In prosperous places scrap is very valuable. For example, in Britain scrap was worth £1250 million in 1972. In that year 60% of lead, 36% of copper and 32% of paper used in Britain came from scrap.

Valuable material, such as clean wastepaper, can be collected separately. Iron and steel can be removed magnetically.

Where labour is freely available, pickers can be employed for a great variety of materials—metal, paper, bones, bottles, broken glass, rags and so on. The sale of this salvage can be more than the wages of the pickers. Unfortunately the market for waste material varies greatly and next year there may be no sale for material which is valuable this year.

Pulverization

This is a quick and relatively simple treatment to give a dense homogeneous and less offensive material (WHO Expert Committee, 1971). Hammer-mills or rotary drums are commonly used. In hammer-mills, free-swinging hammers are placed between discs on a rotor and the pulverized material passes through a grid. Power consumption is 6–10 kWh/tonne of refuse. The most expensive part of the process is replacement of worn hammers. In rotary drums water or sewage sludge is added to reduce the strength of fibrous material; attrition and abrasion in the drum breaks it up.

Refuse can be pulverized before composting, incineration or controlled tipping. In a tip pulverized refuse has many advantages:

(1) Reduced voids, so volume is reduced and less tipping space is required.
(2) More easily controlled in tip.
(3) Less fire risk.
(4) Less attractive to insects and rodents.
(5) Less cover required.
(6) Biological breakdown is quicker, so the land can be re-used sooner.

Compaction

By applying high pressure the density of refuse is increased. Transport costs less and it may be economical to use tips over 100 km from a city. High density bales (compressed refuse contained by chicken-wire or coated with bitumen) have been used to reclaim excavations or to form sea walls. The capital cost is less than incineration plant and large items such as bedsprings or washing machines can be included in the bales.

Incineration

A refuse incinerator was erected in Calcutta in 1863, but caused smoke nuisance. A few years ago 75% of municipal incinerators were unsatisfactory (Davoll, 1972). Incineration leads to air pollution unless the plant is designed, equipped and operated to meet air pollution requirements (WHO Expert Committee, 1971). The temperature must be high to destroy odours; 950–1100°C is normal in modern plant. Dust-arresting equipment must be installed and a high chimney is required to disperse the gases. To satisfy the environmental requirements of clean air the plant must be large, expensive and well-maintained. Incineration should not be considered unless money and technical expertise are readily available.

The advocates of incineration imply that the process is making use of a valuable heat source in refuse. This heat can be used for heating of buildings or for generation of electricity. Either use is only economical under unusual conditions such as the Nottingham district heating scheme in England where a redundant power station was available to provide supplementary heat in winter. The Amsterdam refuse incinerator handles 400 000 tonnes of refuse a year and annually generates 160 000 MWh. The cost of the plant was over £14 million in 1969 and the annual cost is more than four times the income derived from selling electricity and recovered metal. Even working at this scale incineration is an expensive business.

The second plea of the purveyors of incineration plant is that the method eliminates the need for tipping sites, which are difficult to find near some large cities. In fact tips are required. The residue after burning has a volume of about one-tenth of the original refuse. This does not mean that ten times as much tip volume is required when there is no incineration. In a controlled tip refuse is greatly reduced in volume by compaction and degradation of organic matter. The final volume required is only about three times that of incinerator residue; if refuse is pulverized the final volume is only twice that of incinerator residue. If refuse is composted the tip volume required for residues is less than with incineration.

It must also be remembered that the calorific value of refuse in hot countries is usually much lower than that in industrial countries and that the moisture content is usually high after tropical rainfall.

17.9 CONCLUSIONS

Most attention should be given to increasing the efficiency of collection and transport since their cost is about 80% of the total expenditure of dealing with refuse. In hot countries controlled tipping and composting in windrows are the most appropriate methods of disposal, even for the largest cities.

Carefully planned controlled tipping leads to reclamation for valuable purposes of hitherto useless land. Composted refuse is a soil conditioner which is especially useful when the soil structure has deteriorated because of high intensity tropical rainfall.

17.10 REFERENCES

Archarya, C. N. (1939). Comparison of different methods of composting waste materials. *Indian Journal of Agricultural Science*, **9**, 565–572.

Assar, M. (1971). *Guide to Sanitation in Natural Disasters*. Geneva: WHO.

Association of Public Health Inspectors (1972). *Environmental health report 1971*. London: APHI.

Bijlani, H. U., Pande, R. P. and Jain, R. C. (1974). *A Mechanised compost Plant for Delhi*. Mimeograph report. Delhi: City Engineer.

Bijlani, H. U., Pande, R. P., and Jain, R. C. (1975). *A Semi-mechanised Compost Plant for Delhi*. Mimeograph report. Delhi: City Engineer.

British Standards Institution (1959). *Small Incinerators for the Destruction of Hospital Dressings*. London: BSI.

British Standards Institution (1970). BS 3316: *Large Incinerators for the Destruction of Hospital wastes*. London: BSI.

Butcher, H. C. (1973). The problems of industry. In: *Proceedings of Symposium on Disposal of Municipal and Industrial Sludges and Solid Toxic Wastes*. Maidstone: Institute of Water Pollution Control.

Central Public Health Engineering Research Institute (1970). *Feasibility studies for alternate methods of garbage disposal for Calcutta City*. Nagpur: CPHERI.

Central Public Health Engineering Research Institute (1971). *Refuse disposal from multi-storeyed buildings*. (Technical Digest No. 24). Nagpur: CPHERI.

Central Public Health Engineering Research Institute (1973). *Intestinal parasites in refuse*. (Technical Digest No. 37). Nagpur: CPHERI.

Countryside in 1970: Ad Hoc Group (1970). *Refuse disposal*. London: Ad Hoc Group.

Davoll, J. (1972). *Global and ecological aspects of waste disposal*. Paper presented at Conference on Environment 72, London.

Department of the Environment (1971). *Refuse disposal: report of the working party on refuse disposal*. London: HMSO.

Department of the Environment (1974). *Disposal of Awkward Household Waste*. London: HMSO.

Dwyer, D. J. (1975). *People and Housing in Third World Cities*. London: Longman.

Ghate, S. S., Bhide, A. D. and Patwardhan, S. V. (1966). Criteria for assessing the progress of composting. In: *Proceedings of the Symposium on Community Water Supply and Waste Disposal, Nagpur, 1966*, vol II, 68–81. Nagpur: CPHERI.

Ghosh, G., Adhya, A. K. and Radhakrishnan, I. (1964). Research studies on domestic refuse. *Journal of the Institute of Engineer (India)*. **44**, 10, PtPH3, 59–63.

Gotaas, H. B. (1956). *Composting*. (Monograph series no. 31). Geneva: WHO.

Gray, D. A., Mather, J. D. and Harrison, I. B. (1974). Review of groundwater pollution from waste disposal sites in England and Wales, with provisional guidelines for future site selection. *Quarterly Journal Engineering Geology*, **7**, 181–196.

Higginson, A. E. (1973). Future developments in the disposal of domestic refuse and other wastes. In: *Proceedings of the Symposium on Research and Developments in Solid Waste Disposal, Reading, 1973*. London: Institution of Public Health Engineers.

Jeris, J. S. and Regan, R. W. (1973). Controlling environmental parameters for optimum composting. *Compost Science*, **14**, 1, 10–15.

Ministry of Housing and Local Government (1961). *Pollution of Water by Tipped Refuse*. London: HMSO.

Ministry of Housing and Local Government (1967). *Refuse Storage and Collection*. Report of Working Party. London: HMSO.

Ministry of Housing and Local Government (1970). *Disposal of Solid Toxic Wastes*. London: HMSO.

Oluwande, P. A. (1974). Investigations into certain aspects of refuse in Western States of Nigeria. *Solid Waste Management*, 22–34.

Oluyemi, I. O. (1972). *Refuse and Sewage Disposal*. Paper presented to Conference of Nigerian Society of Engineers at Benin City.

Rajagopalan, S. (1974). *Guide to Simple Sanitary Measures for the Control of Enteric Diseases*. Geneva: WHO.

Rao, S. Majumder, N., Ghosh, A. R. and Saha, S. K. (1970). Character and quantity of refuse in rural homes. *Institution of Engineers (India) Journal of Public Health*, **51**, 23–26.

Saxena, S. K. and Patwardhan, S. V. (1965). Natural degradation of raw vegetable matter under aerobic and anaerobic conditions. *University of Roorkee Research Journal*, **8**, 63–67.

Stander, G. J., (1960). Factors which affect the chemistry, bacteriology and biology of surface water supply. In: *Proceedings of the Specialist Meeting on Water Treatment, Pretoria, 1960*.

Surveyor (1958). Mechanical refuse composting system for Bangkok. *Surveyor and Municipal and County Engineer*, **117**, 31–32.

Terman, G. L. and Mays, D. A. (1973). Utilization of municipal solid waste compost. *Compost Science*, **14**, 1, 18–21.

Wilson, D. G., (1974). Problems of solid-waste pollution. In: *Industrial Pollution* (Ed. N. I. Sax). New York: Van Nostrand Reinhold.

WHO Expert Committee (1971). *Solid waste disposal and control* (Technical report series No. 484). Geneva: WHO.

V

Effluent Re-use and Reclamation

18

Domestic Wastes as an Economic Resource: Biogas and Fish Culture

Michael G. McGarry

18.1 THE BIOGAS PLANT

The increasing cost of petroleum-based fuels has given rise to a search for alternative sources of energy. This, coupled with a growing concern for environmental pollution control, has resulted in attention being drawn to a process of methane production by fermentation of farm and human wastes. This fermentation process takes place in a unit which has come to be known as the 'biogas' plant. Simple in design and operation, the biogas plant accepts waste materials which ferment or digest without access to oxygen. The biogas, largely a mixture of methane and carbon dioxide, bubbles out of the liquid, is trapped and may be used as fuel for household lighting or cooking. The digested mixture or slurry can be used on the land as a soil conditioner and fertilizer. There are several other benefits which can be accrued through use of the biogas plant. However, its financial and economic viabilities being difficult to quantify, a comprehensive sensitivity analysis on the process has yet to be carried out. In many instances its financial viability is in doubt; the Indian Government still finds it necessary to provide grants to offset construction costs when propagating the use of biogas in rural areas. There are also social constraints to its acceptance—a reluctance to accept new technologies and a natural preference for traditional values.

Despite these drawbacks, the biogas plant is in use in several countries of Asia. It is estimated that there are over 10 000 plants in operation in India; 29 000 in Korea; 7000 in Taiwan and 80 000 in China. Other countries having a significant number of plants include Pakistan, Bangladesh, the Philippines, Thailand, Tanzania and Fiji. Research is going on in most of these countries and also in Europe, Canada, the US and Gautemala.

There are numerous variations to the biogas plant design. These include the use of single and double digesters; semi-continuous and batch processes; digestion of vegetable waste, nightsoil and/or animal dung; integrated and separate gas collectors; and, a variety of methods for utilizing the effluent

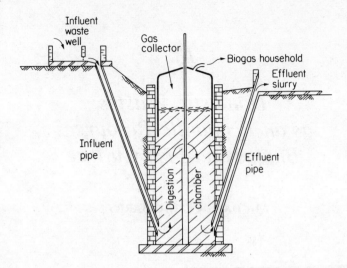

Figure 18.1 Sectional view of a biogas plant

slurry. Basically, it consists of a large chamber constructed partially below ground level and partitioned by a central wall. Daily, the waste material—most often cow dung—is diluted with water (1:1) and fed down the inlet pipe to the bottom of the first of the two partitioned sections. The liquid level in the digester is controlled by the overflow level of the outlet pipe as illustrated in Figure 18.1. While undergoing decomposition by anaerobic digestion, the waste travels up and over the submerged weir and down to the outlet pipe. The theoretical detention time of the slurry in the digester from inlet to outlet is normally 30 to 50 days which allows for gas production and destruction of most of the pathogenic or disease causing organisms. The gas is trapped by an inverted drum placed on the liquid's surface. As gas is produced and trapped, the drum rises acting as a gas storage chamber; the gas is drawn off as needed for lighting and cooking in the household.

The process of anerobic fermentation is a natural one occurring without man's intervention whenever living matter dies and decomposition takes place. The digester is simply a means by which this process can be concentrated, accelerated and its products harvested and put to useful purposes. The wasted matter is broken down by a two-stage bacterial process. Initially the organic matter is degraded by bacteria which produce volatile acids, mainly acetic acid. Care must be taken not to allow the slurry to become acidic to the point whereby the second stage, involving a more sensitive group of bacteria is inhibited. This second group, known as the methane formers, yield methane but multiply slowly and are adversely affected by changes in temperature, low temperature and acid conditions, and die in the presence of oxygen.

Although the process is a natural one, the amount of gas produced and the rate at which it is given off can be increased by creating conditions which are favourable for rapid growth of the micro-organisms. The farmer is very limited in the range of conditions which he can impose on the digester; although continuous feed and constant stirring has been shown to result in greater yields of gas, such conditions cannot easily be achieved on the farm or at the village level. Even if they could, it would be doubtful whether the additional equipment, energy and manpower requirements would be offset by the increased production of gas.

One important variable which the rural farmer does have control over is the quantity, moisture content and type of feed material. A rather crude guide to the suitability of input feed is its carbon to nitrogen content ratio. This ratio has been determined as being best in the vicinity of 30:1. Human excreta is relatively high in nitrogen content (5%–7%) as compared to cow dung (1·7%). Thus, the addition of human excreta, particularly urine (18% N), has the effect of lowering the carbon to nitrogen ratio which results in higher yields of methane. Cattle dung is high in cellulose which the acid forming bacteria find difficult to break down. The yield of biogas from a conventional plant operated solely on cattle dung is about 3 ft³/lb of dung (dry weight) introduced. In contrast, human excreta can be expected to yield double this amount. Most nitrogen is contained in the urine and unless the animal is confined and the urine collected, its nitrogen content is lost. Thus, reported gas yields from pig manure as collected from pens and including urine are higher (6–8 ft³/lb manure dry weight) than from the dung of cattle which are confined only at night.

The biogas

The component gases making up biogas reflect the conditions under which the gas is produced and the chemical characteristics of the feed material. The most valuable component is methane (CH_4) which constitutes 50%–60% of the biogas produced from a typical cattle dung fed plant. Carbon dioxide makes up much of the remainder while small amounts of nitrogen, hydrogen, oxygen, and hydrogen sulphide are to be expected. Higher proportions (60%–65%) of methane in biogas are given off by materials with more balanced feed material such as human and poultry excreta; the proportion of carbon dioxide to methane also reflects pH conditions in the digester, high CO_2 levels being associated with acid conditions in the digesting slurry.

Methane, being the energy source, determines the fuel value of the biogas. The heat value of the biogas has been measured at various levels–from 4·4 to 9·5 kilocalories/l. Normally, as derived from a cattle dung fed digester, it is valued at 4·9 kcal/l. In terms of unit production of gas, the dung from one medium-sized animal (cattle, bullock or buffalo) can produce 500 to 600 l/day while the daily production of gas from one human's waste is only 30 l. It is emphasized that these values have been measured under a variety of field conditions and represent only approximations under normal conditions of plant operation. As stated above, gas yields are sensitive to a variety of conditions such as temperature, mixing, influent feed characteristics and the like. For example, a farmer located in a more temperate zone can expect only a third of the rate of production of gas during the winter months as compared to the summer.

The overall financial objective of plant operation is to maximize the yield from a given quantity of waste to the point whereby additional capital and operating costs on a marginal basis are equal to the value of the gas and effluent slurry produced. This would dictate that the slurry is removed from the digester while still containing some potential for gas production. Under practical conditions, the waste is diluted with water ratios varying from 1:1 in India to 1:10 in the South Pacific and Thailand. Loading rates are normally given as kilograms of volatile solids of wastes per day per cubic metre of digestion chamber volume. Under optimum conditions rates as high as 4 kg/m³-day are reached resulting in detention times of below ten days. Under such optimal conditions gas yields are also considerably improved. However, in rural areas, loading rates are normally below 2·4 kg/m³-day with detention periods above 20 days.

Anaerobic digestion and the rate of gas production may be increased by raising the process temperature. There are two ranges of temperature suitable for digestion: thermophilic (48–60 °C) and mesophilic (30–40 °C). Thermophilic digestion results in greatly increased gas production rates and somewhat improved yields while allowing for a shorter detention time. However, reduction in digester volume and increased yields do not justify the additional cost of energy required to maintain the process temperature at the thermophilic optimum (53 °C). The mesophilic range, having its own optimum at 35 °C (corresponding to a different group of bacteria), is more attractive, particularly in the light of the fact that thermophilic bacteria are very sensitive to changes in their environment and the byproduct sludge at the higher temperature is of poor fertilizer quality and also odorous. Many digesters in the temperate zones of industrialized states are maintained at 35 °C which permits use of lower detention times and smaller unit digester volumes. Under village conditions however, little can be done in practical terms to maintain temperatures much above the ambient and digester temperatures are normally in the 18–30 °C range. It is unfortunate that the methane formers' gas production rate drops off considerably below 18 °C. This has a severe effect on biogas production in temperate zones during the winter months.

The gas is most commonly used for household cooking and lighting. Conventional propane burners are not suitable for use with biogas, the efficiency of energy usage in burning biogas in such a cooker is only 35%; however, this may be increased to 60% through use of a specially designed cooker. The 2-inch to 4-inch burners utilize 225–450 l/hr of biogas while the 100 foot-candle mantle light burns about 100 l/hr. In short, a biogas plant being fed the dung from three to four cattle can supply the fuel needs for cooking and lighting for a Gujarat family of 5 6 persons.

Considerable publicity has been given to the possible use of methane to power automobiles. Unfortunately, biogas cannot be easily liquelified (propane liquefies at about 250 psi; methane requires 5000 psi). Therefore, large storage volumes are required which are not easily transportable. Biogas can be used in converted diesel or petrol engines although the engines are best located close to the source digester to take advantage of continuous gas production and the gas collector's storage capacity. For such purposes, it is advisable to remove the carbon dioxide and hydrogen sulphate components of the biogas before burning. At 25% heat to power conversion efficiency, about 425 l/brake horse-power-hour is required. This holds some promise for village water supply pumps. In order to run a 1 h.p. engine to pump water eight hours a day, about 3·5 m^3 of gas would be required, which would need the contribution of six to seven medium-sized cattle per day. However, the plant would also require skilled maintenance which would not normally be available under village conditions.

The effluent slurry

As the influent waste is diluted and fed into the digester, the effluent or spent slurry is released and channelled away for use as fertilizer (Figure 18.2). On a

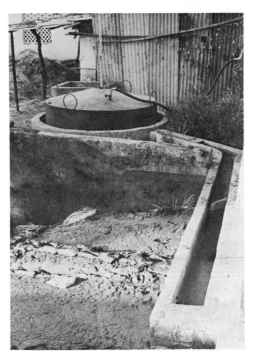

Figure 18.2 An Indian biogas plant successfully operated for over 13 years. The effluent channel leading to the drying pit is illustrated in the foreground [photograph : N. Florida]

dry solids basis, the cattle dung feed is approximately 1·7% of nitrogen whereas the effluent contains about 2% nitrogen. This is not on account of some kind of nitrogen fixation or mysterious nitrogen generation taking place in the digester, but rather a result of a reduction in the total solids which are given off in the form of biogas. In fact, there is invariably an overall loss of nitrogen with gas release. Anaerobic digestion does, however, convert influent plant nutrients such as nitrogen and phosphorous to chemical forms which are more readily taken up by plant life. The slurry is commonly released into sun-drying beds and after drying is spread onto the land. Normally a family-sized digester requires about 20 m² of drying bed area. This method of slurry treatment and use has some drawbacks: (a) the drying area could be otherwise utilized; (b) there is a loss of nitrogen to the atmosphere during drying; and (c) there is considerable difficulty in drying the slurry during the wet season when it must either be stored, used directly on the land or composted. Difficulties associated with transporting the slurry can be alleviated if it can be added to irrigation water before application.

The slurry can be composted with other farm and household wastes by spreading it on a compost pile. The compost is thereby inoculated with a bacterially active organic slurry and nutrients which are beneficial to the process of decomposition. The quantities of slurry which are available normally surpass the farm compost requirements.

Implications for Health

Manure, and in particular human excreta, contain disease causing organisms (pathogens). Direct application of nightsoil to the land can exacerbate the spread of diseases including typhoid, cholera, diarrhoea, whipworm, hookworm, ascariasis, bilharzia, etc. The danger of disease being spread in this way is reduced by natural die-off of pathogens under adverse conditions on the crop or soil and the crop being treated or cooked prior to ingestion. Treating the waste material by anaerobic digestion in the biogas plant before using it as fertilizer lessens the chances of disease transmission as the digester is capable of destroying most pathogens. Studies in China on a biogas plant have illustrated that although the influent feed contained the eggs of the schistosome, the ascarid worm, whipworm and hookworm, only 6·3% of them remained in the effluent. The schistosome ova were completely destroyed and very few hookworm ova managed to survive. On the other hand, the hardiest egg of them all, that of the roundworm or ascarid, managed to pass through relatively unscathed. This egg, with its thick protective albuminous sheath, is remarkable in its capacity to survive longs periods under severe adverse conditions. Under conditions of anaerobic digestion at normal temperatures, six months is required before die-off is assured: the biogas plant normally provides for less than one month. Using the effluent on the aerobic composting pile considerably increases the chances of pathogen kill. If the compost is kept aerobic, the high temperatures reached in the pile are enough to ensure the destruction of even the ascarid. Likewise, using the slurry to enhance algal growth in fish culture ponds also reduces the chances of disease transmission. It can be rightly argued that treatment of wastes in the biogas plant is better than their direct application to the land by indiscriminate defecation or manure spreading, but not enough is known of pathogen transfer through the process nor the ways by which it may be altered to further increase its capacity to destroy pathogens.

Biogas Plant: Costs and Benefits

Social constraints to the acceptance and promulgation of biogas plants have been illustrated by a study conducted by the Indian Agricultural Research Institute (IARI) which installed twelve such digesters and provided maintenance and repair services—all free of charge to the farmer. Technical difficulties encountered during the study included the accumulation of condensation water in the gas line, low moisture content of the digesting sludge reducing gas output and other defects resulting from poor operation. These deficiencies were quickly corrected by the IARI. Despite technical success, seven of the twelve farmers dropped out of the study; reasons for plant closure, apart from apathy and close ties to traditional values, could not be identified. The five plants which continued to function required no further external technical assistance but have not had a multiplier effect resulting in other farmers subscribing to the biogas plant. Difficulties encountered in motivating farmers to improve crop yields by using fertilizers, composts and modern cropping methods also apply to propagation of biogas technology.

The financial viability of the biogas plant has still not been adequately ascertained; there are some conditions under which the plant is definitely not viable. The Indian Government finds it necessary to continue to provide grants and encourages loans to foster the plants' acceptance in rural areas. On the other hand, the numbers of plants in other parts of Asia continue to grow without such incentives. Two financial analysis have been reported in the literature casting biogas in a favourable light; both, however, study the plant under very limited ranges of conditions. Certainly, further analysis required to determine the viability of the plant under a much wider range of conditions. Just as gas production is affected by temperature, mixing conditions, inlet feed characteristics, slurry pH level and water content, etc., so is the financial feasibility of the plant.

Cow dung is a marketable commodity in most parts of India; it is collected, dried in the sun, sold and used as a source of fuel for cooking. There are several disadvantages to this practice: the nutrient content of the dung is not returned to the land and the burning process is very inefficient as most of the heat is lost in copious amounts of odorous smoke. Effective use of cow dung in the biogas plant ensures the return of nutrients to the land and the capture of most of the dung's heat content. Although difficult to quantify, another major benefit may be accrued to public health by attaching the latrine directly to the biogas plant. Without an incentive to utilize human wastes, indiscriminate

354

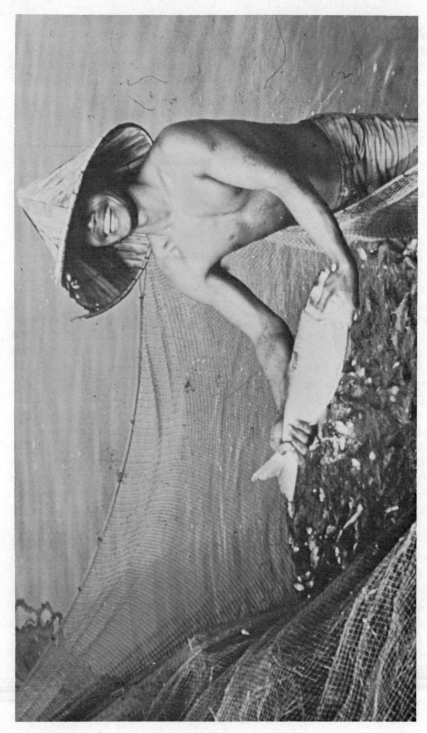

A good catch from a fish pond in south-east Asia (photograph: IDRC, Ottawa)

defecation is the norm in the rural areas and a major cause of the spread of disease (see the editorial introduction to Chapter 16). The biogas plant is therefore propagated by health officials as a means of combating enteric disease; over a third of the Indian plants are fed by human excreta, which has an added effect of increasing gas yields as described above.

The main benefits of the plant are its co-products of gas and fertilizer. Consideration must be given to alternative sources as the plant would not be viable in areas where firewood was plentiful and fertilizer not required. Such conditions are rare but there is some possibility that the use of *both* the effluent slurry as fertilizer and the gas as an alternative fuel is necessary before these benefits outweigh the costs of construction and operation of the plant. It is true, however, that the availability of gas in situations where cow dung is burned as cooking fuel does eliminate smoke and also provides a fuel for lighting and perhaps other purposes. It is noted that the digester is only about 60% effective in recovering the energy theoretically available in the influent cow dung. This, coupled with a 60% burning efficiency of the specially designed cooker, results in an overall capture of 36% of the heat. Use of a conventional cooker can reduce this to 21%. By contrast, the efficiency of heat usage by the traditional method of dried dung burning is only 11%, suggesting that approximately twice the amount of heat is available using the biogas plant. In situations where the effluent slurry is not used, this small amount of gas must be set against the capital and operating costs of the plant. When considering use of the plant for individual families in rural areas of developing countries, one does well to recall that the biogas plant may often cost more to build than the family house itself.

However desirable, a social cost–benefit analysis of the biogas plant is not possible as so many of the benefits are not quantifiable in monetary terms. In particular, there are no means by which one can readily determine the reduction of enteric disease incidence resulting from the proper disposal of excreta in latrines connected to the plant. Likewise, a realistic estimate of the reduced rates of deforestation and soil erosion, consequent upon the introduction of an alternative source of fuel to firewood, would be extremely difficult to make.

18.2 THE RECLAMATION FISH POND

Wastes can be reclaimed as a direct source of feed for fish or as nutrients for the growth of biomass upon which fish can feed. Controlled rearing of fish in ponds is not new; use of a domestic fish pond is illustrated in an Egyptian tomb over four thousand years old; carp culture is reported to have been practised in China 24 centuries ago; and German monks kept records of fish production during the Middle Ages. Fish culture is becoming more popular as food shortages intensify. Likewise, as population pressures increase the need for sanitary wastes disposal, the re-use of human and animal excreta as pond fertilizer or feed makes an attractive proposition.

The waste material which is introduced to a fish pond provides the main source of nutrients for bacterial growth. The byproducts from the wastes' bacterial decomposition, such as ammonia and carbon dioxide, are primary nutrients for the algae which are, in turn, the basic form of food for many of the fish used in pond culture. It would be highly impracticable if not impossible to gain a complete picture of the mass balance of the various elements and energy through the pond's complex ecosystem under natural conditions. The Chinese, over the centuries, have succeeded through trial and error in refining fish culture to a fine art. Their methods include the separate growth of fish fry, use of a variety of waste materials including human excreta, and poly-culture—the stocking of several types of fish in one pond as described below.

The most popular varieties of fish under culture fall into two categories—the Carp and the Tilapia. The silver carp (*Hypophthalmichthys molitrix*), the bighead (*Amstichthys nobilis*), the common carp (*Cyprinus carpio*), the grass carp (*Ctenopharyngodon idella*), and the mud carp (*Cerrhina molitcrella*) are the most commonly stocked carp. The silver carp and the bighead are capable of direct feeding on the plankton. In particular, the silver carp employs gill-rakers by which it can filter out unicellular algae for food. The bighead is able to eat only the larger algal species, while the common carp relies on bottom detritus for food. The carp's popularity is largely due to its rapid growth rate and consequently high productivity under pond conditions. Wide ranges of productivity (kg/ha-yr) are reported in the literature; productivity is sensitive to such factors as competition for food and space, food type and quality, temperature, and other kinds of fish and biota co-inhabiting the pond. One of the strongest influences on productivity is the degree to which the pond culture is controlled and cared for. The addition of excreta to ponds which are otherwise not purposefully fertilized will have a decided effect. Unfertilized and nightsoil fed ponds at the Taoynan Fish Farm in Taiwan were observed to produce averages of 132 kg/ha-year and 619 kg/ha-year of fish respectively. Likewise, the addition of such feed as rice bran, broken rice and peanut cake to excreta-fed ponds also has a beneficial effect. The increased productivity, however, has to be weighed against the cost and availability of such feeds.

In Europe, carp productivities from sewage-fed ponds are reported to range from 400 to 900 kg/ha-year, whereas through careful feeding and mixing of fish species (poly-culture), productivities as high as 5–7000 kg/ha-year have been achieved. Pond productivities of above 1000 kg/ha-year are not uncommon in Asia where nightsoil is applied and the pond is well maintained.

The Tilapias are prolific producers, growing well under a wide variety of conditions and capable of reproduction within the pond. They fall into two groups as defined by their breeding methods. The most common group, the 'brooders' (renamed *Sarotheroden*), gather the newly laid eggs from their nest in their mouths where they are brooded and protected until some weeks old. The brooders include *S. mossambicus* and *S. Niloticus* which use algae as a primary food source; they mature in 6 to 7 weeks and spawn at 2–3 month intervals, thereby posing another problem related to overpopulation in the pond. Productivities in unfertilized ponds of 1000 kg/ha-year are possible but, with fertilization, 2500–3000 kg/ha-year can be achieved. However, under the sub-optimal conditions which are likely to prevail in rural villages, these rates can fall to 220 kg/ha-year.

Over the centuries the Chinese have developed a mode of mixing species in poly-culture to make full use of their range of feeding habits. Thus such species as the silver carp, the bighead, the grass carp, common carp, grey mullet and perch may be stocked in appropriate proportions in one pond. The herbivorous grass carp which utilizes pond weeds and grass is also fed grass and vegetable matter grown for that purpose. Its excreta become the food of the benthal feeding common carp and grey mullet although some rises to the surface to be devoured by the silver carp and bighead. The silver carp and bighead also feed on micro- and macro-plankton respectively. The carnivorous perch is added to reduce the number of second generation fry and unwanted species. The advantages of poly-culture are amply illustrated by experiments carried out at the Fish Culture Station at Dor, Israel, where, with a combination of common carp, silver carp and *Tilapia*, productivities reached over 2300 kg/ha-year, with fertilization, and over 10 000 kg/ha-year when fertilization was supplemented with a protein-rich feed.

Fish Culture Feed and Fertilizer

Cultured fish are a major source of animal protein in China, Japan, Taiwan, Indonesia, the Philippines, Hong Kong and Malaysia; fish farming is also practised in India, Sri Lanka, Thailand, Bangladesh and Pakistan. It is difficult to find any ponds in these countries that are not fed some form of excreta; human or otherwise. In China, Indonesia and Malaysia, latrines are built right over the pond, while in Thailand, Taiwan and Sri Lanka, the nightsoil is collected by cart and delivered to the ponds. Other manures are derived from chicken, cattle, horses, buffaloes, pigs, ducks and even camels. The Chinese method of placing chicken, pig, duck and cattle pens close to or over the pond is practised in Malaysia, Thailand, Indonesia and, of course, China, Hong Kong and Taiwan. Manures and excreta are normally considered fertilizer material for improved algal growth, whereas a host of other feedstuffs act directly as food for the fish; these include oil-seed cakes, vegetable wastes, grass, weeds, rice bran and straw, soya-bean flour, wheat and corn brans, broken rice, fish meal and offal—the amount and variety depending on the kind of fish being cultured and availability of feed material.

Fish Production in Sewage Ponds

In India, raw sewage is fed to fish farms. The largest receives Calcuttan sewage at Bidyadhari in Bengal. Another uses sewage from the Madurai municipality in Madras State. The Calcutta farms provide 10 to 12 tons of fresh fish to the market daily, a fish pond productivity exceeding 900 kg/ha-year. The farmers have learned through trial and error to achieve such productivity levels by skilfully manipulating the raw sewage feed to the ponds. Some difficulties have been encountered through inadvertent shock loading of the ponds with excessive amounts of raw sewage resulting in deoxygenation and fish kill. Treated sewage effluent, still plentiful in nutrients, is the primary source of nutrients for fish in the Munich ponds which provide a form of tertiary or polishing treatment to the city's sewage. There, the carp production rates are in the order of 400–600 kg/ha-year. Similar practices are carried out in Berlin and Kielce, Poland, the latter reporting productivities as high as 1300 kg/ha-year. Common carp production experiments on sewage plant effluent at the Rye Meads near London report productivities in the order of 600–800 kg/ha-year; it is interesting to note that nearly all the rainbow trout sold in England just prior to the Second World War derived from the Munich city sewage-fed pond system.

Whether purposefully stocked or not, oxidation ponds in tropical climates around the world support fish life. In many instances, municipal authorities have turned a blind eye to local farmers harvesting fish from the ponds. Having for the most part been trained in Western universities or in those institutions which are strongly influenced by Western mores, the municipal engineers do not recognize or take advantage of the potential resource and financial return which their ponds represent. Often the ponds are fenced in to keep the public and fish poachers out; municipal employees are paid to cut the grass around the ponds, whereas the same ponds could be leased out to fish farmers who would maintain and manage them as fish farms, thereby providing a means of supporting their families and bringing positive returns to the municipality.

The potential for producing carp in oxidation ponds is amply illustrated by research at the College of Engineering, Guindy, Madras, where the effluent from an oxidation pond was used to feed a fish pond stocked with common carp. Within four months, the fish had reached maturity (initially stocked as 0·3 g fingerlings) and were reproducing by the fifth month. The average fish weight was 620 g during the sixth month; productivity was estimated at 7700 kg/ha-year.

Optimal conditions for sewage treatment and for fish growth are not necessarily identical. Current thought on design of the system tends to be based on its optimization on the basis of sewage treatment—that of minimizing construction, land and operating costs while achieving a given quality of treatment. If sewage-fed fish ponds are indeed an economic proposition, consideration should be given to the design of the treatment process on the basis of optimizing fish production, not sewage treatment. It is highly likely that the fish pond's effluent characteristics would surpass those of conventional oxidation ponds. Pond retention periods would necessarily have to be increased so that full opportunity could be given for nutrient conversion and fish growth. This would have the effect of improving the effluent quality, particularly by fostering pathogen die-off. Land requirements would go up, but such costs would be covered by the overall economic viability of the system. Thus, the approach in design would be to optimize the reclamation potential of a commercially viable process while at the same time achieving a high-quality effluent. This contrasts with current practices of designing for effluent quality at minimum costs without any financial return on investment.

Research in Thailand with reclamation fish ponds has illustrated that it may well be advantageous to design the first sewage-fed pond to optimize algal yield—conventional oxidation pond designs do not achieve this. The effluent of the shallow, high-rate growth pond could then be fed to poly-culture fish ponds.

Nightsoil-Fed Fish Ponds

There are approximately 6000 ha of fish ponds around the city of Tainan, Taiwan. These draw on Tainan for pond fertilizer in the form of nightsoil which is regarded as a marketable commodity—truly a liquid asset. Nightsoil

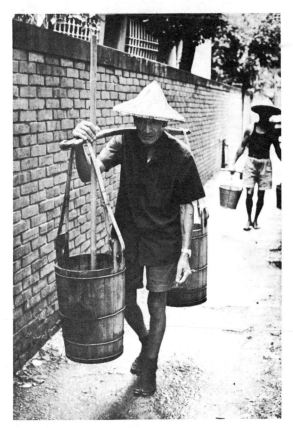

Figure 18.3 The Municipal Collector makes his rounds in the early morning hours using dipper and bucket for cartage and transfer to animal-drawn carts
[photograph: M. G. McGarry]

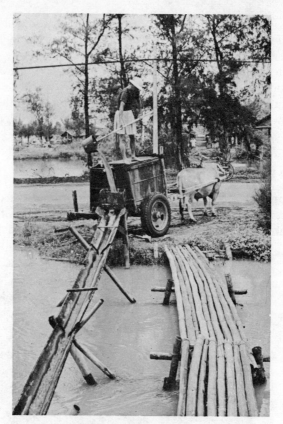

Figure 18.4 After purchase, the nightsoil is transported to the fish farm and fed down channels to the pond as fish feed and pond fertilizer [photograph: M. G. McGarry]

is collected in the early morning hours by municipal collectors, purchased by the farmers, and fed to the ponds (Figure 18.3 and 18.4). During the peak season, when nightsoil is at a premium, it is 'stolen' from the vaults before the municipal collection is made and sold in what can be rightly called a black-market in nightsoil. Nightsoil is added as a means of introducing both macro- and micro-nutrients for algal growth. Attempts are being made to propagate the use of inorganic fertilizers in ponds, but the farmers are reluctant to rely upon such methods in the face of rising costs of chemical fertilizers when they have developed the use of excreta to a fine art over the centuries. Even where commercial fertilizers are employed, the micro-elements continue to be added in the form of manure or nightsoil. Nightsoil can also be regarded as a feed: at the appropriate time, the fish gather in expectation at the pond's input point and feed voraciously on the material as it is let into the pond. In Java, thousands of community and household ponds are used to reclaim household and human wastes while acting as a source of protein for the local population. There, the latrines are located directly above the pond.

River Fish Culture in Cages

The River Tijibunut receives nightsoil and sewage from Bandung city in Indonesia. Fisherman have developed the practice of growing carp in cages (karambas) which are partially submerged in the river's two branches. The western branch is densely populated with karambas. The heavily polluted water flows through the cage which has 1–4 cm bar spaces on its sides for the purpose. The karambas are normally stocked with 200 to 400 carp (8–12 cm sized) for fattening and removed some 2 to 3 months later yielding 50 to 75 kg of fish per karamba. The fish have usually more than doubled their weight in that short time within the karamba volume of just over 1 m^3. The fish are not normally given any other food than what is in the river itself. As in many heavily polluted running waters, masses of *Sphaerotilis* and *Zooglea* grow, can be found attached to surfaces of the cage and undoubtedly serve as food for the fish, although larvae of the *Tendipedide* taken from the cage bottoms predominate in the fish guts.

Brackish Water Fish Culture

Our understanding of the ecosystem of fish ponds is very limited, consequently it is extremely difficult to maintain one algal bloom under out door conditions; it is nearly impossible to pre-select an algal bloom and provide conditions so that it will remain the majority species. The milkfish (*Chanos chanos*), prized as a delicacy, is grown in brackish water ponds along the western coastal belt of Taiwan, and has a strong preference for bottom-growing algae such as *Lyngbya*, *Phormidium* and *Oscillatoria*. The 16 000 ha of milkfish ponds in Taiwan represent less than 3% of the total area of such ponds in the world. At the end of the growing season, the farmer dries out his pond and fertilizes it by mixing nightsoil collected from the nearby town and rice bran into the bottom muds. The pond is then filled to 15 cm and again allowed to dry. This is repeated three or four times. The procedure fosters growth of the benthic algae and inhibits the proliferation of nanoplankton such as *Chlorella* and *Scenedesmus* which, by causing turbidity, would decrease the amount of sunlight reaching the benthic algae.

Industrial Wastewater Fish Culture

Industrial wastes have also been used in fish culture. Research with the use of daily, sugar mill, abattoir and starch mill waste has been conducted in Czechoslovakia and practised by an Austrian starch mill. The rubber processing wastes of Malaysia hold particular potential in ponds. Ammonia, added to prevent premature coagulation of the serum from the trees, is wasted with the effluent and can be used as a basis of algal protein production. Fish culture on such industrial wastes circumvents the possibility of disease transmission which may prevail where domestic sewage or nightsoil is used.

Implications for Health

Not enough is known about the transfer of pathogens from excreta through the fish to the consumer. Dissection of fish grown on raw excreta in Indonesian river cages revealed numerous eggs of parasites, including the roundworm *Ascaris*. On the other hand, where the pond is used to culture fish, the pond itself provides a buffer by fostering a rapid die-off of bacteria and breaking the transmission chain of such parasites as the hookworm. The hardy ascarid ova itself is either ingested by the fish and secreted or settles to the bottom of the pond. Fortunately, the fish cannot act as intermediary hosts to the vast majority of human parasitic agents and the only way transmission may be effected is by direct transfer from the pond on the fish's scales or in its gut. A further buffer is provided by cooking the fish before eating.

Chlonorchiasis, a disease of the liver, is caused by *Clonorchis sinensis* which is transmitted from the faeces through snails and then to certain fish of the carp family. It would at first appear unlikely that the disease being so particular in its mode of transmission could find its way to man. The carp hosts, however, are regarded as a delicacy and are eaten raw on auspicious occasions. The disease is a public health problem in several parts of Asia and particularly in the north-east of Thailand. Likewise the cat liver fluke, of lesser public health importance, utilizes snails and the carp as intermediary hosts *en route* to its final destination, man. The oriental lung fluke causes paragonimiasis in man, its eggs reach the pond in man's faeces. *Paragonimus* then uses snails and certain freshwater crayfish or crabs as intermediary hosts. Unfortunately these crabs are delicious, especially when eaten raw after being saturated in wine or crushed to make a paste sauce. The fourth parasite of concern is *Diphyllobothrium*, the fish tapeworm, which grows sometimes to enormous lengths after attaching itself to the small intestine and causing anaemia. Its intermediary hosts are crustaceans and a variety of freshwater fish. All of the above diseases can be curtailed by ensuring that the final intermediary hosts are properly cooked, transmission relying heavily on the crab or fish being eaten raw or partially cooked.

European fish culture practice recommends that if sewage-grown fish are to be sold for human consumption, they should be kept in a clear water (ostensibly unpolluted) pond for a month or at least two to three weeks prior to marketing. This is the practice at Munich. It would be pointless to discourage or attempt to ban the direct application of nightsoil to ponds on the basis of public health. Use of nightsoil as pond fertilizer has been practised in most Asian ponds for centuries. Literally millions rely on this method of waste reclamation as a means of income generation and protein supply. However, more data is needed on the potential for spread of disease through fish culture and on the definition of methods by which the transmission chain can be broken while continuing to encourage the practice of waste re-use through reclamation fish ponds.

It is interesting to note that both biogas plant and reclamation fish pond technologies have been developed in the developing countries, and that scientists of the industrialized states have only become aware of the potential for such systems during the past decade—largely as a consequence of the so-called environmental crisis. Oxidation ponds have been designed primarily as a means of treating sewage and fish culture ponds have utilized excreta and manure for purposes of pond fertilization; little attention has been given to the use of oxidation ponds as a source of fish protein nor to fish ponds for disposal of urban nightsoil for purposes of public health and environmental protection.

18.3 BIOGAS BIBLIOGRAPHY

Anon. (1974). Digestion of night-soil for destruction of parasite ova, Szechwan Research Institute of Antiparasitic Diseases and Mienchu County Antischistomiasis Office, Szechwan. *Chinese Medical Journal*, No. 2, Feb.

Anon. (1975). Popularizing the use of marshy gas in rural areas. *Peking Review*, 30, July 1975.

Anon. (1975). Report on the workshop of biogas technology and utilization, New Delhi, 28 July–2 August, 1975. Economic and Social Commission for Asia and the Pacific, Report No. IHT/BG/(2)/3.

Florida, N. (1973). Small-scale biogas plants. *Appropriate Technology Series*, CUSO, 151 Slater Street, Ottawa.

Fry, L. J. and Merrill, R. (1973). Methane digesters for fuel and fertilizer. *New Alchemy Institute Newsletter*, No. 3, Spring. Box 432, Woods Hole, Mass., 02543 USA.

K & Vic (1973). Gobar gas (methane) industry, *Commerce*, January 13, India.

K & VIC (1975). *Gobar gas, How and Why*. Publ. Directorate of Gobar Gas Scheme, Khadi and Village Industries Commission, Gramodaya, Irla Road, Ville Parle (West), Bombay 400056, India.

Lapp, H. M. (1975). *Travel Report of a Study of Methane from Animal Wastes by Anaerobic Processes in Scotland, England, Germany, Norway and Denmark*. Unpublished, Department of Agricultural Engineering, University of Manitoba, Winnipeg, Manitoba.

Lapp, H. M., Schulte, D. D. and Buchanan, L. C. (1974). *Methane Gas Production from Animal Wastes*. Publ. Canada Department of Agriculture, Ottawa K1A OC7, Canada.

McGarry, M. G. (1975). *Developing Country Sanitation*. Report to the International Development Research Centre, Ottawa.

Nagar, B. R. (1975). Biogar plants based on night-soil and/or animal dung. *IRCWD News*, June, Ueberlandstrasse 133, CH-8600, Dubendorf, Switzerland.

Po, Chung (1973). Production of methane gas from manure. *Proceedings of the International Biomass Energy Conference*, May 13–15, Winnipeg.

Prasad, C. R., Krishna Prasad, K. and Reddy, A. K. N. (1974). Biogas plants: Prospects, problems and tasks. *Economic and Political Weekly*, **IX**, 32–34, Special Number, India.

Singh, R. B. (1974). *Biogas Plant*. Publ. Gobar Gas Research Station, Ajitmal, Etawah (U.P.), India.

18.4 FISH CULTURE BIBLIOGRAPHY

Allen, G. H. (1969). A preliminary bibliography on the utilization of sewage in fish culture. *FAO Fisheries Circular*, No. 308, Document No. FR:/L308. Food and Agricultural Organization, Rome.

Allen, G. H. (1970). The constructive use of sewage, with particular reference to fish culture. Paper No. FIR:MP/70/R-13, December 1, 1970. *Proceedings of the FAO Technical Conference on Marine Pollution and its Effects on Living Resources and Fishing,* Rome.

Jayangondar, I. S. and Ganagi, S. V. (1965). Some observations on the use of sewage stabilization lagoons in India. *Hydrobiologia. Acta Hydrobiologica, Limnogica et Protistologia,* The Hague, 126 (3/4): pp. 331–348.

Lin, Shu-yen (1968). Pond fish culture and the economy of inorganic fertilizer application. *Fisheries Report Series No. 6.* Chinese–American Joint Commission on Rural Reconstruction, Taipei.

McGarry, M. G. (1972). *Sewage as a Natural Resource: Economic Disposal of Domestic Wastewaters.* Paper presented at the Environmental Pollution Control Symposium, March, Kuala Lumpur.

Muthuswamy, S., Govindan, S. and Sundaresan, B. B. (1974). Productivity of *Cyprinus Carpio* in stabilization pond Effluents. *Indian Journal of Environmental Health,* **16**, 4, 370–379.

Noble, R. (1975). Growing fish in sewage. *New Scientist,* July 31, 259–261.

Payne, I. (1975). Tilapia—a fish of culture. *New Scientist,* July 31, 256–258.

Prowse, G. A. (1966). A review of the methods of fertilizing warm-water fish ponds in Asia and the Far East. *Proceedings of the World Symposium on Warm-Water Pond Fish Culture.* FAO Report No. 44, Vol. 3, pp. 7–12, Rome.

Rabanal, H. R. (1966). Stock manipulation and other biological methods of increasing production of fish culture in Asia and the Far East. *Proceedings of the FAO World Symposium on Warm-Water Fish Culture.* Paper No. FR V/R-3, Rome.

19

Public Health Considerations
in Wastewater and Excreta Re-use
for Agriculture

H. I. Shuval

19.1 INTRODUCTION

Water shortages are becoming an increasingly important problem in arid zones as well as in areas considered to have plentiful water resources. Growing population and industrialization coupled with the introduction of modern intensive agricultural techniques involving irrigation are causing increasingly heavy demands on water resources. The re-use of municipal and industrial wastewater has become an attractive option for increasing water reserves in such areas. Re-use of wastewater for agricultural purposes may be particularly attractive, since this may allow for the expansion of intensive agriculture while preserving limited resources of good quality drinking water for the rapid urban development that is taking place in most regions of the world. In addition to the amounts of water provided by wastewater re-use in agriculture, many agronomists see the advantage of using such water, since it is rich in organic content and can be expected in many cases to supply part or even all of the nitrogen required to fertilize the fields as well as some of the other essential nutrients. The direct agricultural application of human excreta ('nightsoil') has been widely practised in many areas of the world primarily for its fertilizer value.

However, in planning wastewater re-use high priority must be given to the public health considerations since wastewater carries a potentially dangerous load of pathogenic micro-organisms that can be infectious to man. Health criteria must be established in the early planning stages of any wastewater re-use programme so as to ensure that the benefits gained by additional water resources are not negated by unreasonable public health risks to agricultural workers and the public at large.

This chapter presents a review of the main public health problems associated with wastewater and excreta re-use in agriculture.

This chapter is based in part on material published in *Water Renovation and Reuse* (edited by H. I. Shuval) by permission of the publishers, Academic Press Inc., New York.

19.2 TYPES OF CONTAMINANTS

The degree of concern about the various types of potential contaminants is of course dependent on the type of water re-use being considered. Such concern from the health point of view might be quite minimal for most microbial and chemical contaminants in the case of surface irrigation of industrial crops and would become extremely acute in the case of any planned re-use for edible crops. What follows is a brief review of the main microbial and chemical contaminants that may appear in wastewater which bear some relationship to various re-use strategies.

Microbiological contaminants

Since John Snow's classical investigations of cholera in London in 1854, it has been understood that water can serve as an efficient vector of human pathogenic micro-organisms of sewage origin. We know today that the raw wastewater of a community usually carries the full spectrum of pathogenic bacteria, viruses, protozoa and helminths associated with the enteric diseases endemic in the community which are excreted by clinical cases and carriers. During periods of epidemics of enteric diseases the concentration of pathogens can increase many times over.

It is worth noting that the pathogenic agents of diseases not known to exist in the community can at times be detected in excreta or wastewater, since the organisms may be excreted in quite high concentrations on a regular basis by undetected carriers. In a study of the appearance of *Salmonella* organisms in 96 samples of wastewater and polluted water in Tel Aviv, we were able to isolate 229 *Salmonella* strains which included 34 serotypes (Yoshpe-Purer and Shuval, 1970). The dominant type was *S. paratyphi B*. Many of the isolated organisms were rare in the community while a number had never been isolated from human cases in Tel Aviv. In another study carried out during the cholera outbreak in Jerusalem in 1970 we were able to detect *Cholera vibrio* in wastewater samples from neighbourhoods where no clinical cases of the disease had then been reported.

Such findings provide further support to the premise that human excreta and raw wastewater must be considered most serious potential sources of a wide variety of enteric pathogens, regardless of whether serious enteric disease epidemics are present in the community or not.

Kehr and Butterfield (1943) pointed out that while the level of coliforms found in community wastewater is fairly constant, the ratio of typhoid organisms to coliforms is a function of the endemic disease rate in the community. Thus for any given concentration of coliforms found in wastewater the risk of pathogens being present would be 10- or 100-fold greater in certain Mediterranean, South American or Asian countries than in the United States, since some such countries have 10 or even 100 times greater enteric disease rates. The risks associated with wastewater re-use using equivalent treatment processes would be correspondingly greater in such countries.

Enteroviruses present a particularly difficult problem since studies indicate that viruses are more resistant to inactivation by natural factors in the water environment and to most water and wastewater treatment process than are coliforms. This means that under many circumstances a low coliform count in an effluent destined for re-use may not provide a clear assurance that the effluent is free of potentially infectious enteric viruses which have survived the treatment processes.

Our studies (Shuval, 1970) and the work of others indicate that domestic sewage carries from 1–100 enteric viruses per millilitre. Enteroviruses found in wastewater may include more than sixty types, all of them considered pathogenic to man. These viruses include poliovirus, echo viruses and coxsackie viruses. Adenoviruses and reoviruses clinically considered respiratory have been found in wastewater. Most important of all is probably the virus of infectious hepatitis, which has been shown by epidemiological studies to have caused over 50 waterborne epidemics. Although techniques for detecting this virus in water are now being developed, it has not been possible to do so in the past.

Methods have now been developed for detecting low levels of viruses in large volumes of water (Shuval and Katzenelson, 1972). It is likely that in the future routine virus assays of wastewater for some high levels of re-use will be required since coliform tests appear inadequate, at least in certain cases.

Factors affecting the degree of risk

The degree of risk of infection from sewage-borne pathogens in any re-use project depends on many factors, including the efficiency of wastewater treatment processes in removing or inactivating the pathogens, the survival of the pathogens in the wastewater effluent, in soil and on crops in the case of agricultural re-use, and the infectivity, or minimal infectious dose, required to cause infection in man.

Removal by treatment processes

While it is well accepted that conventional biological wastewater treatment processes provide only minimal removal of enteric bacteria, disinfection can often provide very high levels of bacterial inactivation. It is possible by optimal combinations of wastewater treatment and chemical disinfection to achieve coliforms counts in treated effluent consistently lower than 100/100 ml. Enteric viruses are, however, usually many times more resistant to chlorination than are coliforms (Shuval, 1975). Ozone is a most effective virocidal agent. Our studies (Katzenelson *et al.*, 1974) indicate that under controlled conditions a 99% kill of poliovirus can be achieved with 0·1 mg/l of ozone residual in under 10 seconds while the same concentration of chlorine residual would require 10 minutes and iodine 100 minutes to achieve the same results.

If effluent re-use for certain purposes calls for total effective removal of pathogens it now appears to be within the limits of developing technology to achieve this goal. However, in developing countries with limited resources and shortages of the skilled technicians required to operate such a system, it would be justifiable only under unusual conditions to aim at achieving such a high-quality effluent. Under most conditions lower levels of treatment for restricted wastewater re-use with low health risk crops would be a more practical approach. Alternatively a properly designed system of waste stabilization (including maturation) ponds might be more effectively used (see Chapter 14).

The question of microbial survival in soil and on crops will be discussed later.

Minimal infective dose

With the possibility of obtaining significant reductions in the number of pathogens by active treatment processes or by die-off in the soil or on crops, one must ascertain how many pathogens must be ingested to cause infection or disease in man. It has been established that for certain salmonella infections a person must ingest many millions of viable organisms in order to become infected. For this reason, such salmonella infections are most often associated with certain contaminated foods held at room temperature for periods of many hours, thus enabling the massive multiplication of the initial inoculum of the pathogen. On the other hand, the ingestion of a few typhoid bacilli appears to be sufficient to cause infection in a certain percentage of susceptible humans who have a low level of resistance. Very low levels of enteroviruses in water or on crops may also present a potential health risk. It has been experimentally established that ingestion of as little as one tissue culture infectious dose of poliovirus (Plotkin and Katz, 1967) and other enteroviruses is sufficient to infect a percentage of susceptible persons. The minimal infective dose for infectious hepatitis has not been determined, but epidemiological evidence seems to indicate that the ingestion of but a few organisms might be sufficient to cause infection in some persons. The ingestion of a relatively small number of cholera organisms may also lead to human infection. Similarly infection with protozoan or helminthic pathogens may occur with a small number of ingested organisms as well.

With the above considerations in mind it becomes apparent that very high removals of enteric pathogens are essential in any type of water re-use associated with human consumption of crops, body contact sports or consumption as drinking water. The same goes for any form of re-use where the effluent is sprayed into the air and microbial aerosols can be dispersed over relatively wide areas, particularly in the vicinity of residential zones. It has been demonstrated that inhaled enteric bacteria can cause human infections in doses many times lower than when ingested (Sorber and Guter, 1975). Inhaled salmonellae for example are 1000 times more infective.

Since we cannot determine in advance the exact type of communicable disease organisms that may at times be present in the wastewater stream destined for re-use, it is reasonable to assume that it is a distinct possibility that highly infectious disease agents will indeed be present and that the ingestion of a very few of such organisms may cause human infection. Health criteria for different forms of water re-use must be based on this conservative assumption.

Chemical contaminants

The unbridled increase in the use of hundreds of new, and often structurally complex, synthetic compounds in industry and agriculture has resulted in the appearance of many of these potentially toxic materials in municipal and industrial wastewater streams. Many of these chemicals which appear in wastewater are known not only for their acute toxic effects but also for their chronic effects which can be detected only after long periods of exposure. Materials having carcinogenic, mutagenic as well as teratogenic effects have been isolated in wastewater, polluted surface water and drinking water obtained from surface sources. Trace metals which may at times reach toxic concentrations have also been found on many occasions in wastewater streams, particularly those carrying a high percentage of industrial wastes (Shuval, 1962).

Certain chemicals found in wastewater can be harmful to agriculture. Of particular concern is boron whose compounds are often including in various forms of synthetic detergents. It is beyond the scope of this chapter to deal with chemicals deleterious to the soil and to the plants themselves. There is evidence, however, that organic and inorganic chemicals in wastewater used for irrigation can under certain circumstances accumulate in the plants and present potential toxic risks to consumers of the agricultural products. This factor should be given consideration in planning wastewater re-use of industrial effluents which may contain toxic compounds.

19.3 HEALTH ASPECTS OF VARIOUS TYPES OF AGRICULTURAL RE-USE

Each form of wastewater re-use in agriculture presents its own specific health problems. This section will review the problems associated with each type of re-use.

The World Health Organization (WHO, 1973) has presented a comprehensive and authoritative report on the health aspects of various forms of re-use. The WHO report has suggested treatment processes to meet the given health criteria for wastewater re-use which is reproduced here as Table 19.1. The rationale behind the health criteria and the treatment processes required to meet them is presented in the following sections.

The application of human faeces as an agricultural manure has been widely practised in the Far East for many centuries, while the re-use of municipal wastewater for agricultural irrigation is one of the oldest forms of water reclamation. At the end of the last century, major land irrigation projects were developed in Germany and in England. It should be pointed out, however, that the primary motivation of these early European projects was essentially

370

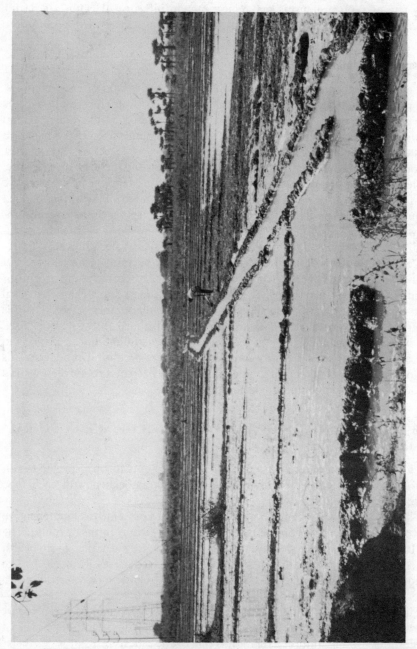

Crop irrigation using effluent from oxidation ponds (photograph: IDRC)

Table 19.1 Suggested treatment processes to meet the given health criteria for wastewater Re-use

Health criteria (see below for explanation of symbols)	Irrigation			Recreation		Industrial	Municipal re-use	
	Crops not for direct human consumption	Crops eaten cooked; fish culture	Crops eaten raw	No contact	re-use		Non-potable	Potable
	A + F	B + F or D + F	D + F	B	D + G	C or D	C	E
Primary treatment	●●●	●●●	●●●	●●●	●●●	●●●	●●●	●●
Secondary treatment		●●●	●●●	●●●	●●●	●●●	●●●	●●
Sand filtration or equivalent polishing methods		●	●		●	●	●	●
Nitrification						●		●●●
Denitrification								●●
Chemical clarification								●●
Carbon absorption								●●
Ion exchange or other means of removing ions		●				●		●●
Disinfection		●	●●●	●	●●●	●	●●●	●●

Health criteria:
A Freedom from gross solids; significant removal of parasite eggs.
B As A, plus significant removal of bacteria.
C As A, plus more effective removal of bacteria, plus some removal of viruses.
D Not more than 100 coliform organisms per 100 ml in 80% of samples.
E No faecal coliform organisms in 100 ml, plus no virus particles in 1000 ml, plus no toxic effects on man, and other drinking-water criteria.
F No chemicals that lead to undesirable residues in crops or fish.
G No chemicals that lead to irritation of mucous membranes and skin.

In order to meet the given health criteria, processes marked ●●● will be essential. In addition, one or more processes marked ●● will also be essential, and further processes marked ● may sometimes be required.
[a]Free chlorine after 1 hour.

Reproduced by permission of the World Health Organization from 'Reuse of effluents: methods of wastewater treatment and health safeguards'. *WHO Technical Report Series No. 517*, Geneva, 1973.

treatment and disposal of municipal wastewater rather than water conservation and recycling. For example, the first Royal Commission on Sewage Disposal in England concluded in its report in 1865 that 'the right way to dispose of town sewage is to apply it continuously to the land, and it is by such application that the pollution of rivers can be avoided'.

It is important here to review the possible health risks associated with various forms of water re-use and excreta applications in agriculture. The degree of risk involved may vary greatly. Such re-use may be directed solely to the irrigation of industrial or other crops not for direct human consumption while on the other hand it may involve highly health-sensitive crops such as fruits or vegetables generally consumed uncooked. In either case, the health risks to agricultural workers must be evaluated as well as the possible dispersion of aerosolized pathogens by spray irrigation in the vicinity of residential areas.

Contamination of crops with pathogens

Although public health authorities have long ago pointed out the risks of using human faeces as a manure on vegetable crops, systematic scientific studies on the survival of enteric pathogens in soil and on crops began to appear in the literature only in the 1920s. One of the earliest studies on survival of enteric pathogens in soil was made in 1921 by Kligler who was the founder of the Department of Hygiene at the Hebrew University of Jerusalem. He showed that typhoid bacilli could survive for months in moist subsoil contaminated with faeces although the movement of the bacteria through the soil was very restricted. McClesky and Christopher (1941) studied pathogen survival on strawberries while Falk (1949) studied the survival of enteric bacteria sprayed on tomatoes. His work at Rutgers was followed up by the extensive classical study together with colleagues on the health risks associated with growing vegetables in sewage contaminated soil (Rudolfs et al., 1950 and 1951).

These studies indicated that bacteria, protozoa and helminths do not penetrate healthy undamaged surfaces of vegetables, and die away rapidly on crop surfaces exposed to sunlight. However, pathogens can survive for extended periods inside leafy vegetables or in protected cracks or stem areas. We initiated our first studies with colleagues in Israel in the early 1950s on the health problems associated with sewage irrigation (Shuval, 1951). Bregner-Rabinowitz (1965) detected numerous pathogens in the raw sewage of Jerusalem destined for irrigation including Salmonella spp., Shigella dysenteriae, parasitic eggs of Ascaris, Trichuris, Trichstrongylus, Taenia hymenolepis and cysts of Giardia lamblia and Entamoeba. In the effluent of a trickling filter plant used for one of our sewage irrigation studies (Rigbi et al., 1956), the same pathogens were detected but less frequently and in smaller numbers.

In these studies the survival of Salmonella tennessee organisms inoculated into the effluent was studied in sewage-irrigated soil. In winter the bacteria could not be detected by the 46th day on the surface of the soil, but only dis-

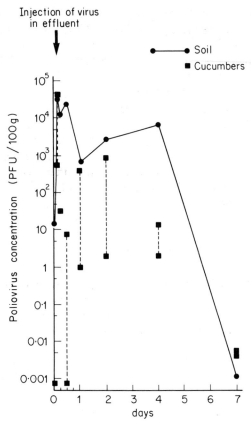

Figure 19.1 Virus concentration in soil and on cucumbers irrigated with effluent inoculated with poliovirus (unpublished data of B. Fattal and E. Katzenelson, Environmental Health Laboratory, Hebrew University of Jerusalem, 1975)

appeared from the moist subsoil on the 70th day; whereas in summer they disappeared on the 23rd day on the surface and 37th day at a depth of 8 inches. In all cases however, there was, about a 99% reduction within the first week.

Dunlop *et al.* (1951) found that although salmonellae could be recovered from a large number of samples of sewage-contaminated irrigation water, they were unable to recover these pathogens from samples of vegetables irrigated with this water.

In our own recent studies in Israel we have investigated the survival of poliovirus in sewage-irrigated soil and on crops. We have been able to show that poliovirus inoculated into the sewage could be detected in the irrigated soil for 7 days and it was possible to recover the virus from the cucumbers 7 days after initial irrigation (Figure 19.1).

It is quite clear from the many studies to date that pathogens are present in sewage and excreta in great quantity and variety and can survive for periods in the soil or on crops (Benarde, 1973). However, the viability of such micro-organisms varies greatly, depending on the type of organisms and various environmental factors such as climatic conditions, soil moisture, soil pH and the amount of protection provided by the crops.

In his review of this problem Dunlop (1952) went so far as to say that despite the known presence and viability of pathogens in wastewater and soil, he knew of no disease outbreaks or epidemics that had been related to, or were known to be caused by, irrigation with properly treated sewage. He concluded that if effluents were properly treated, it was safe from the microbial point of view to harvest crops for human consumption within 4 hours of irrigation. Dunlop did not define the degree of treatment or disinfection he would require.

A dramatic demonstration that pathogens in untreated sewage used for irrigation could in fact remain viable on the vegetables long enough to cause a cholera outbreak, occurred in Jerusalem in 1970 (Cohen et al., 1971). When cholera cases first appeared in the city it was quickly ascertained that the drinking water supply derived from deep protected wells and chlorinated before distribution was not the vector. However, during the outbreak we demonstrated the presence of *Cholera vibrio* of the El tor type in the main sewage lines in various parts of the city and in the soil of some agricultural plots illegally irrigated with raw sewage used for growing vegetables supplied to the Jerusalem market. The pathogens were later recovered from the sewage-irrigated vegetables. This illegal sewage irrigation was stopped and the epidemic quickly came to an end. The freshly sewage-irrigated, leafy vegetables widely sold in Jerusalem undoubtedly provided the main secondary pathway for the spread of the disease after a few carriers or clinical cases entered the city from neighbouring countries where cholera outbreaks were in progress.

From the foregoing it is apparent that irrigation of health-sensitive crops including fruits and vegetables eaten uncooked with raw or partially treated wastewater can present real health risks. Even effluent from conventional biological wastewater treatment plants or waste stabilization ponds cannot generally be considered absolutely safe. For these reasons health authorities in many countries have established regulations restricting the types of crops that can be grown with effluent that has not undergone a high degree of disinfection. Irrigation with non-disinfected effluent of industrial crops, seed crops, tree nurseries and other crops not destined for direct human consumption are usually allowed.

The use of raw sewage is generally not considered desirable for irrigation of any kind, both for aesthetic reasons and so as to avoid the presence of aggregates of faecal matter on the fields which may serve as a source of direct contamination of workers or mechanical transmission by flies and other vectors.

Even sewage irrigation of crops usually consumed cooked, such as potatoes or beets, should not be considered free of risks since the contaminated surfaces of the vegetables may introduce pathogens into kitchens where working surfaces and utensils may become contaminated thus infecting other foods.

Unrestricted agricultural utilization

Certain agricultural and economic conditions may warrant the treatment of wastewater to such an extent that it can be used for unrestricted irrigation of all agricultural crops. Farmers find some difficulty in carrying out the normally desirable crop rotation regimes if restrictions on the types of crops that may be grown are too onerous. This also may become a serious public health problem since it is not administratively possible in many cases to control the types of crops that are in fact grown by farmers who are supposedly required to limit themselves to certain 'safe' crops. The economic temptation to grow high-value salad crops even if the effluent quality does not warrant this is difficult to overcome. These considerations have led to the development of treatment procedures and standards to overcome such problems.

If wastewater is to be used for the irrigation of agricultural crops in an unrestricted manner, including fruits and vegetables usually consumed uncooked, a high degree of disinfection is necessary to inactivate the pathogens. Additional processes may be required to remove certain resistant protozoans or helminths. The World Health Organization (WHO, 1973) meeting of experts on this subject has recommended that crops eaten raw should be irrigated only with biologically treated effluent that has been disinfected to achieve a coliform level of not more than 100 organisms per 100 ml in 80% of the samples. It has been demonstrated that it is technically feasible to effectively disinfect a good quality wastewater effluent so as to achieve such low coliform counts (Shuval, 1975).

The World Health Organization also states that in certain situations sand filtration or equivalent polishing methods may be required. This relates in particular to the need to remove helminths in those areas of the world where such parasitic diseases are endemic. A defined and tested technology for the removal of protozoans or helminths generally resistant to chemical disinfection is yet to be established but microstrainers have been proposed to meet this requirement. Slow sand filtration should be effective but may not be economically feasible in many situations.

A number of problems arise in meeting the objectives of effluent disinfection for unrestricted irrigation. The problem of the greater resistance of enteroviruses to chlorination has not been fully overcome. Our studies (Shuval, 1975) have shown that it is quite feasible to achieve a coliform count of around 100/100 ml by applying as little as 5 mg/l of chlorine to the effluent of a high-rate biological filter plant. However, when we inoculated poliovirus type 1 into the same disinfection system, only about a 90% reduction was achieved in one hour. In our studies we have shown that with a 1-hour contact time, about 10 times as much chlorine is required to achieve the same degree of disinfection for poliovirus as is required for coliforms. Besides the cost, the formation of potentially toxic organohalide compounds by such high doses of chlorine might rule out such treatment (Beller et al., 1974). Our recent studies on ozone (Katzenelson et al., 1974) indicate that this powerful oxidant inactivates

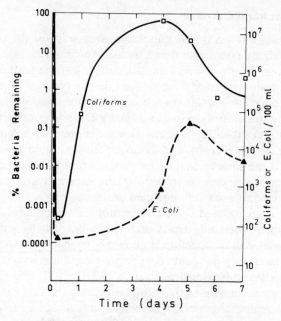

Figure 19.2 Regrowth of coliforms and *E. coli* in effluent at 20 °C after inactivation with 5 mg/l of applied chlorine and no dechlorination

viruses many times more rapidly than chlorine and may hold out promise for the effective disinfection required for re-use purposes.

Another problem is the regrowth of coliforms after chlorination. This phenomenon was first reported upon by Rudolfs and Gehm (1936). In our studies of disinfection of the effluent of a high-rate biofiltration plant in Jerusalem we were able to show that coliform counts lower than 100/100 ml could be achieved on a regular basis within 15 minutes after chlorination at doses of some 10 mg/l. However, after storage for 3 days in an operational reservoir prior to agricultural irrigation, coliform counts increased 10-fold on the average. In laboratory studies we were able to demonstrate massive regrowth of coliforms and faecal coli 3–4 days after chlorination (Figure 19.2). The hygienic significance of the high coliform counts in such cases is difficult to determine since it is not clear whether pathogens can regrow after initial partial disinfection in a like manner. The State Health Department in California (State of California, 1973) has recognized this problem and specifically states that the bacteriological standard is considered to be fulfilled if 'at some point in the treatment process' the required coliform count is achieved. However, since information on the regrowth ability of enteric pathogenic bacteria in dilute substrates such as polluted water or wastewater effluent is lacking, the California formulation should be considered as a tentative one.

Health of workers and public

Little attention has been paid in the past to the potential health risks to workers in wastewater irrigation projects or to the public who may live in adjacent residential areas or who may pass through on public highways.

Direct contamination

One early study in the United States on the health of workers at sewage treatment plants did not reveal any excessive risks of communicable disease including infectious hepatitis in this group. However, it has been reported from India that hookworm infections are much more common among workers on sewage farms than among the farming population in general. The low levels of personal hygiene and the local custom of walking barefoot are undoubtedly major contributory factors to the disease situation among sewage farm workers in India.

The potential health risk to workers may be derived from direct contact with wastewater which may contaminate hands which later contaminate food. Appropriate sanitary facilities for washing and eating and good personal hygiene can go a long way to reduce this risk.

Dispersion of microbial aerosols

Another problem is the possible inhalation of aerosolized sewage containing pathogens from spray irrigation. Our laboratory in Jerusalem has initiated studies to evaluate this problem (Katzenelson and Teltch, 1975) and in preliminary studies have been able to recover enteric bacteria including *Salmonella* spp. 100–350 m downwind of a field, spray irrigated with non-disinfected effluent. The size of the viable aerosol particles were determined with an Anderson cascade sampler and it could be shown that a significant percentage of the recovered bacteria were associated with particles in the 1–4 μm range which can be inhaled into the lungs and can be considered potentially infectious. Our estimates indicate that somewhere between 0·1% and 1% of the sewage sprayed into the air forms aerosols which are capable of being carried considerable distances by the wind. The rate of die-off and reduction in the concentration of pathogens incorporated in the aerosols is a function of wind speed, temperature, relative humidity, ultra violet radiation and local topographic features. Sorber *et al.* (1974) made some theoretical calculations as to the potential dispersion of bacteria or viruses aerosolized by sewage spray and suggested that a buffer zone of up to one mile would be advisable to prevent infections in adjacent residential areas. Although there is as yet no sound scientific basis for establishing such buffer zones, there is already sufficient data to indicate that an area of some 500 m from spray irrigation with sewage can carry infectious bacteria in the air. The limits of the buffer zone including some safety factor should surely be beyond this range. Here one must also reconsider the health risks to workers moving directly in the zone of spray in such irrigation projects. Although no epidemiological evidence is available as yet, it does appear from existing evidence that there is a real risk of inhalation of aerosolized pathogens. It would seem advisable to consider the heavy disinfection of all effluents used for any form of spray irrigation regardless of the crops irrigated or the proximity of residential areas.

There is undoubtedly need for further investigation of this question and such studies are in progress in a number of places. Until such time as a firmer scientific basis is available, caution should prevail in the protection of agricultural workers and the public from any risks that may be associated spray irrigation.

Irrigation of pasture land

The risks to the health of animals and potentially to man associated with cattle grazing on sewage-irrigated pasture have been studied by a number of authors. Greenberg and Kupka (1957) in their review of the transmission of tuberculosis by wastewater point out that the wastes from institutions treating tuberculosis patients or industries such as dairies or slaughterhouses handling tuberculous animals will almost always contain large numbers of tubercule bacilli. The bacilli will not be removed by conventional biological treatment but only after very heavy chlorination.

Animals grazing on sewage-irrigated pasture or drinking such sewage can become infected. In another review Greenberg and Dean (1958) point out that a number of authors reported that cattle grazing on pastures irrigated with sewage often show significant increases in beef tapeworm infections of *Cysticercus bovis* which can infect persons who consume the beef with the adult stage of the tapeworm *Taenia saginata*. The disease is widely distributed throughout the world in both animals and man, and is still considered a serious health problem in many areas. Reports indicate that conventional sewage treatment is inadequate to completely eliminate tapeworm eggs from sewage or sludge. Sand filtration or microstraining are suggested processes for effective removal of the eggs (Silverman and Griffiths, 1955). Microstraining has been shown to remove about 90% of the *T. saginata* eggs. However, it is recognized that these methods may not be technically feasible in many countries.

Some regulations for sewage irrigation of pasture lands have recommended allowing the grazing of cattle after the fields are completely dry. The efficacy of this procedure is open to question in light of the findings of Jepsen and Roth (1952) who showed that the eggs of *T. saginata* may remain viable under natural conditions for months—'long enough to permit protracted contamination of fields and crops'. It appears that in areas where this disease is endemic, sewage irrigation of pasture lands should be avoided unless special treatment facilities for removal of the pathogens are provided.

Fish ponds

Wastewater has been used to add nutrients to fish ponds which are used for growing fish for human consumption in some areas. In an area such as Israel, where this is practised, the potential danger of transmission of helminthic infections to pond workers exists. Reference should be made to Chapter 15 for a detailed discussion of this point.

Although fish cannot become biologically infected with human bacterial pathogens, they can become mechanically contaminated and in that way introduce pathogens into kitchens and cause human infections. Although there is little epidemiological evidence on actual disease transmission, the risk exists. Holding fish in clean water ponds for some period before marketing may reduce the extent of contamination. The question of accumulation of toxic chemicals and off-tastes in fish grown in wastewater has not been studied but reports on taste problems have been made.

19.4 SUMMARY AND CONCLUSIONS

Wastewater re-use in agriculture is becoming an ever more attractive method of increasing water resources utilization, particularly in the more arid portions of the world. In addition to the value of the reclaimed water itself, the nutrients contributed to the soil and to the crops by use of such water, rich in organic matter and micronutrients, cannot be overlooked, particularly in a period of rapidly increasing costs of chemical fertilizers.

The use of human excreta or 'nightsoil' for crop fertilization has been widely practised for years in many regions of the world. While the improvement in soil productivity is of vital importance, the public health risks caused by disease transmission to agricultural workers or to be consumers of vegetable crops eaten raw must be carefully considered, for in certain cases such risks may counterbalance the economic and social benefits of improved soil fertility.

Human excreta and raw municipal wastewater have been shown to carry the full spectrum of pathogenic micro-organisms endemic in the community. Most conventional wastewater or excreta treatment processes can only partially remove such pathogens. There is evidence that despite natural die off in the fields and on crops due to the sun's rays, desiccation and other hostile environmental factors, pathogens from wastewater or excreta used in agriculture can survive long enough to infect potential consumer of those vegetable crops normally eaten raw. While advanced highly complex wastewater and excreta treatment processes are available today which are capable of totally removing *all* pathogens, it is doubtful that such high degree of treatment would be technologically feasible or economically justifiable under normal circumstances in most developing countries.

The use of lower levels of treatment and restricting the type of crops to those that may cause less risk of disease transmission to consumers may be the only practical approach for utilizing wastewater and excreta in agriculture in such developing countries. It must be recognized that governmental restrictions on the type of crop grown are in some cases not easily enforced, particularly where economic incentives may lead farmers to grow more profitable, but higher-risk vegetable crops.

380

In developing a programme for wastewater and excreta re-use in agriculture in an economy in dire need of more water and soil nutrients to feed its growing population, careful consideration must be given to the benefits and risks involved. While the economic and social benefits of recycling such vital resources cannot be achieved at zero risk, the risks of increased communicable disease transmission, with its possible heavy economic and social burden of lowered productivity and increased human suffering, can often negate the apparent benefits.

A balanced approach combining low-cost waste treatment methods capable of providing reasonable, although not complete, reductions in pathogen levels with restriction of crops to those presenting a low level of public health risk appears to be the most prudent policy to achieve the maximum social benefits from waste re-use.

19.5 REFERENCES

Bellar, T. A., Lichenberg, J. J. and Kroner, R. C. (1974). The occurrence of organohalides in chlorinated drinking waters. *Journal of the American Water Works Association*, **66**, 703–706.

Benarde, M. A. (1973). Land disposal of sewage effluents: appraisal of health effects of pathogenic organisms. *Journal of the American Water Works Association*, **65**, 432–440.

Bregner-Rabinowitz, S. (1956). The survival of coliforms, *St. faecalis* and *Sa. tennesse* in the soil and climate of Israel. *Applied Microbiology*, **4**, 101.

Cohen, J., Schwartz, T., Kalazmer, R., Pridan, D., Ghalayini, H. and Davies, A. M. (1971). Epidemiological aspects of cholera el Tor outbreak in a non-endemic area. *The Lancet*, July 10, 86–89.

Dunlop, S. G. (1952). The irrigation of truck crops with sewage-contaminated water. *Sanitarian, Los Angeles*, **15**, 107.

Dunlop, S. G., Twedt, R. M. and Wang, W. L. L. (1951). *Salmonella* in irrigation water. *Sewage and Industrial Wastes*, **23**, 1118.

Falk, L. (1949). Bacterial contamination of tomatoes grown in polluted soil. *American Journal of Public Health*, **39**, 1338–1342.

Greenberg, A. E. and Dean, B. H. (1958). The beef tapeworm, measly beef, and sewage: a review. *Sewage and Industrial Wastes*, **30**, 262.

Greenberg, A. E. and Kupka, E. (1957). Tuberculosis transmission by wastewaters—a review. *Sewage and Industrial Wastes*, **29**, 524–537.

Jepsen, A. and Roth, H. (1952). Epizootiology of *Cysticercus bovis*: Resistence of the eggs of *Taenia saginata*. In: *Report of the 14th International Veterinary Congress, London 1949*, **2**, 49.

Katzenelson, E. and Teltch, B. (1975). Dispersion of enteric bacteria in the air as a result of sewage spray irrigation and treatment processes. *Journal of the Water Pollution Control Federation (in press)*.

Katzenelson, E., Kletter, B. and Shuval, H. I. (1974). Inactivation kinetics of viruses and bacteria in water by use of ozone. *Journal of the American Water Works Association*, **66**, 725–729.

Kehr, R. W. and Butterfield, C. T. (1943). Notes on the relationship between coliform and enteric pathogens. *Public Health Reports*, **58**, 589–607.

Kliger, I. J. (1921) Investigations of soil pollution and the relation of various types of privies to the spread of intestinal infections. *International Health Board Monograph No. 5*, p.4. Rockefeller Institute of Medical Research.

McClesky, C. A. and Christopher, W. (1941). The longevity of certain pathogens on strawberries. *Journal of Bacteriology*, **41**, 98.

Plotkin, S. A. and Katz, M. (1967). Minimal infective doses of virus for man by the oral route. In: *Transmission of Viruses by the Water Route* (Ed. G. Berg). New York: Interscience.

Rigbi, M. Aramy, A. and Shuval, H. (1956). Efficiency of a small high-rate trickling filter plant at Jerusalem, Israel. *Sewage and Industrial Wastes*, **28**, 852,

Rudolfs, W. and Gehm, H. W. (1936). Sewage chlorination studies. *Bulletin 601*. New Jersey Agricultural Experiment Station, New Brunswick, N. J.

Rudolfs, W., Falk, L. L. and Ragotzkie, R. A. (1950). Literature review of the occurrence and survival of enteric, pathogenic and related organisms in soil, water, sewage and sludges, and on vegetation. I. Bacterial and virus diseases; II, Animal parasites. *Sewage and Industrial Wastes*, **22**, 1261 and 1471.

Rudolfs, W., Falk, L. L. and Ragotzkie, R. A. (1951). Contamination of vegetables grown in polluted soil. I. Bacterial contamination. *Sewage and Industrial Wastes*, **23**, 253.

Shuval, H. I. (1951). Public health aspects of sewage irrigation. *Journal of the Israel Association of Architects and Engineers*, September.

Shuval, H. I. (1962). The public health significance of trace chemicals in waste water utilization. *Bulletin of the World Health Organization*, **27**, 791.

Shuval, H. I. (1970). Detection and control of enteroviruses in the water environment. In: *Developments in Water Quality Research* (Ed. H. I. Shuval). Ann Arbor: Ann Arbor–Humphrey Science Publishers.

Shuval, H. I. (1975). Disinfection of wastewater for agricultural utilization. In: *Advances in Water Pollution Research* (Ed. S. H. Jenkins). Oxford: Pergamon Press.

Shuval, H. I. and Katzenelson, E. (1972). Detection of enteric viruses in the water environment. In: *Water Pollution Microbiology* (Ed. R. Mitchel). New York: Wiley.

Silverman, P. H. and Griffiths, R. B. (1955). Review of methods of sewage disposal in Great Britain with special reference to the epizootiology of *Cysticercus bovis*. *Annals of Tropical Medicine and Parasitology*, **49**, 436.

Sorber, C. A., Schaub, S. A. and Bausum, H. T. (1974). Virus survival following wastewater spray irrigation of sandy soils. In: *Virus Survival in Water and Wastewater Systems*. Austin: University of Texas Press.

Sorber, C. A. and Guter, K. J. (1975). Health and hygiene aspects of spray irrigation. *American Journal of Public Health*, **65**, 47–52.

State of California (1973). Statewide standards for the direct use of reclaimed water for irrigation and recreational impoundments. *California Administrative Code, Title 17, Public Health*.

WHO (1973). Reuse of effluents: Methods of wastewater treatment and health safeguards. *Technical Report Series No. 517*. Geneva: World Health Organization.

Yoshpe-Purer, Y. and Shuval, H. I. (1970). Salmonellae and bacterial indicator organisms in polluted coastal water and their hygienic significance. *Proceedings of the FAO Technical Conference on Marine Pollution and its Effects on Living Resources and Fishing*. Rome: Food and Agriculture Organization.

Problems of Domestic Wastewater Reclamation: Editorial Introduction

A substantial number of developing countries are arid or partly arid for some or all of the year. Water for domestic needs may therefore be in very short supply and costly to obtain. In such situations in urban areas, it is tempting to consider wastewater reclamation schemes which will permit the recycling of domestic water. The technology for this is available and has been applied in arid countries such as Israel, Namibia and South Africa.

Wastewater reclamation, though technically feasible, is an extremely expensive and sophisticated procedure. In addition, it is a very dubious practice when the overall logic of the system is considered. Imagine you are a Martian visiting earth for the first time and that you have no preconceived ideas about water and wastewater engineering. You visit the town of Windhoek in Namibia and you note that the area is extremely arid and that water is in very short supply. You enquire further and you discover that the strange earthlings who inhabit Windhoek do not try by every means possible to reduce water usage. Instead they obtain, at substantial cost, additional volumes of water, over and above those strictly necessary for drinking, washing and industrial processes, which they employ to move waste matter along pipes. This strange use of scarce resources they call a 'sewerage system' which they regard with pride and consider to be technologically clever. This system produces large volumes of very dirty water which the earthlings treat at great cost and eventually produce a water of a very high quality—in fact, clean enough to drink. This reclaimed water they then re-use—not only to drink, but to move wastes along pipes again and so produce more large volumes of dirty water which need more costly treatment. Why, you will wonder do the people of Windhoek not use their wastes to some productive purpose (like fish farming or agricultural fertilization), save their scarce water for strictly necessary purposes and invent a better way of moving wastes about than washing them down pipes in a stream of drinking water?

The chapter by Stander and Clayton which follows is included in this volume for completeness and as a cautionary tale. The reclamation of water up to, but not exceeding, a quality necessary for its re-use in some industrial process may be an economically viable strategy in water-scarce areas. However, in most situations in developing countries, the reclamation and recycling of domestic wastewater will be too expensive, too technologically sophisticated, too prone to breakdown and, in the eyes of a puzzled Martian, too silly.

20

Planning and Construction of Wastewater Reclamation Schemes as an Integral Part of Water Supply

G. J. STANDER *and* A. J. CLAYTON

20.1 INTRODUCTION

Quantitively, South Africa's available surface and underground water resources are a weak link in its future socio-economic development. According to current information, the assured yield of these resources which could effectively be harnessed is estimated at $60\,000 \times 10^3\,\mathrm{m}^3/\mathrm{d}$, which is equivalent to $3.6\,\mathrm{m}^3/$ hd-d for the country's present total population. With improved engineering techniques for impounding surface waters and tapping of, as yet, unknown underground sources, this quantity could be increased to $75\,000 \times 10^3\,\mathrm{m}^3/\mathrm{d}$ which is equivalent to $4.5\,\mathrm{m}^3/\mathrm{hd}\text{-}\mathrm{d}$. This small quantity of water, namely $4.5\,\mathrm{m}^3/$ hd-d, compared with $22.5\,\mathrm{m}^3/\mathrm{hd}\text{-}\mathrm{d}$ in the United States, must provide man and animal with their daily water needs, keep the wheels of industry turning, and quench the thirst of irrigation schemes.

A breakdown of current usage of water in the Republic shows that: (a) the current total water usage by all sectors amounts to $29\,500 \times 10^3\,\mathrm{m}^3/\mathrm{d}$, i.e. 40% of the total estimated assured yield of surface and underground sources; (b) irrigation farming is responsible for 80% of the aforementioned consumption and represents 32% of the estimated assured yield of surface and underground water resources; cattle, sheep and dry-land farming are responsible for a negligible fraction of this consumption, probably about $270 \times 10^3\,\mathrm{m}^3/\mathrm{d}$; (c) cities, towns, industry, mining and power generation are responsible for 17% of the current daily water consumption, and represent only 7% of the estimated assured yield of surface and underground water resources. This is a modest consumption if one considers that industry and mining today produce 40% of the country's gross national product.

Let us look into the future—at that magic year 2000 adopted almost in every country in the world! (1) It is estimated that the total population of the Republic

This paper was originally published in *Water Pollution Control*, volume 70, pp. 228–234, 1971. It is reproduced here by permission of the Institute of Water Pollution Control. © Institute of Water Pollution Control, 1971.

of South Africa will be in excess of 40 million. (2) The standard of living will be higher and the country will be heavily industrialized. (3) A greater proportion of the population will be concentrated in towns and cities—of the order of 80% at the turn of the century as compared with the current 48%.

These factors will be responsible for a total water demand of $45\,500 \times 10^3$ m^3/d by towns, cities, industries, mines and power stations. Furthermore, agricultural demand, essentially irrigation farming, is estimated at $35\,400 \times 10^3$ m^3/d. The total demand will thus be $80\,000 \times 10^3\,m^3/d$, i.e. $500 \times 10^3\,m^3/d$ in excess of the maximum potential yield of surface and underground waters, viz. $75\,000 \times 10^3\,m^3/d$.

These statistics broadly indicate that the country is heading for a substantial water shortage on a basis of current usage technology. Seen regionally, the problem becomes more accentuated, and in certain industrialized areas of the country socio-economic progress is already prejudiced by water shortages. Furthermore, the available fresh water in the hydrologic cycle is a fixed quantity. Consequently, our most constructive course of action calls for a critical appraisal of our present philosophies and technologies of water resources development and utilization. The challenges posed by this situation have forced the acceptance of the inevitable fact that water supply, beneficial use and re-use of water, wastewater management and reclamation, and the control of pollution are inseparable components in a broad water conservation plan for every metropolitan area as well as for the country as a whole. This concept has stimulated scientists and engineers in the Republic to some remarkable achievements in water resources optimization which show that the country's future development will not so much be curtailed by actual quantities of fresh water available, but rather by our water resources management.

20.2 INTERNAL RE-USE OF WATER BY INDUSTRIES

Current advances in unit production processes and wastewater technology have placed in the hands of the industrial and chemical engineer a wide range of versatile techniques for practising multiple internal circulation of water and effluents in manufacturing processes. The reclamation of effluents from the unit processes in a factory is today recognized as an effective and economic means of augmenting the water required for increased production output and for reducing water consumption per unit of production. Depending on the nature of the manufacturing plant, a saving in water consumption of between 50% and 95% can be achieved, as seen from the examples recorded in Table 20.1.

It is in industry's own interest to practise water re-use and effluent reclamation as an integral part of industrial water supply. By doing this it will not only justify its continued existence, but also ensure the future expansion of its production programme. The benefits which could accrue from the planned re-use of water and reclamation are illustrated in the case of a key chemical industry in the Pretoria/Witwatersrand/Vereeniging complex. This particular factory has, since 1962, increased its production by as much as 70% and reduced

Table 20.1 Water savings effected by planned reclamation of process
waters for internal re-use

Industry	Water requirements (m³/tonne)	
	Without reclamation and re-use	With reclamation and re-use
Fruit and vegetable canning	11·2	5·4
Kraft paper pulp	201	4·0–11·2
Newsprint	116	27
Hardboard	67	33·5
Soaps, fats and oils	54	10·7
Steel	246	5·4–6·7
Glass containers	1·8	0·7

its water intake from the Rand Water Board by $182 \times 10^3 m^3$ per month. Furthermore, 36·6 and 19·3 tonnes per month of ammonia and urea respectively are recovered, and the final effluent which is discharged into a river is of suitable quality to serve as a source of raw water for future development in the area.

The extent to which water consumption is reduced by internal recirculation of process waters by some major industries is shown in Table 20.2.

The small volume of intake water is mainly used to replace consumptive losses through evaporation of cooling water.

In general it can be said that the major industries in the Republic are already water-conscious, and that these industries are trying their best to modernize their factories and to keep abreast with new developments in order to cut down effluent pollution and water consumption. Unfortunately, however, this awareness is largely lacking among industries which discharge their effluents into municipal sewers. The basic reasons for apathy towards a planned water economy in a factory stem from the fact that water is a cheap raw material and that regulations for the discharge of effluents into municipal sewers discourage a water awareness among water users.

Table 20.2 Ratio of intake water to water in recirculation for some
major industries in South Africa

Product	Water recirculated (10^3 m³/d)	Water intake (10^3 m³/d)	Ratio (%)
Steel	732	21·2	2·9
Thermal power[a]	3928	98·0	2·5
Oil from coal	823	63·6	7·8
Chemicals	491	17·2	3·5
Total	5974	200	3·3

[a]All inland power stations employ natural draught wet cooling towers.

20.3 RECLAMATION OF EFFLUENTS

As indicated earlier, cities, towns, industries, mining and power generation are responsible for a modest 17% of the current total daily water usage in the Republic, generating 40% of the gross national product. Because of this high value of water, and since the water intake by these sectors is largely non-consumptive—as much as 60% to 100% reaching the sewage treatment facilities of industrialized urban areas—it is both economically and strategically sound for a water-short country to exploit treated effluents to the full as sources of water supply.

Only 20% of over 455×10^3 m^3 of purified effluent available in the Pretoria/Witwatersrand/Vereeniging complex is re-used directly in industry and in power generation. By the year 2000, about 2700×10^3 m^3 of purified effluent will be available in this area; for the metropolitan area of Johannesburg alone, 85% of the estimated daily water consumption of 1130×10^3 m^3 will end up as effluent in sewage-treatment plants. It is beyond imagination that this fact should be ignored in the planning and development of new water resources for this and other industrial complexes.

It must be accepted that over 80% of any new water imported into an area will become reclaimable effluent. Because this new water will become increasingly expensive, because the costs of reclaiming effluents by modern advanced techniques have become competitive with that of freshwater supplies, and because water is the life-blood of sustained socio-economic development of the Republic or any particular area, re-use of water by the industrial sector and reclamation of effluents for redistribution must be planned and managed as an inseparable component of the water household of all existing and new industrialized areas in the Republic. The case history of the city of Windhoek, capital of Namibia, proves that by the dynamic and progressive harnessing of existing information on water technology, and of new developments generated by scientific and engineering enterprise, future progress will not be jeopardized by limited water resources but rather by the way we plan and utilize those resources. It is here where critical path planning, water resources management and intensive applied research should be forged together into an effective task force.

As early as 1954 it was realized that the future economic progress of Windhoek depended on the utilization of reclaimed water. It was further recognized that it would be both an economically and strategically sound policy to exploit the reclamation of treated sewage effluent as an integral part of the freshwater household of Windhoek.

Figure 20.1 shows the necessity of reclaiming water in the critical period before the Swakop scheme comes into operation. In order to meet this demand and to obviate the immediate problems during the critical period when the Goreangab Dam storage dropped to 20% of its capacity in September 1968, it was imperative that the commissioning of the reclamation plant and the integration of this source into the bulk supply system should be effected in the

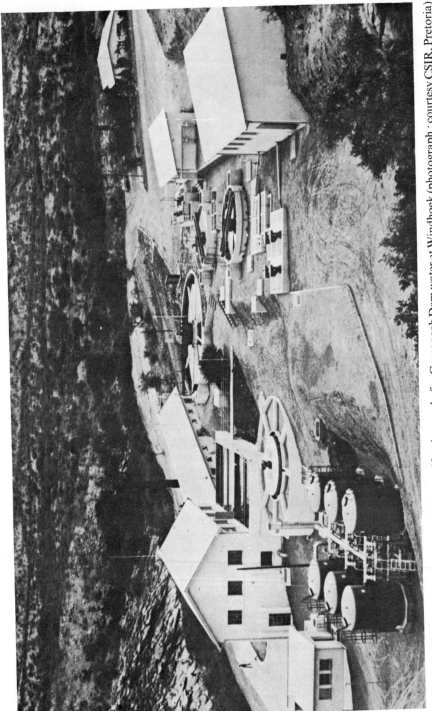

Integrated water reclamation plant and water purification works for Goreangab Dam water at Windhoek (photograph : courtesy CSIR, Pretoria)

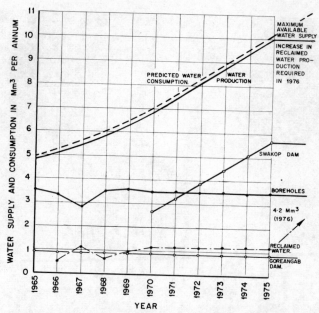

Figure 20.1 Predicted water consumption and production patterns

shortest possible time. Immediate steps were therefore taken to ensure that the final product would conform to the health quality requirements, particularly with respect to the microbiological standards.

Additional reclamation capacity will have to be commissioned by 1976. From past records it has been established that approximately 35% of the water production is returned to the main outfall of the Gammams sewage works as sewage. Thus, by 1977 there will be a total potential for reclamation of $4200 \times 10^3 \, m^3$ per annum. As the existing plant can produce $1200 \times 10^3 \, m^3$ per annum, additional reclamation facilities with a design capacity of approximately 3000×10^3 will be required.

The water reclamation facility for Windhoek has now been successfully in operation for extended periods and has, therefore, come to stay as a future water augmentation system in its own right. With commendable foresight, the city's sewage treatment plant was constructed in the catchment of the freshwater supply dam and near the water treatment plant, thereby facilitating the integration of the reclaimed water with the freshwater reticulation.

The total capital cost of the reclamation works amounts to R221 300. This sum does not include the cost of five additional maturation ponds which were constructed at the Gammams sewage works as these are considered to be part of sewage treatment. In the following calculation of the production cost of reclaimed water it is therefore assumed that maturation pond effluent is supplied to the new works at no charge and that the interest and redemption costs of the existing water treatment facilities at Goreangab are also not charged to the reclaimed water. Labour and pumping costs are shared in proportion to the respective quantities of dam water and maturation pond effluent treated. Costs are calculated on the basis that 1200×10^3 m³ of effluent plus 1200×10^3 m³ Goreangab Dam water are treated annually.

Total treatment costs (in South African cents) per cubic metre

	cents	cents
Aluminium sulphate at 160 mg/l (6·07 cents/kg)	0·97	
Carbon dioxide at 36 mg/l as L.P. gas (18·52 cents/kg)	0·70	
Lime at 30 mg/l (1·60 cents/kg)	0·05	
Chlorine at 12 mg/l (28·66 cents/kg)	0·35	
Activated carbon	2·90	
		4·97
Electricity: blowers, mechanical equipment and recarbonators (2·5 cents/kWh)	1·20	
Pumping to reservoirs	2·22	
Labour ($\frac{1}{2} \times$ R16 224 p.a.)	0·67	
Interest and redemption on loan ($3\frac{1}{2}\%$ for 20 years) R15 478·64 p.a.	1·29	6·38
		10·35
10% maintenance and overheads		1·04
		11.39

The corresponding total cost for the purified Goreangab dam water is 10·7 cents/m³. The former cost figure for carbon treatment is expected to be reduced by 1·4 cents/m³ when regeneration of the spent carbon becomes feasible, resulting in a total cost of 10 cents/m³. It should be noted that chemical and labour costs in Windhoek are considerably higher than for the Pretoria/Johannesburg area; consequently, the production of reclaimed water could be expected to be considerably less. Further cost reductions can be expected with the new lime softening flotation-ammonia stripping system for the Pretoria plant.

The practical experience gained in Windhoek and the new advanced purification techniques developed by the National Institute for Water Research with the $4·54 \times 10^3$ m³/d demonstration plant at Pretoria (Figure 20.2) have proved that modern waste water technology makes it practicable to supply 50% of the water demand of urbanized industrialized areas by practising reclamation of effluents as an integral part of the domestic water supply, and that with two cycles of re-use it is possible to make available water to the extent of 75% of the original freshwater intake. For South Africa, this means that the estimated demand of $45 500 \times 10^3$ m³/d mentioned earlier for freshwater

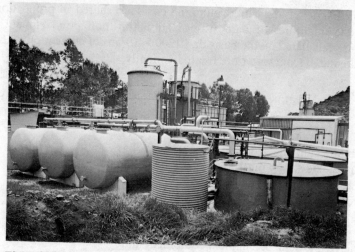

Figure 20.2 Demonstration water reclamation plant (capacity 4.5×10^3 m^3/d) at Pretoria sewage treatment works

by municipalities and industries by the year 2000 could be reduced by $19\,500 \times 10^3\,m^3/d$ by the planned reclamation of effluent as an integral part of the fresh-water supply.

20.4 CONCLUSIONS

South Africa is already moving along a critical path with respect to its available water resources. Within the next generation, water demand will exceed freshwater supplies and future socio-economic development will depend on our ability to use and re-use available water resources efficiently. The optimization of wastewater rehabilitation and the management and re-use of water requires, at national level, as much, if not in fact greater, far-sighted research, planning and financial input than the development of freshwater supplies. A practical demonstration of this is afforded by Windhoek, the capital of Namibia, which became at the end of 1968 the first city in the world to practise large-scale and continuous reclamation of wastewater as an integral part of domestic water supply. Research is therefore being pursued at an undiminished rate to improve the economics and efficiency of wastewater reclamation plants. The $4.54 \times 10^3\,m^3/d$ demonstration plant, currently operating at the Pretoria sewage works, will provide engineers and authorities with the necessary data and criteria for the planning, construction and operation of reclamation plants throughout the country.

Central and local government and regional water supply authorities now have at their disposal readily available data and expertise on which they can forge industrial water supply and wastewater management policies which will encourage industry to contribute its share in the optimization of the country's water resources. The achievement of this objective, coupled with the fact that industry consumes only 15% of the total water intake of a local authority serving an industrialized area, will ensure unhampered industrial development without prejudice to the water economy of the area concerned; the real problem is the increasing water requirements of the residential areas to accommodate a rising population. Consequently, the reclamation of sewage effluents as a source of water supply must constitute an integral part of industrial development. Only then will it be possible to maintain a stable equilibrium between water supply and demand.

The writing is on the wall for both water-short and water-plentiful areas in South Africa. In the future it will be more advantageous to subsidize local authorities to reclaim their effluents than to develop new water schemes involving the piping of water over long distances.

Index